Dermatology Pearls

ELEANOR E. SAHN, MD
Associate Professor of Dermatology
  and Pediatrics
Department of Dermatology
Medical University of South Carolina
Charleston, South Carolina

Series Editors

STEVEN A. SAHN, MD
Professor of Medicine and Director
Division of Pulmonary and
  Critical Care Medicine
Medical University of South Carolina
Charleston, South Carolina

JOHN E. HEFFNER, MD
Professor and Vice Chairman
Department of Medicine
Medical University of South Carolina
Charleston, South Carolina

HANLEY & BELFUS, INC./Philadelphia

Publisher: HANLEY & BELFUS, INC.
Medical Publishers
210 S. 13th Street
Philadelphia, PA 19107
(215) 546-7293, 800-962-1892
FAX (215) 790-9330
Website: http://www.hanleyandbelfus.com

Library of Congress Cataloging-in-Publication Data

Dermatology pearls / by Eleanor E. Sahn.
     p.   cm.—(The Pearls Series®)
    Includes bibliographical references and index.
    ISBN 1-56053-315-3 (alk. paper)
    1. Skin—Diseases Case studies.   2. Skin—Diseases Atlases.
  I. Sahn, Eleanor E. II. Series.
    [DNLM: 1. Skin Diseases—diagnosis Case Report. 2. Skin
Diseases—pathology Case Report.   WR 141 D435 1999]
RL98.D47   1999
616.5—dc21
DNLM/DLC
for Library of Congress   99-20512
                                               CIP

DERMATOLOGY PEARLS   ISBN 1-56053-315-3

Last digit is the print number: 9 8 7 6 5 4 3 2 1

CONTENTS

FOREWORD

Problem-based learning has become highly valued in the medical school curriculum. In fact, some schools have abandoned the traditional lecture-based curriculum and turned entirely to focusing on the patient as the primary stimulus for all medical learning. Many of the subjects that I know best are those that I learned mostly by myself, through independent study. This book allows us to return to the patient and motivates us with actual clinical problems to continue our pursuit of life-long learning at our own pace.

Dr. Eleanor Sahn has drawn from her extensive clinical experience and knowledge of pediatric and adult dermatology to select cases that traverse the broad spectrum of dermatology—from developmental defects to inflammatory diseases to cutaneous neoplasms. Each problem is introduced by a clinical vignette and a color illustration of the cutaneous findings, by which the reader can exercise his or her diagnostic skills. Dr. Sahn then leads the reader by the hand through the diagnostic features, pathophysiology, and management of each problem. This is an exciting way to learn and a fun way to improve one's clinical skill in dermatology. For those who are interested in exploring these conditions even further, Dr. Sahn has provided carefully chosen references that contain our best information.

Dermatology Pearls is an engaging book. Dr. Sahn has a delightfully readable style that makes learning enjoyable. These "pearls" can be put to good use by each one of us in the care of our patients who have skin disease.

JOHN C. MAIZE, MD
Professor of Dermatology and Pathology
Chairman, Department of Dermatology
Medical University of South Carolina
Charleston, South Carolina

EDITORS' FOREWORD

The ability to walk into an examination room and make an immediate diagnosis has always fascinated physicians. In our medical world of highly sophisticated diagnostic testing, the physician who can combine clues gained from careful bedside observations with clear medical reasoning to arrive at a diagnosis is perhaps closest to the ideal that first drew many of us into medicine. Dermatologic disorders represent the greatest opportunity for skilled clinicians to arrive at an accurate differential diagnosis from the patient exam. These diagnoses often extend beyond primary cutaneous conditions and provide the sentinel signs and keys to understanding systemic disorders. Patients benefit greatly from clinicians sufficiently skilled to observe and correctly interpret the cutaneous manifestations of disease.

In *Dermatology Pearls,* Dr. Eleanor Sahn provides a unique approach for preparing physicians to recognize important dermatologic disorders. The 100 patients presented in a case history format comprise an extensive atlas of skin signs representing the major cutaneous disorders. Fundamental approaches to care, combined with the most recent advances in dermatologic science, are emphasized. Consequently, *Dermatology Pearls* provides an opportunity for general clinicians to gain an understanding of skin disease and practicing dermatologists to hone their skills with an up-to-date review.

We thank Dr. Sahn for lending us her expertise in writing the 12th book in The Pearls Series.® We anticipate that *Dermatology Pearls* will extend the skills of physicians who seek to maximize the diagnostic value of the clinical exam.

STEVEN A. SAHN, MD
JOHN E. HEFFNER, MD
Series Editors

PREFACE

When I switched from internal medicine to dermatology 14 years ago, I began a new "pocket brain." In it, I recorded common and not so common pearls of wisdom from my teachers and the literature. I also began photographing typical as well as unusual skin lesions that I encountered in my daily practice. From this material, *Dermatology Pearls* has emerged.

The 100 cases presented in this book are clinical vignettes of patients seen over 10 years in a busy dermatology practice within an academic medical center. Some diseases are common but with an unusual twist, while others are rare. After the initial clinical description is read, the reader can formulate a differential diagnosis and plan. The diagnosis is revealed and discussed on the following page, with exploration of the clinical findings, differential diagnosis, pathogenesis, histopathology, and therapeutic options. Pertinent information from the current literature is included. The discussion concludes with brief take-home messages, or pearls, highlighting fundamentally important concepts and recent advances in care.

This volume is directed toward dermatology residents preparing for their board examinations, practitioners wishing to learn more dermatology or preparing for recertification exams, and physicians wishing to improve their diagnostic skills in dermatology.

I gratefully acknowledge the invaluable and always cheerful assistance of my secretary, Kathy Suggs. I wish to thank my dermatology teachers and mentors: Dr. Richard Dobson, who first enticed me into dermatology and later opened the door to pediatric dermatology; Dr. John Maize, who provided helpful suggestions for the book; Dr. Pearon Lang; and Dr. Bruce Thiers. Finally, I want to express my appreciation to my past and present dermatology residents who have contributed both directly and indirectly to the evolution of this book with their questions, insights, and enthusiasm.

ELEANOR E. SAHN, MD

DEDICATION

To my children—Jim, Mike, and Rachel

Sharing in the first part of your lives has been my greatest joy.

PATIENT 1

A 3-year-old child with fever, meningismus, and purpuric skin lesions

A previously healthy 3-year-old girl presented with 1 day of fever, lethargy, and stiff neck followed by 6 hours of rapidly progressive purpura.

Physical Examination: Temperature 40°C; pulse 160; respirations 50; blood pressure 60/40. Neurologic: lethargy and meningismus. Skin: reticulated purpuric macules and necrosis over legs, lower abdomen, and buttocks (see figure).

Laboratory Findings: WBC 45,000/µl with 90% bands; platelet count 90,000/µl. Coagulation panel: PT 17 sec, APTT 45 sec, fibrinogen 150 mg/dl, decreased factors V and VIII, D-dimers 8 mg/ml, protein C 30% (normal 77–124%), protein S 40% (normal 62–117%). Skin biopsy: fibrin thrombi in small blood vessels with necrosis and hemorrhage; no inflammatory opacities. CSF analysis: protein 100 mg/dl, nucleated cells 500/µl, 75% neutrophils, glucose 20 mg/dl, Gram stain revealed G-diplococci. Blood and spinal fluid cultures: pending.

Question: What diagnosis is most compatible with the clinical presentation?

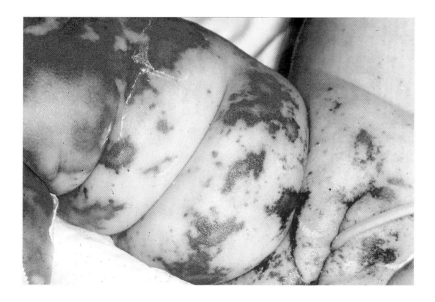

Diagnosis: Purpura fulminans with meningococcal meningitis

Discussion: A previously healthy child presenting with fever, hypotension, lethargy, meningismus, and progressive purpura suggests the diagnosis of purpura fulminans (PF). PF is a term used to describe the skin findings in a heterogeneous group of diseases. Purpura, hemorrhage, necrosis, and gangrene result from disseminated intravascular coagulation (DIC) with widespread thrombosis in small capillaries and venules and resultant hemorrhagic infarction. The brain, bladder, eye, and intestines also may be affected.

Purpura fulminans is seen in **three clinical settings**. Overwhelming bacterial sepsis is the most common setting, most often due to meningococcemia. Other bacteria that have been reported in association with purpura fulminans include *Staphylococcus aureus*, β-hemolytic streptococcus, *Streptococcus pneumoniae*, *Hemophilus influenzae*, and *Hemophilus aegyptius*.

PF is seen in a second group of patients, usually children and young infants, who have inherited deficiencies of protein C, protein S, or antithrombin III. Resistance to activated protein C may play a major role in neonatal PF. This resistance is associated with increased risk of thrombosis and is the result of a mutation in the gene coding for coagulation factor VR506-CQ. Approximately 3–5% of the general population have this mutation, and 25–50% of individuals with venous thrombosis show this mutation. Relative protein C and S deficiencies also occur in overwhelming sepsis and may initiate PF.

The third clinical setting is idiopathic or postinfectious, also seen most often in children. In these cases, PF occurs following a febrile illness, typically varicella or streptococcal infection. An autoimmune-acquired protein S deficiency may be the initiating event, since anti-protein S antibodies have been found in several patients.

Diagnosis of PF depends upon the clinical setting as well as the results of the skin biopsy and laboratory evaluation. The *differential diagnosis* of a skin biopsy specimen that shows fibrin thrombi, hemorrhage, and cutaneous necrosis without neutrophilic or lymphohistiocytic infiltrate includes, in addition to DIC, cryoglobulinemia, coumadin necrosis, hemolytic uremic syndrome, antiphospholipid antibody syndrome (lupus anticoagulant syndrome), thrombotic thrombocytopenic purpura, and protein C or S deficiency.

The mortality rate in PF is high, estimated at 20–50%. Successful management includes early, aggressive treatment of the underlying cause if one can be elicited, appropriate antibiotics, volume replacement, fresh frozen plasma, and heparin. Treatment of protein S or C deficiencies with protein C concentrate may be necessary. Tissue-type plasminogen activator has been used to limit thromboembolic complications. In patients with autoantibodies to protein S, additional therapies such as plasmapheresis and immunosuppression currently are being evaluated. Significant morbidity occurs in survivors who sustain major organ dysfunction as a result of thromboembolic phenomenon. **Peripheral gangrene** frequently necessitates amputations, and epiphyseal injuries may produce long-term limb-length deficiencies.

The present patient's blood and CSF cultures were positive for *Neisseria meningitides*. She responded to large doses of IV antibiotics and fluid, with resolution of symptoms over several weeks. However, peripheral gangrene necessitated amputation of three toes on the left foot.

Clinical Pearls

1. Rapidly spreading purpura and fever suggest bacterial sepsis and prompt treatment.
2. Meningococcemia is the most common cause of bacterial sepsis associated with PF.
3. Acquired or congenital deficiencies of protein C, protein S, or antithrombin III may be pathogenic in a multitude of thrombotic syndromes.
4. If there is no response to replacement of protein C, an autoantibody should be suspected and plasmapheresis should be instituted.

REFERENCES

1. Levin M, Eley BS, Louis J, et al: Postinfectious purpura fulminans caused by an autoantibody directed against protein S. J Pediatr 127:355–363, 1995.
2. Rivard GE, David M, Farrell C, et al: Treatment of purpura fulminans in meningococcemia with protein C concentrate. J Pediatr 126:646–652, 1995.
3. Pipe SW, Schmaier A, Nichols WC, et al: Neonatal purpura fulminans in association with factor V R506Q mutation. J Pediatr 128:706–709, 1996.
4. Sheridan RL, Briggs SE, Remensnyder JP, et al: Management strategy in purpura fulminans with multiple organ failure in children. Burns 22:53–56, 1996.

PATIENT 2

A 27-year-old woman with fever, diarrhea, hypotension, and macular erythema

A 27-year-old woman sustained an open tibial fracture in an automobile accident. She underwent open reduction and did well for 3 weeks postoperatively. Then a high fever, headache, weakness, diarrhea, and a sunburn-like facial rash developed. Two days later, she became confused and lost consciousness.

Physical Examination: Temperature 40.3°C; pulse 135; blood pressure 60/0. HEENT: strawberry tongue. Neurologic: barely arousable. Skin: Diffuse erythroderma, desquamation of palms and soles, with facial and limb edema (see figure); 3-cm fluctuant nodule over left tibial surgical wound. Gastrointestinal: guarding on palpation of abdomen; watery diarrhea.

Laboratory Findings: WBC 19,500/μl with 60% segmented neutrophils, 10% bands. AST and bilirubin: twice normal. BUN 48 mg/dl, creatinine 2.5 mg/dl. Urine: 3+ proteinuria. Cultures of blood, CSF and urine: sterile. Culture of fluctuant leg nodule: *Staphylococcus aureus*. Antistreptolysin O titer: less than 100 IU/ml.

Question: What is the most likely diagnosis?

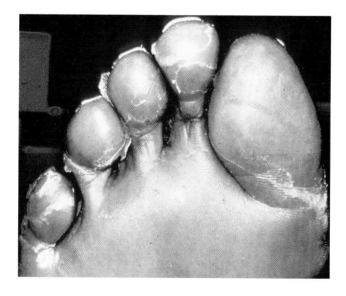

Diagnosis: Toxic shock syndrome resulting from staphylococcal abscess at open fracture site

Discussion: Toxic shock syndrome, first described in 1978, is caused by a toxin produced by *Staphylococcus aureus*, phage group 1, types 16, 29, 35, 36, and 52. These toxins are termed toxic shock syndrome toxin-1 (previously known as enterotoxin F) and toxic shock syndrome-1 negative toxins, and they include Staphylococcus enterotoxins A–E. Almost all menstrual and some nonmenstrual cases are caused by toxic shock syndrome toxin-1.

In 1987, toxic shock-*like* syndrome was described secondary to group A beta-hemolytic streptococcus. Certain invasive pyrogenic group A streptococci produce exotoxins A, B, and C, which can cause toxic shock–like syndrome (most often, enterotoxin A is causative). Marked biologic similarities exist between streptococcal exotoxins A, B, and C (the same exotoxins that cause scarlet fever) and the toxic shock syndrome toxins produced by *S. aureus*. There may be a **synergistic effect** between toxic shock syndrome toxin-1 produced by Staphylococcus and pyrogenic exotoxin C produced by Streptococcus when these infections are identified together in a single patient. These potent toxins are capable of multisystem injury by acting as superantigens, which leads to massive polyclonal T-cell stimulation with production of inflammatory mediators and cytokines. These cytokines (TNF-alpha, IL 1-B, and IL 6) mediate fever, shock, and tissue injury.

Staphylococcal toxic shock syndrome occurs in young, menstruating females in approximately half of the cases, often related to polyacrylate rayon tampon use. The other 50% of cases are seen in males and neonates in the following situations: (1) postoperative wound infections, (2) skin grafts, (3) burns, (4) abscesses, and (5) nasal packing. Patients present with fever greater than 39°C for longer than 5 days, hypotension, and scarlatiniform macular erythema over the entire skin surface. The erythema resembles an acute sunburn and resolves with fine scale and then desquamation of the palms and soles at 1 to 2 weeks, as in the present patient. Palmar and facial edema and multiorgan involvement of the GI, musculoskeletal, mucous membrane (including tongue and conjunctiva), renal, hepatic, hematologic, and neurologic systems also can occur.

The mortality rate in staphylococcal toxic shock syndrome is less than 5%, whereas in streptococcal toxic shock–like syndrome it approaches 30%. The increased mortality is believed to result from the extremely virulent strains of Streptococcus that have emerged in recent years. In addition to desquamative macular erythroderma, the streptococcal organisms produce bullae and soft tissue infection with necrotizing fasciitis or myositis in a high percentage of patients, leading to the higher morbidity and mortality. Similarly, blood cultures are positive in less than 15% of cases of toxic shock syndrome due to *S. aureus*, whereas they are positive in greater than 50% of the cases of streptococcal toxic shock–like syndrome.

The *differential diagnosis* of toxic shock syndrome includes streptococcal scarlet fever, leptospirosis, Rocky Mountain spotted fever, rubella, and viral exanthems.

Therapy of toxic shock syndrome includes appropriate antibiotic coverage and supportive care in an intensive care unit. Aggressive surgical intervention may be necessary to provide adequate drainage for localized infections in staphylococcal toxic shock syndrome or to excise areas of necrotizing fasciitis or myositis in streptococcal toxic shock–like syndrome. Other therapies that have been used include antagonists of TNF-alpha and IL 1, antitoxin antibodies, and high-dose immunoglobulins to neutralize toxin.

Clinical Pearls

1. The resurgence of Group A beta-hemolytic streptococcal infections is producing an increasing incidence of toxic shock–like syndrome.

2. Invasive Group A beta-hemolytic Streptococcus that produces toxic shock–like syndrome may be genetically related to the virulent strains of *Staphylococcus aureus* that produce toxic shock syndrome.

3. If a patient does not develop antibodies against erythrogenic toxins during the recovery period of streptococcal toxic shock–like syndrome, he or she will remain susceptible to severe streptococcal infections in the future.

REFERENCES

1. Todd J, Fishaut M, Kapral F, et al: Toxic shock syndrome associated with phage-group 1 Staphylococci. Lancet 2:1116–1118, 1978.
2. Smith RJ, Schlievert PM, Himelright IM, et al: Dual infections with *Staphylococcus aureus* and *Streptococcus pyogenes* causing toxic shock syndrome: Possible synergistic effects of toxic syndrome toxin-1 and streptococcal pyrogenic exotoxin C. Diagn Microbiol Infect Dis 19:245–247, 1994.
3. Leung DYM, Travers JB, Norris DA: The role of superantigens in skin disease. J Invest Dermatol 105:375–425, 1995.
4. Wolf JE, Rabinowitz LG: Streptococcal toxic shock-like syndrome. Arch Dermatol 131:73–77, 1995.
5. Jorup-Ronstrom C, Hofling M, Lundberg C, et al: Streptococcal toxic shock syndrome in a postpartum woman: Case report and review of the literature. Infection 24:164–167, 1996.

PATIENT 3

A 21-year-old man with an erythematous, vesicular eruption

A 21-year-old marine recruit was treated for a sore throat with trimethoprim-sulfamethoxazole (TMP-SMX). Two days later, an erythematous, macular eruption developed on his extremities, followed by vesicles and bullae on his lips and intraoral mucous membranes (see figures). He had been treated with TMP-SMX 5 years previously without a reaction.

Physical Examination: Temperature 39°C; pulse 120; respirations 30; blood pressure 120/78. Skin: widely disseminated, erythematous, round macules, some with a papule or vesicle in center, characterized by three rings of color—a central purpuric or vesicular part, a middle edematous and pale area, and a peripheral erythematous ring; numerous vesicles and bullae on lips and extending into mouth, producing erosion on buccal and gingival mucosa.

Laboratory Findings: CBC, LFT, renal function, chest radiograph, and urinalysis: normal. Skin biopsy: vacuolar change in basal cell layer, with necrotic keratinocytes in clumps and individually; marked subepidermal edema with a sparse lymphohistiocytic dermal infiltrate.

Questions: What type of drug reaction does this represent? How would you manage it?

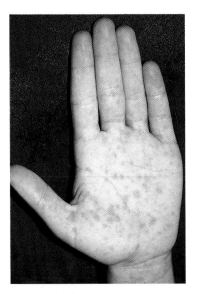

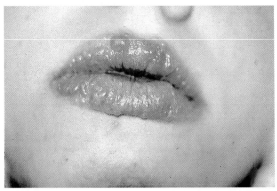

Diagnosis: Stevens-Johnson syndrome due to trimethoprim-sulfamethoxazole

Discussion: Stevens-Johnson syndrome is one of three related diseases characterized by epidermal injury and similar clinical, etiologic, and histopathologic findings. **Erythema multiforme** consists of individual erythematous macules with typical or atypical target (iris) morphology, as described in this patient. There is no or minimal mucous membrane involvement, and less than 20% of the body area is involved in the reaction. **Erythema multiforme major** (Stevens-Johnson syndrome) consists of the clinical findings in erythema multiforme plus more severe mucous membrane involvement, with 10–20% of the body surface area affected. There is fever and blistering of the lips and intraoral mucosa, as occurred in this patient. **Toxic epidermal necrolysis** (TEN) involves over 20–30% of the body area, with confluent tender erythema that rapidly progresses to bullae formation and erosions. Severe mucous membrane involvement and fever also are present. There is no consensus at present as to how best to classify this spectrum of diseases.

The cause of Stevens-Johnson syndrome and TEN is thought to be an immune reaction to a foreign antigen, most often a drug. Cytotoxic T-cells release cytokines, which result in keratinocyte degeneration. Herpes simplex virus has been implicated, particularly in recurrent erythema multiforme. This type of erythema multiforme may have a better prognosis than that not associated with herpes simplex virus. Drugs most often associated with the Stevens-Johnson syndrome and TEN are sulfonamides, oxicam, nonsteroidal anti-inflammatories, chlormezanone, anticonvulsants, and allopurinol. Surprisingly, corticosteroids recently have been added to this list. Immediate cessation of the offending drug, while advocated, will probably not alter the course.

The incidence of Stevens-Johnson syndrome is estimated at one to six cases per million persons per year. The timing of drug intake is critical in associating it with Stevens-Johnson syndrome or TEN. On first exposure to a drug, a reaction will occur 7–21 days after the initial dose. On re-exposure, a severe reaction can begin within 2 days, as occurred in the present patient.

Supportive care is the mainstay of treatment for both Stevens-Johnson syndrome and TEN. Large areas of skin involvement with blisters and erosions require careful dressing and isolation techniques, intravenous fluid and electrolyte management, and prompt treatment of infection. These patients are best managed in the hospital burn unit. The offending drug should be discontinued and no drugs from that family should be reinstituted. In very severe involvement, multi-organ failure can occur, with lymphopenia, neutropenia, gastrointestinal hemorrhage, liver failure, and pulmonary compromise. The use of systemic corticosteroids in the treatment of Stevens-Johnson syndrome and TEN remains controversial. Since most of the deaths are related to overwhelming infection or fluid and electrolyte imbalance, many believe that systemic corticosteroids are contraindicated. There are some small studies, however, that advocate their use in short courses. Since the diseases are self-limited once the offending drug is discontinued, there rarely would be an indication for using systemic corticosteroids.

In the present patient, skin involvement was 20%, requiring treatment in the burn unit. The TMP-SMX was immediately stopped. With aggressive fluid and electrolyte management and topical care of the denuded areas, he eventually recovered with minimal scarring.

Clinical Pearls

1. Erythema multiforme, Stevens-Johnson syndrome, and toxic epidermal necrolysis form a continuum of similar clinical, etiologic, and histopathologic features, but the disorders vary in the severity of epidermal injury.

2. Implication of a drug suspected of causing Stevens-Johnson syndrome is based on timing of first exposure. The drug started 7–21 days prior to symptoms is more likely to be the offender than drugs the patient has been taking for months or years.

3. Immediate discontinuation of the offending drug in Stevens-Johnson syndrome probably will not alter the course.

4. Systemic corticosteroid use in Stevens Johnson syndrome is controversial. If used, it should be given as a short burst only (5–10 days).

REFERENCES

1. Chan HL, Stern RS, Arndt KA, et al: The incidence of erythema multiforme, Stevens-Johnson syndrome, and toxic epidermal necrolysis. Arch Dermatol 126:43–47, 1990.
2. Schopf E, Stuhmer A, Rzany B, et al: Toxic epidermal necrolysis and Stevens-Johnson syndrome. Arch Dermatol 127:839–842, 1991.
3. Bastuji-Garin S, Rzany B, Stern R, et al: Clinical classification of cases of toxic epidermal necrolysis, Stevens-Johnson syndrome, and erythema multiforme. Arch Dermatol 129:92–96, 1993.
4. Rasmussen JE: Erythema multiforme. Arch Dermatol 131:726–728, 1995.
5. Roujeau JC, Kelly JP, Naldi L, et al: Medication use and the risk of Stevens-Johnson syndrome or toxic epidermal necrolysis. N Engl J Med 333:1600–1608, 1995.
6. Ka Kourou T, Klontza D, Soteropoulou, et al: Corticosteroid treatment of erythema multiforme major (Stevens-Johnson syndrome) in children. Eur J Pediatr 156:90–93, 1997.

PATIENT 4

A 57-year-old diabetic man with fever, productive cough, and purple nodules

A 57-year-old man with insulin-dependent diabetes mellitus and chronic obstructive pulmonary disease developed a productive cough, fever, and malaise. He was treated with oral tetracycline, but 5 days later tender, purple nodules on erythematous bases developed over his trunk and extremities.

Physical Examination: Temperature 40.6°C; pulse 140; respirations 32; blood pressure 90/60. Chest: bronchial breath sounds right axilla. Skin: erythematous, purple, tender nodules, 0.5- to 2-cm in diameter, scattered over lower trunk and extremities (see figure).

Laboratory Findings: WBC 22,000/μl with 80% neutrophils, 6% bands. Glucose: 380 mg/dl. Sputum Gram stain: many gram-negative rods. Chest radiograph: right middle lobe pneumonia. Blood and sputum cultures: pending.

Questions: What is the underlying diagnosis? What is your immediate course of action?

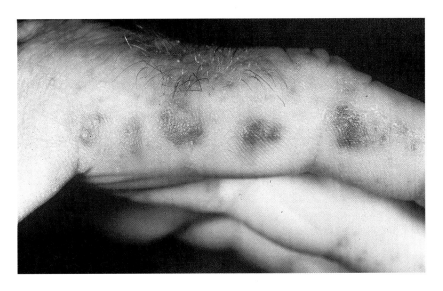

Diagnosis: Ecthyma gangrenosum associated with pseudomonas pneumonia and septicemia

Discussion: Ecthyma gangrenosum is a true **dermatologic emergency**, since it is virtually pathognomonic of pseudomonas septicemia. It is present in 30% of cases of pseudomonas sepsis. Had the present patient not been treated immediately and aggressively for gram-negative sepsis, he might not have survived until the blood and sputum cultures grew *Pseudomonas aeruginosa.*

Ecthyma gangrenosum is a vasculitis characterized by relatively few neutrophils but an intense bacillary infiltrate of the medial and adventitial layers of the vessel wall, with relative sparing of the intimal layer. Circulating immune complexes and bacterial exotoxins or endotoxins also may be pathogenic.

The clinical picture features erythematous, purpuric macules or nodules that may have vesicles, bullae, or hemorrhagic bullae superimposed. The vesicles or bullae evolve into necrotic ulcers, often with a black eschar in the center of an erythematous plaque. Other clinical presentations include blastomycosis-like pyoderma, erysipelas-like indurated plaques, and nodular cellulitis. The most common sites of ecthyma gangrenosum are the axillae and anogenital areas, where the skin is moist; however, the lesions can be seen on any part of the skin.

While *P. aeruginosa* was the originally described cause, other organisms such as *Staphylococcus aureus, Serratia marcescens, Escherichia coli,* klebsiella, candida, aspergillus, *Aeromonas hydrophilia,* and *Stenotrophomonas maltophilia* have been implicated. *P. aeruginosa* is a saprophytic, ubiquitous, intestinal gram-negative rod that requires a portal of entry—usually skin fissures or erosions, venipuncture sites, nasogastric or endotracheal tubes, urinary catheters, the umbilical cord in neonates, or the respiratory tract when a lung infection is present, as in the current case.

Pseudomonas sepsis is seen most often in the following situations: (1) prolonged antibiotic, chemotherapy, or steroid use; (2) diabetes mellitus; (3) neutropenia; (4) hypocomplementemia; (5) hypoimmunoglobulinemia; (6) malignancy; and (7) renal transplant. The *differential diagnosis* of the skin lesions includes cryoglobulinemia, drug eruption, periarteritis nodosa, necrotizing vasculitis, Sweet's syndrome, and chloroma.

Ecthyma gangrenosum portends a poor prognosis, with the mortality rate estimated at 30–70%. Three factors worsen the prognosis: neutropenia, multiple lesions, and increased time from diagnosis to institution of therapy. Thus, it is critical to recognize the skin lesions and institute appropriate therapy promptly. If conventional antibiotic therapy fails, some success has been reported in severe ecthyma gangrenosum with granulocyte-macrophage colony stimulating factor.

The present patient was treated with piperacillin, tobromycin, fluids, and vasopressor agents, and he eventually recovered.

Clinical Pearls

1. Severe bacterial infections in neutropenic hosts may be successfully treated by adding granulocyte-macrophage colony stimulating factor to an unsuccessful antibiotic regimen.

2. Ecthyma gangrenosum often is misdiagnosed initially, which results in delay of diagnosis and treatment of pseudomonas sepsis and increased mortality.

3. Patients at risk of pseudomonas sepsis should avoid exposure to pseudomonas species by avoiding under-chlorinated swimming pools, whirlpools, and hot tubs, as well as poorly washed raw vegetables.

REFERENCES

1. Greene SL, Su WPD, Muller SA: Ecthyma gangrenosum: Report of clinical, histopathologic, and bacteriologic aspects of eight cases. J Am Acad Dermatol 11:781–787, 1984.
2. Fleming MG, Milburn PB, Prose NS: Pseudomonas septicemia with nodules and bullae. Pediatr Dermatol 4:18–20, 1987.
3. Sevinsky LD, Viecens C, Ballesteros DA, et al: Ecthyma gangrenosum: A cutaneous manifestation of *Pseudomonas aeruginosa* sepsis. J Am Acad Dermatol 29:104–105, 1993.
4. Agger WA, Mardan A: *Pseudomonas aeruginosa* infections of intact skin. Clin Infect Dis 20:302–308, 1995.
5. Becherel PA, Chosidow O, Berger E, et al: Granulocyte-macrophage colony–stimulating factor in the management of severe ecthyma gangrenosum related to myelodysplastic syndrome. Arch Dermatol 131:892–894, 1995.

PATIENT 5

A 3-month-old infant with facial dermatitis and irritability

After 2 months of irritability, poor feeding, and almost continuous crying while awake, a totally breast-fed 3-month-old male infant suffered a facial and perianal eruption with diarrhea.

Physical Examination: General: crying and irritable; vital signs normal; weight 10.2 pounds (30th percentile). Skin: sharply demarcated, erythematous, scaly papules and plaques around the mouth, eyes, and thigh (see figure, *top*); moist, erythematous, partially eroded plaques in perianal distribution (see figure, *bottom*); nails and hair normal.

Laboratory Findings: Potassium hydroxide (KOH) examination: negative for hyphae. CBC, serum chemistries, Westergren ESR, antinuclear antibody: normal. Biopsy of thigh plaque: pending.

Questions: What is the most likely diagnosis? What is your immediate course of action?

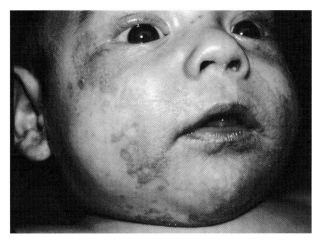

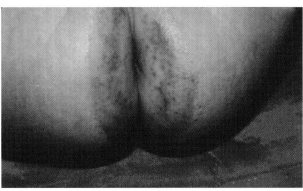

Diagnosis: Acrodermatitis enteropathica or other zinc deficiency

Discussion: Acrodermatitis enteropathica (AE) is an autosomal recessive disorder characterized by periorificial and acral dermatitis, alopecia, diarrhea, irritability, and depression. Physical examination is significant for erythematous patches and plaques of dry, scaly, eczematous skin, which may evolve into crusted, vesiculobullous, erosive, and pustular lesions. Paronychia as well as loss of scalp hair, eyebrows, and eyelashes may occur. Lesions may become secondarily infected with *Staphylococcus aureus* and *Candida albicans.* Withdrawal, depression, photophobia, and loss of appetite often are seen.

Symptoms of AE occur within the first few months after birth and may appear shortly after discontinuation of breast feeding. This phenomenon has led many to believe that human milk has a beneficial ligand that bovine milk lacks. The protein concentration of human milk may affect **zinc bioavailability**. The AE mutation produces decreased intestinal zinc absorption and/or transport, but the precise nature of the metabolic defect is unknown.

AE can be accurately diagnosed only after attempts to remove zinc supplements have failed. Thereafter, the patient with AE must remain on zinc supplements for life. Differentiating AE from acquired zinc deficiency can be difficult since the presentation is the same. Studies have shown that low zinc levels in the mother's milk may produce an acquired zinc deficiency in full-term, breast-fed infants. These levels may be due to a defect in mammary zinc secretion. Acquired zinc deficiency also may occur in premature infants, regardless of maternal zinc levels, due to the infant's greater bodily demand and lower bodily stores of zinc.

The *differential diagnosis* includes: atopic dermatitis, psoriasis, seborrheic dermatitis, kwashiorkor, cystic fibrosis, glucagonoma syndrome, essential fatty acid deficiencies, mucocutaneous candidiasis, histiocytosis X, neonatal lupus erythematosus, epidermolysis bullosa, biotin and multiple carboxylase deficiencies, and acquired zinc deficiencies.

The diagnosis is made clinically and histopathologically. Plasma, hair, urine, parotid saliva zinc, and serum alkaline phosphatase (which may be low) levels can be helpful. Zinc concentrations in maternal breast milk also can help differentiate AE from acquired zinc deficiency. Treatment involves oral zinc supplementation for life in a dose of 2–5 mg/kg/day.

In the present patient, histopathologic examination of the skin biopsy specimen revealed prominent parakeratosis at the stratum corneum, irregular epidermal hyperplasia, and scattered individual dyskeratotic keratinocytes. The papillary dermis was edematous, with prominent tortuous capillaries. There were perivascular and interstitial inflammatory infiltrates composed of lymphocytes and histiocytes. This finding was consistent with AE.

A plasma zinc level was obtained, and the child was immediately begun on oral zinc sulfate supplement at a dose of 5 mg/kg/day. The initial plasma zinc level was 1.2 mcg/dl (normal 68–130). The infant's attitude improved almost immediately, with decreased crying and irritability. Normal smiling behavior appeared for the first time, and a plasma zinc level was normal 1 month later. An attempt to wean the child off oral zinc therapy at the age of 1 year resulted in recurrence of the face rash and irritability. He again was placed on oral zinc supplement and continues to do well as he approaches his fourth birthday.

Clinical Pearls

1. Untreated AE can lead to severe failure to thrive and death.

2. The AE mutation affects intestinal zinc absorption/transport. In addition, human fibroblasts from patients with AE show abnormal zinc metabolism and lower zinc transport compared to normal patients.

3. Zinc deficiency rarely is seen in totally breast-fed infants.

4. Periorificial dermatitis and zinc deficiency may be the presenting findings in cystic fibrosis.

REFERENCES

1. Schmidt CP, Tunnessen W: Cystic fibrosis presenting with periorificial dermatitis. J Am Acad Dermatol 25:896–897, 1991.
2. Ando K, Goto Y, Matsumoto Y, et al: Acquired zinc deficiency in a breast-fed mature infant: A possible case of acquired maternal decreased zinc uptake by the mammary gland. J Am Acad Dermatol 29:111–112, 1993.
3. Grider A, Young EM: The acrodermatitis enteropathica mutation transiently affects zinc metabolism in human fibroblasts. J Nutr 126:19–24, 1996.

PATIENT 6

A 63-year-old woman with a pruritic, photodistributed eruption

A 63-year-old woman developed an erythematous eruption on the face following sun exposure 6 weeks previously. The eruption was extremely pruritic and spread to the extensor surfaces of her forearms and hands. She felt well otherwise. Past history revealed a total hysterectomy for ovarian cancer 17 years previously and a radical mastectomy for breast cancer 4 years previously. Her only medications were tamoxifen for 4 years, glyburide for 3 years, and acetaminophen occasionally.

Physical Examination: General: healthy appearing, normal vital signs. Skin: photodistributed, erythematous, scaly eruption covering face, V of neck (see figure, *left*), extensor forearms, and upper back; erythematous plaques limited to skin over joints on dorsal hands (see figure, *right*); posterior nail fold capillary dilatations and infarcts; well-healed mastectomy scar. Lymph nodes: normal. Abdomen: normal.

Laboratory Findings: CBC, sequential multiple analysis-20, creatine phosphokinase, electromyogram: normal. Chest radiograph: no evidence of metastatic disease. Skin biopsies of dorsal hand and extensor forearm: pending.

Questions: What is your diagnosis? What is the most appropriate work-up?

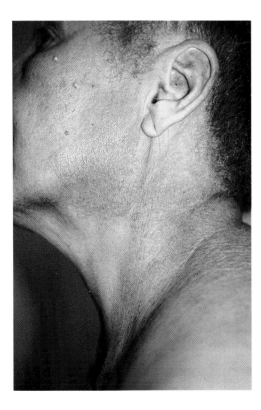 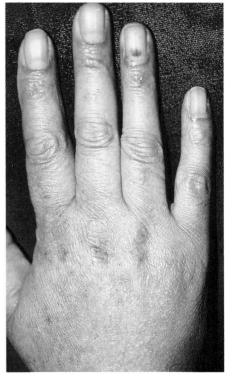

Diagnosis: Paraneoplastic dermatomyositis with recurrent breast cancer

Discussion: Paraneoplastic dermatomyositis is dermatomyositis occurring in **association with internal malignancy**. The reported incidence in patients with dermatomyositis is 8–45%. The malignancy may precede, be concurrent with, or follow the diagnosis of dermatomyositis. After several years with dermatomyositis, a patient's risk of malignancy is similar to that of the normal population. Increased risk of malignancy has been reported in dermatomyositis sine myositis, polymyositis, and juvenile dermatomyositis, as well as in dermatomyositis itself.

The most common types of malignancy reported in association with dermatomyositis are lung, breast, gastrointestinal, ovarian, and cervical cancers, and malignant melanoma and leukemia have been reported. The prognosis for these malignancies appears to be worse in those with myositis and malignancy. One study noted that **cutaneous necrosis** in association with dermatomyositis was a predictor of malignancy.

Other paraneoplastic dermatologic diseases or findings that should prompt an investigation for malignancy include: acanthosis nigricans, tripe palms, dermatitis herpetiformis, extramammary Paget's disease, hypertrophic pulmonary osteoarthropathy, clubbing, pemphigus vulgaris, unexplained pruritus, pyoderma gangrenosum, Sweet's syndrome, reactive erythemas such as erythema gyratum repens, necrolytic migratory erythema, multicentric reticulohistiocytosis, palmar hyperkeratosis, acquired ichthyosis, Bazex's syndrome, florid cutaneous papillomatosis, the sign of Leser-Trelat, and hypertrichosis lanuginosa acquisita.

The evaluation of the newly diagnosed patient with dermatomyositis should include a thorough history and physical examination, routine laboratory tests and screens, including CBC, blood chemistries, chest radiograph, stool for occult blood, and mammograms. If there is a past history of malignancy, as in the present patient, a more extensive examination for recurrent or metastatic disease should be undertaken. Otherwise, any further testing should be based on the findings from the routine examinations.

In the present patient, histopathologic examination of skin showed a superficial perivascular infiltrate with a vacuolar interface dermatitis. A colloidal iron stain was positive for dermal mucin, but a periodic acid–Schiff stain was negative for basement membrane thickening. The lack of a deep infiltrate or basement membrane thickening made lupus erythematosus less likely. The presence of mucin made a drug eruption less likely.

The patient was found to have a carcinoma of the opposite breast on mammography. A lumpectomy was performed, followed by 6 weeks of radiation therapy. Her eruption gradually improved with emollients, topical corticosteroid cream, and sun avoidance over this time period.

Clinical Pearls

1. Newly diagnosed dermatomyositis may be a marker of internal malignancy. A thorough history, physical examination, and age-appropriate laboratory screenings are warranted.

2. Diagnostic criteria for dermatomyositis and paraneoplastic dermatomyositis are the same, and include characteristic clinical and histopathologic skin changes as well as muscle findings (weakness; biopsy changes; elevated creatine phosphokinase, alanine aminotransferase, and aldolase) if myositis is present.

3. Cutaneous necrosis in dermatomyositis may be a marker of malignancy.

REFERENCES

1. Callen JP: Dermatomyositis and malignancy. Clin Dermatol 11(1):61–65, 1993.
2. Callen JP: Relationship of cancer to inflammatory muscle diseases: Dermatomyositis, polymyositis, and inclusion body myositis. Rheum Dis Clin North Am 20(4):943–953, 1994.
3. Chow WH, Gridley G, Mellemkjaer L, et al: Cancer risk following polymyositis and dermatomyositis: A nationwide study in Denmark. Cancer Causes Control 6(1):9–13, 1995.
4. Kurzrock R, Cohen PR: Cutaneous paraneoplastic syndromes in solid tumors. Am J Med 99(6):662–671, 1995.
5. Whitmore SE, Watson R, Rosenshein NB, et al: Dermatomyositis sine myositis: Association with malignancy. J Rheumatol 23(1):101–105, 1996.

PATIENT 7

A 3-month-old infant with hypomelanosis and seizures

A 3-month-old African-American girl was noted at birth to have white patches on the extremities and trunk. At $2^1/_2$ months of age, she had a grand mal seizure following a paroxysm of coughing. The diagnosis at that time was reflux-related hypoxic seizure disorder.

Physical Examination: Vital signs: normal. General: developmentally normal. Skin: hypopigmentation—linear streaks on extremities, checkerboard patches on abdomen, whorls and swirls on back (see figure).

Laboratory Findings: Karyotype: 46 XX. MRI of brain: normal for age.

Pediatric Ophthalmologic Examination: Hyperopia, but no evidence of strabismus or cataracts.

Question: What are the underlying diagnosis and the prognosis for this child?

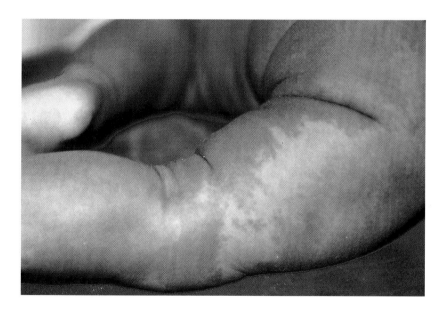

Diagnosis: Hypomelanosis of Ito (incontinentia pigmenti acromians, systemized nevus depigmentosus)

Discussion: Hypomelanosis of Ito (HI) is a congenital syndrome consisting of hypopigmented patches, which follow the developmental lines of Blaschko, and systemic manifestations, most often neurologic or ophthalmologic. Reported association with systemic involvement varies from 30% to 75%. Current data suggest that earlier reports exaggerated the incidence of underlying abnormalities.

The hypopigmented patches may not be noted at birth, but are seen in early childhood. They usually are bilateral, but may be unilateral. Blaschko's developmental lines tend to produce a pattern that is linear on the extremities, marbled with whorls and swirls on the trunk, and V-shaped over the spine.

Neurologic abnormalities found in association with HI include structural brain anomalies, seizure disorders, mental retardation, and developmental delay. Associated ophthalmologic abnormalities include strabismus and cataracts. Other systemic findings reported with HI include musculoskeletal anomalies, such as skeletal or hemifacial hypoplasia, autism, precocious puberty, language disabilities, neuroblastoma, cerebellar ataxia, and palmoplantar keratoderma.

The *differential diagnosis* of congenital hypopigmentation following the lines of Blaschko includes fourth-stage **incontinentia pigmenti**, which is hypopigmented and usually atrophic. Typically there is a history of blistering, verrucous lesions and hyperpigmentation. **Goltz syndrome** can show hypopigmented streaks, but also multiple other findings, including atrophy, papillomas, nail dystrophy, and characteristic musculoskeletal findings. Early systemized **epidermal nevus** can appear as faint hypopigmented streaks or patches which subsequently become hyperkeratotic. **Nevus depigmentosus** can present with an identical pattern of hypopigmentation, but no associated systemic involvement. There may be a difference in the histopathologic findings between nevus depigmentosus and HI, but some authors believe that HI is, in fact, systemized nevus depigmentosus. Linear and whorled hypermelanosis and the third stage of incontinentia pigmenti present with hyperpigmented streaks, swirls, and patches in a pattern identical to HI. It may be difficult to determine whether the primary pigmentary abnormality is *hypo*pigmentation or *hyper*pigmentation.

On histopathologic examination, HI-affected skin shows decreased melanocytes, some of which are abnormally shaped. There appears to be a nearly normal content of melanosomes in the melanocytes which are present. Nevus depigmentosus is thought to represent a functional defect in melanocytes, with a normal number of melanocytes and melanosomes but a decreased transfer of melanosomes to keratinocytes, thereby producing the hypopigmented appearance of the skin.

The present patient had no further seizure activity by 1 year of age and is being followed by the pediatric neurology and dermatology services. She is not being treated with medication.

Clinical Pearls

1. Hypomelanosis following Blaschko's lines is an uncommon finding in dermatology and warrants a precise evaluation to exclude hypomelanosis of Ito, incontinentia pigmenti (fourth stage), Goltz syndrome, linear epidermal nevus (early), nevus depigmentosus, chimerism, mosaicism, and associated systemic involvement.

2. Hypomelanosis of Ito probably represents a heterogeneous group of genetic disorders and may be a description rather than a diagnosis.

3. Many patients with HI show chromosomal mosaicism. There is a subgroup of girls with hypomelanosis of Ito due to X; autosome translocation. Genetic clarification is ongoing.

4. The evaluation of the infant with hypomelanosis of Ito includes pediatric neurologic and ophthalmologic examinations, brain MRI, and karyotyping.

REFERENCES

1. Sybert VP: Hypomelanosis of Ito: A description, not a diagnosis. J Invest Dermatol 103(5 Suppl):141S–143S, 1994.
2. Cavallari V, Ussia AF, Siragusa M, et al: Hypomelanosis of Ito: electron microscopical observations on two new cases. J Dermatol Sci 13:87–92, 1996.
3. Hatchwell E: Hypomelanosis of Ito and X; autosome translocations: A unifying hypothesis. J Med Genet 33:177–183, 1996.
4. Nehal KS, Pe Benito R, Orlow SJ: Analysis of 54 cases of hypopigmentation and hyperpigmentation along the lines of Blaschko. Arch Dermatol 132:1167–1170, 1996.
5. Steiner J, Adamsbaum C, Desguerres I, et al: Hypomelanosis of Ito and brain abnormalities: MRI findings and literature review. Pediatr Radiol 26(11):763–768, 1996.

PATIENT 8

A 4-month-old girl with a photodistributed face eruption

A 4-month-old girl suffered an asymptomatic facial eruption at 6 weeks of age following brief sun exposure. Her mother brought her in when the rash failed to dissipate after 2 months. The child was the product of a normal pregnancy and delivery, was in good health, and had an older sibling also in good health. The patient's mother denied joint pains, weight loss, and rashes, but had noted dry eyes in recent months.

Physical Examination: Pulse: 140 and regular. Skin: erythematous, scaly plaques with raised borders and telangiectasias encircling eyes and covering top of cheeks and bridge of nose (see figure); cutis marmorata pattern over legs. Abdomen: no organomegaly. Extremities: pulses 2+ bilaterally. Cardiac: regular rate and rhythm, no murmurs.

Laboratory Findings: CBC, Chem-20, and urinalysis: normal. Antinuclear antibody (ANA): negative. Extractable nuclear antigen screen positive: anti-RNP antibody inconclusive, anti-Smith and anti-La antibodies negative, anti-Ro antibody strongly positive at a titer greater than 80 units (normal 0–19). Electrocardiogram: normal. **Mother's laboratory findings:** WBC 4.0/µl (normal 4.8–10.8); ANA 1:1280 (speckled pattern); anti-DNA negative; rheumatoid factor 377 (normal 0–20 IU/ml). Extractable nuclear antigen screen positive: anti-Ro antibody 161, anti-La antibody 124 (normals for both 0–19 units), anti-Smith and anti-RNP antibodies negative.

Questions: What is the underlying diagnosis? What is the appropriate follow-up in this family?

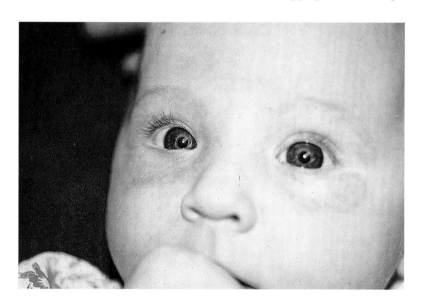

Diagnosis: Neonatal lupus erythematosus

Discussion: Neonatal lupus erythematosus (NLE) is a transplacentally acquired autoimmune disease that presents at or before birth with heart block, or in early infancy with a photodistributed skin eruption. The eruption is transient and spontaneously resolves at 6–8 months of age when maternal antibody clears from the child's system; on rare occasions it persists to 15 months. Maternal autoantibodies that have been implicated include Ro, La, U₁RNP, nDNA, cardiolipin, ANA, and rheumatoid factor. Later development of systemic lupus erythematosus (SLE) or other connective tissue in the child is reported, but extremely rare.

Only 25% of mothers of infants with NLE fulfill the diagnostic criteria for SLE. Therefore, NLE is a misnomer. Asymptomatic mothers who later develop SLE usually have a nonlife-threatening variety. Other connective tissue diseases seen in mothers of infants with NLE include subacute cutaneous lupus erythematosus, Sjögren syndrome, Raynaud's phenomenon, and sicca syndrome. Photosensitivity and arthritis also are noted.

In addition to the risks to the mother of developing connective tissue disease, future pregnancies are at risk. There is an increased incidence of spontaneous abortion, a 15% incidence of recurrence of congenital heart block, and a 25% incidence of a subsequent child affected with either the cutaneous or cardiac manifestations of NLE. Congenital heart block carries a mortality rate of 15–30%, and two-thirds of children who survive require permanent pacemakers. There is some evidence that congenital heart block diagnosed in utero can be successfully treated with **dexamethasone**.

The cutaneous disease of NLE typically presents with photodistributed papules and plaques, which may be annular or polycyclic, on the face, scalp, and (less likely) on the trunk and extremities. The lesions most closely resemble those of subacute cutaneous lupus erythematosus. Features of discoid lupus erythematosus, such as follicular plugging, atrophy, and telangiectasias, are seen less commonly. Occasionally erosions or targetoid lesions resembling erythema multiforme may be seen. One patient presented with the findings of cutis marmorata telangiectatica congenita (persistent livedo reticularis pattern on legs, telangiectasia, and superficial ulcerations) who was found to have NLE.

The *differential diagnosis* of the facial eruption of NLE includes seborrheic dermatitis, tinea corporis, viral exanthem, granuloma annulare, atypical erythema multiforme, erythema annulare centrifugum, syphilis, psoriasis, atopic dermatitis, nevus flammeus (port-wine stain), and photosensitive genodermatoses such as Bloom or Rothmund-Thomson syndrome.

The eruption in this infant resolved over the subsequent 2 months with the use of a mild topical steroid cream and vigorous photoprotection including daily sunscreens and sun avoidance. The mother was referred for rheumatologic work-up and diagnosed with connective tissue disease–unspecified type, with close follow-up suggested. Risk of recurrence in subsequent pregnancies was discussed with both parents. The likelihood of this infant developing progressive disease or a different connective tissue disease is low.

Clinical Pearls

1. Neonatal lupus erythematosus is caused by maternal autoantibodies transferred transplacentally. These autoantibodies include: Ro, La, U₁RNP, nDNA, cardiolipin, ANA, and RF. Smith autoantibody has not been reported in NLE.

2. NLE is a misnomer since only 25% of mothers fulfill the criteria for SLE.

3. NLE may present with a livedo pattern and ulcerations that resemble cutis marmorata telangiectatica congenita.

4. The recurrence rate of congenital heart block in NLE is 15% in subsequent pregnancies, a three-fold increase over the rate in a prima gravida with the same autoantibody pattern.

REFERENCES

1. Lee LA, Norris DA, Weston WL: Neonatal lupus and the pathogenesis of cutaneous lupus. Pediatr Dermatol 3:491–497, 1986.
2. Provost TT, Watson R, Gammon WR, et al: The neonatal lupus syndrome associated with U₁RNP antibodies. N Engl J Med 316:1135–1138, 1987.
3. Neidenbach PJ, Sahn ES: La (SS-B)-positive neonatal lupus erythematosus: Report of a case with unusual features. J Am Acad Dermatol 29:848–852, 1993.
4. Buyon JP: Neonatal lupus: Bedside to bench and back. Scand J Rheumatol 25:271–276, 1996.
5. Carrascosa JM, Ribera M, Bielsa I, et al: Cutis marmorata telangiectatica congenita or neonatal lupus? Pediatr Dermatol May-Jun 13:230–232, 1996.

PATIENT 9

A 15-year-old girl with erosions on the lower lip

A 15-year-old girl sustained painful erosions primarily located on the middle of the lower lip. These persisted for 6 weeks despite treatment with topical antifungal agents, topical steroids, and emollients as well as the discontinuation of all irritants including lipstick, sunscreen, toothpaste, and spices. Her only medication was erythromycin 500 mg b.i.d. for 2 years for acne vulgaris.

Physical Examination: General: healthy appearance. Skin: an erythematous eroded plaque over middle of lower lip, with similar smaller lesions on mid upper and lateral lip; no extension onto vermilion border nor onto intraoral mucosa; hair, nails, lymph nodes normal.

Laboratory Findings: CBC and blood glucose: normal. KOH examination of lower lip: hyphal elements and spores.

Questions: What is the diagnosis? How would you treat it?

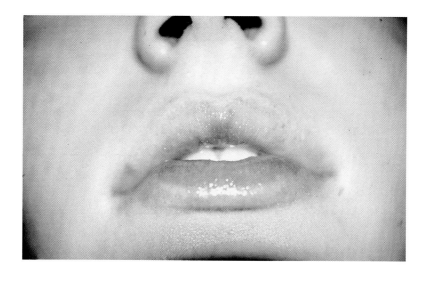

Diagnosis: Erosive Candida cheilitis

Discussion: Candida cheilitis was described by Jansen, et al. in 1963 and has been rarely reported since that time. It represents Candida infection of the lip alone, without intraoral thrush or involvement of the labial commissures (angular cheilitis or perleche). Jansen divided Candida cheilitis into **two clinical types**: erosive candida cheilitis, in which there are bright red erosions of the middle lower lip, sometimes with desquamation or hyperkeratosis, and granular cheilitis, in which the vermilion border and lip have a granular appearance.

Candida cheilitis also has been termed cheilocandidosis or juvenile juxtavermilion candidiasis. In some reports, intraoral Candida infection and/or angular cheilitis occurred simultaneously. Precipitating or associated factors in the etiology of Candida cheilitis include compulsive lip licking, Sjögren's syndrome, actinic lip damage, diabetes mellitus, hematologic abnormalities, poor dental hygiene, smoking, drug therapy, malocclusion due to decreased vertical height or malfitting dentures, drooling due to a deepened commissure produced by aging facial muscles, contact dermatitis, wind burn, chapping, and squamous cell carcinoma.

The *differential diagnosis* of an erythematous, eroded plaque on the lower lip includes allergic contact dermatitis, irritant contact dermatitis, cheilitis granularis, granulomatous cheilitis (Milkerson-Rosenthal syndrome), cutaneous Crohn's disease, atopic cheilitis (lip-licker dermatitis), herpes simplex infection, and squamous cell carcinoma.

The present patient was treated with **fluconazole** 200 mg daily for 2 weeks with resolution of all symptoms. Chronic antibiotic therapy for treatment of acne vulgaris may have played a contributory role in this case.

Clinical Pearls

1. Candida cheilitis is rare and is frequently misdiagnosed as contact dermatitis.

2. It is not necessary to perform an elaborate search for underlying disease in a healthy patient with one episode of Candida cheilitis that responds to oral antifungal agents.

3. A positive Candida culture does not indicate pathogenic significance, since many normal individuals demonstrate growth of *Candida albicans* from the oral mucosa. A positive KOH examination of the lip erosion is necessary to confirm the diagnosis of Candida cheilitis.

REFERENCES

1. Jansen GT, Dillaha CJ, Honeycutt WM: Candida cheilitis. Arch Dermatol 88:141–145, 1963.
2. Reade PC, Rich AM, Hay KD, et al: Cheilocandidosis: A possible clinical entity. Report of five cases. Br Dent J 152:305–308, 1982.
3. Bouquot JE, Fenton SJ: Juvenile juxtavermilion candidiasis yet another form of an old disease? J Am Dent Assoc 116:187–192, 1988.

PATIENT 10

A 16-year-old girl with a reticulated, violaceous skin eruption

A 16-year-old girl first experienced an eruption on the dorsum of the feet at the age of 10. The rash spread to involve all four extremities and the trunk over the subsequent 6 years. She was asymptomatic and in good health, with a negative review of systems. She was on no medications and took no nonprescription medications or drugs. She did not smoke.

Physical Examination:　Vital signs: normal. Skin: violaceous, reticulated, mottled patches most pronounced over dorsum of feet and anterior legs (see figure), but also present on forearms, palms, and lower trunk; erythema blanched on diascopy, leaving a hemosiderin stain; no nodular or palpable lesions; posterior nail fold capillaries normal. Remainder of physical examination: normal.

Laboratory Findings:　CBC with differential, platelet count, ESR: normal. Amylase and lipase: normal. Rapid plasmin reagin: negative. Skin biopsy: pending.

Questions:　What is this reaction pattern termed? How would you arrive at a specific diagnosis?

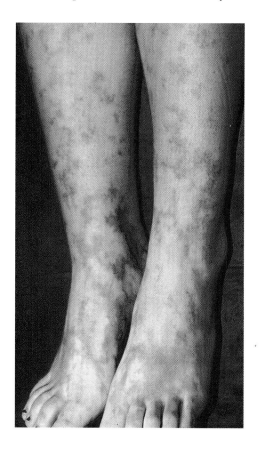

Diagnosis: Livedo reticularis (primary or idiopathic)

Discussion: Livedo reticularis is a vascular reaction pattern that is produced by a multitude of underlying conditions or diseases. The violaceous, net-like pattern is due to dilatation of the venous plexus in the subpapillary dermis. Dilatation can result from hyperviscosity of the blood, decreased blood outflow from the skin, or small vessel abnormalities, such as vasculitis or vasospasm.

The *differential diagnosis* of livedo reticularis can be divided into congenital, which includes cutis marmorata telangiectatica congenita, and acquired, which includes physiologic (cutis marmorata), idiopathic, and a large group of conditions and diseases. Secondary causes of livedo reticularis include connective tissue diseases (mixed systemic lupus erythematosus, scleroderma, dermatomyositis, rheumatoid arthritis, and cutaneous or systemic polyarteritis nodosa); vasculitis (leukocytoclastic vasculitis, granulomatous arteritis of Churg-Strauss, and livedoid vasculitis); paraproteinemia (cold agglutininemia or cryoglobulinemia); intravascular occlusion (disseminated intravascular coagulation [DIC], protein C and S deficiencies, antithrombin III deficiency, thrombocythemia, polycythemia vera, thrombotic thrombocytopenic purpura, macroglobulinemia, and cholesterol emboli); infections (syphilis, meningococcemia, endocarditis, tuberculosis); drugs (amantadine, catacholamines, quinidine, and minocycline); and conditions such as antiphospholipid syndrome, pancreatitis, eosinophilia myalgia syndrome, carcinoid, pheochromocytoma, hypothyroidism, mycosis fungoides, and hyperparathyroidism with hypercalcemia. For patients with persistent livedo reticularis in whom an underlying cause is not found, as in the present patient, the diagnosis is considered idiopathic or primary.

The histopathologic findings in livedo reticularis are variable and depend on the duration and severity of the condition. In the mildest forms, only dilatation of superficial capillaries may be seen. Other cases may feature DIC or vasculitis with intimal proliferation and arterial thrombi.

Idiopathic acquired livedo reticularis is asymptomatic, diffuse, and symmetric. It most commonly affects young women aged 25–45. Occasionally, these patients develop small, painful ulcerations in the winter (livedo reticularis with winter ulcerations) or in the summer (livedo reticularis with summer ulcerations). Therapies tried with varying success for painful ulcerations include antiplatelet agents such as dipyridamole, ticlopidine, and low-dose aspirin. Pentoxifylline, which decreases blood viscosity by increasing erythrocyte flexibility, can be helpful. Bed rest is necessary for ulcer healing. Agents that enhance fibrinolysis, such as stanozolol, have been helpful as well.

In the present patient, the biopsy specimen revealed fibrin thrombi in the small blood vessels with secondary sweat gland necrosis and a sparse perivascular lymphocytic infiltrate. The following additional blood work was found to be normal or negative: antinuclear antibody, anti-DNA, hepatitis B surface antigen, cryoglobulins, cold agglutinins, creatine phosphokinase, antithrombin III, lupus anticoagulant, protein S, protein C, antiphospholipid antibody, and fibrin monomers. She was placed on 325 mg of aspirin per day and instructed to avoid cold exposure, cigarette smoking, and birth control pills or hormones, since these can increase intravascular coagulation. After 2 months on low-dose aspirin therapy, the eruption faded somewhat. She will be closely followed.

Clinical Pearls

1. Livedo reticularis is a vascular reaction pattern that requires methodical evaluation to arrive at a precise diagnosis.

2. Livedo reticularis results from dilatation of the venous plexus in the subpapillary dermis. This dilatation can be produced by hyperviscosity of the blood, decreased blood outflow, or vessel abnormalities such as vasculitis or vasospasm.

3. Patients with idiopathic livedo reticularis should avoid cold and medications or conditions known to increase blood viscosity or coagulability (e.g., smoking, birth control pills).

4. Drugs may be overlooked as a cause of livedo reticularis.

REFERENCES

1. Weir NU, Snowden JA, Greaves M, et al: Livedo reticularis associated with hereditary protein C deficiency and recurrent thromboembolism. Br J Dermatol 132:283–285, 1995.
2. Elkayam O, Yaron M, Caspi D: Minocycline-induced arthritis associated with fever, livedo reticularis, and pANCA. Ann Rheum Dis 55:769–771, 1996.
3. Morell A, Botella R, Silvestre JF, et al: Livedo reticularis and thrombotic purpura related to the use of diphenhydramine associated with pyrithyldione. Dermatology 193:50–51, 1996.

PATIENT 11

A 7-year-old boy with a scaly eruption and abnormal tongue

A 7-year-old boy with a fever and a sore throat was treated with amoxicillin. Two days later, an erythematous eruption developed on his neck, accompanied by a tongue abnormality. The amoxicillin was discontinued. One week later, the eruption had faded, but was replaced by diffuse desquamation.

Physical Examination: Temperature 40.5°C; pulse 130; blood pressure 100/70. Skin: diffuse erythema with fine desquamation over face and upper trunk, with circumoral sparing; linear streaks of petechiae in antecubital fossae. Intraoral exam: enlarged tonsils with purulence; tongue coated white with protrusions of enlarged red papillae (see figure). Nodes: enlarged (1- to 2-cm) lymph nodes in anterior cervical chains and submandibular areas bilaterally.

Laboratory Findings: WBC 15,500/µl with 80% neutrophils. Antistreptolysin O titer and throat culture: pending.

Questions: What is your diagnosis? What therapeutic options would you consider?

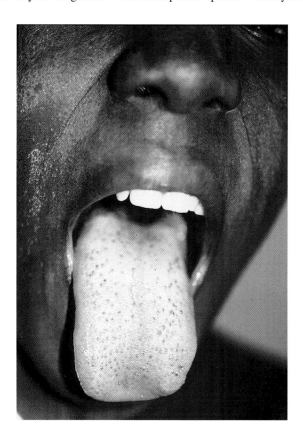

Diagnosis: Scarlet fever due to streptococcal pharyngitis

Discussion: Scarlet fever is an infectious disease affecting children between the ages of 4 and 8 that is caused by pyrogenic exotoxins produced by group A beta-hemolytic streptococci (GABHS). These exotoxins, termed A, B, and C, occasionally are produced by groups of beta-hemolytic streptococci other than group A. The source of the streptococcal infection usually is the tonsils or pharynx, but occasionally skin infections or surgical wounds harbor the streptococcus. Most adults have antibodies to these streptococcal exotoxins and, therefore, are not susceptible to scarlet fever. For this reason, it is extremely unlikely for a child to have a recurrent attack of scarlet fever.

Fever and pharyngitis usually precede the appearance of the eruption by 1–4 days, as in this child. The rash characteristically begins on the neck or face and spreads downward, with pronounced circumoral pallor or sparing and sparing of the palms and soles. There are three diagnostic signs: **Pastia's sign** represents accentuation of erythema and/or petechiae in the skin folds due to capillary fragility; **tiny rough papules** produce a sandpaper feel to the skin of the trunk; and **strawberry tongue**.

Strawberry tongue refers to a thick, white coat over the tongue with erythematous, enlarged papillae protruding (white strawberry tongue). This finding is noted early in the illness. Later, the white coating is shed, and a bright red, shiny, glistening tongue with swollen papillae remains (red strawberry tongue). Strawberry tongue is classically seen in three diseases: scarlet fever, toxic shock syndrome, and Kawasaki's disease.

The *differential diagnosis* of scarlet fever includes staphylococcal scarlet fever, which usually does not feature a strawberry tongue; staphylococcal scalded-skin syndrome, which has no enanthem; toxic shock syndrome, which has specific diagnostic criteria; Kawasaki's disease; streptococcal toxic shock–like syndrome; drug eruptions, especially those due to anticonvulsants; and certain viral illnesses (e.g., infectious mononucleosis, rubella, and enteroviral infections).

The diagnosis is made clinically, with support obtained from a throat culture positive for GABHS. A rising ASO titer also is supportive. The incidence of rheumatic fever following scarlet fever is decreased by the prompt institution of therapy, but the incidence of post-streptococcal glomerulonephritis is not decreased. Therefore, it is imperative that the urinalysis be followed for several months after resolution of the illness.

The present patient was treated with a 10-day course of oral penicillin, with resolution of all signs and symptoms. A repeat urinalysis at 2 months was negative for microscopic hematuria.

Clinical Pearls

1. Strawberry tongue is part of the enanthem seen in scarlet fever, Kawasaki's disease, and toxic shock syndrome.

2. The incidence of scarlet fever, along with other more invasive streptococcal diseases such as necrotizing fasciitis, is increasing after several decades of decline.

3. Prompt treatment of scarlet fever decreases the incidence of rheumatic fever, but does not decrease the incidence of post-streptococcal glomerulonephritis. Follow-up urinalysis is necessary.

REFERENCES

1. Stevens DL: Invasive group A streptococcal infections: The past, present, and future. Pediatr Infect Dis J 13:561–566, 1994.
2. Hsueh PR, Teng LJ, Lee PI, et al: Outbreak of scarlet fever at a hospital day care centre: Analysis of strain relatedness with phenotypic and genotypic characteristics. J Hosp Infect 36(3):191–200, 1997.
3. Halsey NA, Abramson JS, Chesney PJ, et al: Severe invasive group A streptococcal infections: A subject review. Pediatr 101:136–140, 1998.

PATIENT 12

A 13-year-old girl with photosensitivity and face rash

A 13-year-old girl developed a face rash following sun exposure 2 years ago. The rash gradually worsened over the ensuing months, and small pitted scars developed over her cheeks. Treatment with topical corticosteroid cream and ointment, an antifungal agent, antibiotics, and griseofulvin resulted in no improvement. She was in good health with no systemic symptoms. Family history revealed a maternal aunt with systemic lupus erythematosus requiring renal dialysis.

Physical Examination: Skin: erythematous, scaly plaques over cheeks, nose, chin, temples, and mid-forehead in a photodistribution (see figure); plaques contain atrophic pits with some follicular plugging; erythema on dorsum of hands, sparing the proximal interphalangeal joints. HEENT: pinnae showed follicular plugs; scalp hair diffusely thin in parietal, occipital, and frontal areas, with short thin hairs at the frontal hairline. Nails: posterior nail fold capillaries normal. Remainder of physical examination: normal.

Laboratory Findings: CBC, chemistry profile, urinalysis, antinuclear antibody (ANA), anti-double-stranded DNA, and Westergren sedimentation rate: all normal or negative. Potassium hydroxide (KOH) examination: negative. Punch biopsy of skin from right lateral malar area: pending.

Questions: What is your diagnosis? How would you treat this condition?

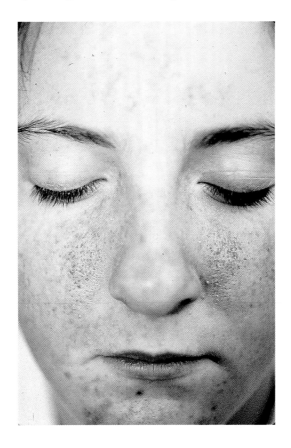

Diagnosis: Cutaneous lupus erythematosus

Discussion: Cutaneous lupus erythematosus (LE) is a chronic inflammatory disease that often results in scarring. It also is termed discoid LE or benign limited LE as opposed to systemic LE, which involves multiple organ systems and is diagnosed based on a set of strict criteria established by the American College of Rheumatology. Patients with systemic LE have a 15% incidence of discoid LE lesions. Of those patients who have only cutaneous manifestations with negative serologies at diagnosis, 5–10% will experience systemic disease in the future.

Cutaneous LE typically demonstrates classic discoid (disc-shaped or coin-shaped) plaques, but also may lead to papulosquamous or urticaria-like plaques. There are varying degrees of scale, telangiectasia, follicular plugging, alopecia, hyperpigmentation (usually early), and hypopigmentation (usually later and in scarred areas). An erythematous plaque characteristically enlargens, leaving central scarring and atrophy.

The pathogenesis of LE involves multiple immunologic abnormalities, with defects in helper T-cells and T-cell cytokines implicated. One recent study attempted to identify the T-cell cytokine profile in cutaneous LE using messenger RNA extracted from punch biopsy specimens. There was an over-representation of IL-5 messenger RNA in cutaneous LE versus normal controls, suggesting that IL-5, in combination with locally produced IFN-γ, may play a pathogenic role.

The *differential diagnosis* of an erythematous, photodistributed facial eruption includes: seborrheic dermatitis, dermatomyositis, drug eruption, atopic dermatitis, contact dermatitis, and keratosis pilaris atrophicans faciei.

Three types of alopecia are seen in patients with LE: discoid LE involvement of the scalp can directly destroy follicles, resulting in a **scarring alopecia**; **telogen effluvium**, which is seen more frequently in children, can occur with the acute onset of systemic LE; and so-called **lupus hair**, which features thin, short, fragile hairs around the periphery of the scalp, particularly at the temporal and frontal areas, may result from the catabolic effects of the disease process producing weakened hairs.

Therapy for scarring lesions of cutaneous LE includes topical, intralesional, or oral corticosteroids, (TB skin test must be done first). In photosensitive cutaneous LE, hydroxychloroquine often is successful. Other therapies which are currently used in more severe disease, including systemic LE, include immunosuppressive agents such as azathioprine and cyclophosphamide, clofazamine, retinoids, and thalidomide. Strict sun avoidance and the daily use of a sunscreen with an SPF 15 or higher are mandatory in all patients with LE.

In the present patient, histopathologic examination showed compact orthohyperkeratosis with follicular plugging. There was thinning of the epidermis and diffuse vacuolar alteration of the basement membrane zone, with scattered necrotic keratinocytes. Thickening of the basement membrane was confirmed on periodic acid–Schiff stain. A moderately dense, superficial and deep, perivascular and periadnexal infiltrate consisted of lymphocytes and macrophages. The dermal collagen bundles were separated by a stringy, basophilic material consistent with mucin, and the superficial dermis showed telangiectasia. Direct immunofluorescence of lesional skin revealed granular deposits of IgG, IgM, C_1q, and C_3. These findings were consistent with LE.

Further work-up in this child—CH_{50} and an extractable nuclear antigen screen (Smith, RNP, SS-A, and SS-B autoantibodies)—excluded ANA-negative systemic LE.

Treatment was begun with 200 mg hydroxychloroquine PO b.i.d. The cutaneous LE cleared dramatically over the ensuing 6 months.

Clinical Pearls

1. Benign cutaneous LE and systemic LE can both feature discoid lesions. The incidence of discoid lesions in systemic LE is about 15%.

2. The work-up of a new patient with biopsy-proven cutaneous LE includes a Westergren ESR, ANA, urinalysis, CBC with differential and platelet count, and chemistry profile. Further work-up is determined by the complete history and physical examination, as well as the results of the screening laboratory tests.

3. Both UVA (long-wave) and UVB (short-wave) light can initiate or aggravate cutaneous lupus lesions.

4. Patients with anti-ds DNA antibodies and hypocomplementemia also frequently suffer severe renal disease.

5. The serum complement level should be followed in systemic LE because a decrease often precedes development of renal disease.

REFERENCES

1. Laitman RS, Glichklich D, Sablay LB, et al: Effective long-arm normalization of serum complement levels on the course of lupus nephritis. Am J Med 87:132, 1989.
2. Lehmann P, Holt ZE, Kind P, et al: Experimental reproduction of skin lesions in lupus erythematosus by UV-A and UV-B radiation. J Am Acad Dermatol 22:181, 1990.
3. Schachner LA, Hansen RC (ed): Pediatric Dermatology, 2nd ed. New York, Churchill-Livingstone, 1995, pp 1105–1112.
4. Stein LF, Saed GM, Fivenson DP: T-cell cytokine network in cutaneous lupus erythematosus. J Am Acad Dermatol 36:191–196, 1997.

PATIENT 13

A 5-month-old child with cleft palate, eyelid fusion, facial anomalies, and scalp dermatitis

A 5-month-old girl was born with bilateral cleft palate and lip and bilateral ankyloblepharon filiforme adnatum (partial fusion of the eyelids with epithelial bands). She also had decreased scalp hair, eyebrows, and eyelashes. At 1 month of age, eroded plaques developed on her scalp, and these persisted. There was no family history of similar abnormalities.

Physical Examination: Face: partial surgical repair of bilateral cleft palate and cleft lip; flattened and broad nasal bridge; prominent mandible; scant eyebrow and eyelash hair (see figure, *left*). Scalp: hair short and scant; crusted, eroded, erythematous plaques. Ears: small, cup-shaped, and posteriorly rotated auricles (see figure, *right*). Nails: thin and hypoplastic.

Laboratory Findings: Chromosomal analysis, CBC, serum protein electrophoresis, and quantitative immunoglobulins: normal. Culture of scalp erosions: small to moderate growth of mixed flora, including group A beta-hemolytic streptococcus and *Staphylococcus aureus*.

Questions: What is the underlying syndrome? What are the primary concerns in management and follow-up?

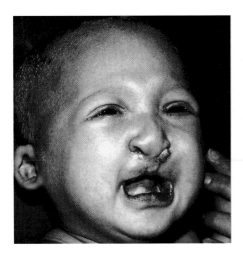 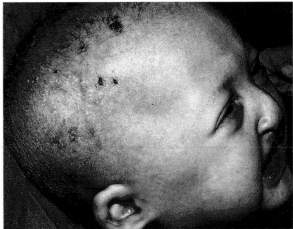

Diagnosis: Ankyloblepharon, ectodermal dysplasia, and cleft lip and palate (AEC syndrome, Hay-Wells syndrome)

Discussion: AEC syndrome is one of over a hundred types of ectodermal dysplasia that have been described. Ectodermal dysplasia refers to a diverse group of inherited disorders with abnormalities in epidermal appendages (hair, teeth, nails, and eccrine sweat glands) as well as in other organs. Hay and Wells first described AEC in 1976 as an autosomal, dominant, ectodermal dysplasia with cleft lip and palate as well as ankyloblepharon (which may be incomplete—ankyloblepharon filiforme adnatum). Other features often seen in AEC include decreased or absent hair of lashes, brows, and scalp; dystrophic nails; decreased or absent teeth; and severe, chronic scalp dermatitis.

The *differential diagnosis* of AEC in an infant includes two other types of ectodermal dysplasia that share overlapping features. The first is ectrodactyly-ectodermal dysplasia-clefting (EEC) syndrome, which consists of ectodermal dysplasia, ectrodactyly in the form of the lobster-claw deformity of the hand, and cleft lip and palate. The second is Rapp-Hodgkin syndrome, which consists of ectodermal dysplasia, cleft lip and palate, and characteristic midfacial and craniofacial abnormalities. In boys, hypospadias may be seen. If infants with AEC are born with large areas of dermatitis, hyperkeratosis, peeling skin, or skin erosion, then congenital ichthyoses such as epidermolytic hyperkeratosis and certain types of epidermolysis bullosa also must be considered.

Management of these patients requires input from multiple subspecialties. Surgical correction of facial abnormalities is necessary. Chronic conjunctivitis and lacrimal duct abnormalities requiring ophthalmologic care may occur after repair of ankyloblepharon. Scalp dermatitis can present the biggest challenge to the dermatologist caring for the patient with AEC syndrome. Frequent bacterial infections of the scalp require oral antistaphylococcal antibiotics. Some of these children have the hypohidrotic or anhidrotic type of ectodermal dysplasia, and therefore need to avoid overheating. Since patients with AEC often have dental abnormalities, they should be followed by a pediatric dentist so that appropriate cosmetic dental procedures for small, absent, or pointed teeth can be performed.

In the present patient, sporadic occurrence of AEC was assumed, but as with all autosomal dominant conditions, genetic counseling is appropriate. Surgical correction of the fused eyelids was performed at 5 days of age, and the cleft palate and lip abnormalities were repaired soon thereafter. No unexplained fevers had occurred, and sweating appeared to be normal; therefore, the ectodermal dysplasia was not anhidrotic. The scalp was helped by tap water compresses, mineral oil soaks, shampooing, and gentle debridement of crusts. Topical emollients and antibiotics also were used daily, with occasional courses of systemic antibiotics.

Clinical Pearls

1. The three types of ectodermal dysplasia that involve cleft lip and palate include AEC syndrome, EEC syndrome, and Rapp-Hodgkin syndrome.

2. Because of the widespread dermatitis that may be seen at birth in AEC syndrome, other diagnoses, such as epidermolysis bullosa and congenital ichthyosis, should be considered.

3. Chronic, refractory scalp dermatitis often is the major clinical concern in patients with AEC syndrome.

REFERENCES

1. Shwayder TA, Lane AT, Miller ME: Hay-Wells syndrome. Pediatr Dermatol 3:399–402, 1986.
2. Felding IB, Björklund LJ: Rapp-Hodgkin ectodermal dysplasia. Pediatr Dermatol 7:126–131, 1990.
3. Fosko SW, Stenn KS, Bolognia JL: Ectodermal dysplasias associated with clefting: Significance of scalp dermatitis. J Am Acad Dermatol 27:249–256, 1992.
4. Vanderhooft SL, Stephan MJ, Sybert VP: Severe skin erosions and scalp infections in AEC syndrome. Pediatr Dermatol 10:355–340, 1993.
5. Mallory SB, Krafchik BR: What syndrome is this? Ectrodactyly, ectodermal dysplasia, and cleft palate (EEC) syndrome. Pediatr Dermatol 14:239–240, 1997.
6. Mallory SB, Krafchik BR: What syndrome is this? Ankyloblepharon-ectodermal defects-cleft lip and palate (Hay-Wells) syndrome. Pediatr Dermatol 14:403–405, 1997.

PATIENT 14

A 1-year-old girl with vascular and lymphatic abnormalities and limb hypertrophy

A 1-year-old girl was born with a port-wine stain affecting the right buttock, leg, and foot; gigantism of the right leg; and macrodactyly of the first three toes on the right foot and the second and third toes of the left foot. She had several episodes of sepsis during the past 6 months, requiring IV antibiotic therapy. Grouped, fixed vesicles appeared on the right buttock 6 months previously.

Physical Examination: General: active, healthy appearing. Skin: large port-wine stain extending from top of right buttock to right toes; clear, blood-filled vesicles consistent with lymphangioma circumscriptum within port-wine stain on right buttock (see figures, *left* and *middle*). Extremities: right leg 4 cm longer and significantly larger in circumference than left leg; macrodactyly of some toes (see figure, *right*).

Laboratory Findings: CBC and coagulation profiles: normal. Radiograph of feet: distal phalangeal bones larger than the interphalangeal bones bilaterally. MRI of right leg: numerous vascular anomalies, including abnormal deep venules and an AV malformation of right thigh; lymphangioma circumscriptum of right buttock showed deep connections to underlying vascular channels.

Questions: What is the differential diagnosis? What are your treatment options?

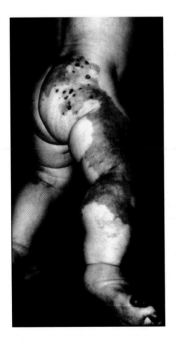 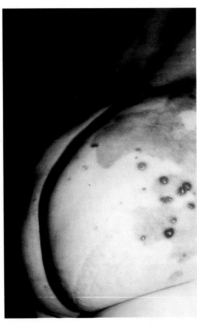 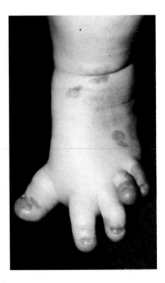

Diagnosis: Klippel-Trénaunay-Weber syndrome

Discussion: Klippel-Trénaunay-Weber (KTW) syndrome is the combination of complex vascular malformations with limb hypertrophy (gigantism). The nomenclature of complex vascular malformations such as KTW syndrome currently is in a state of flux. Historically, KTW syndrome referred to a combination of capillary, lymphatic, venous, and arteriovenous malformations along with limb hypertrophy. KTW was later divided into Klippel-Trénaunay (angio-osteohypertrophy) syndrome, consisting of capillary, lymphatic, and venous malformations along with limb hypertrophy, and Parks-Weber syndrome, in which similar combined vascular anomalies are seen, but arteriovenous fistulae or shunts also are present.

An entire upper or lower limb is involved in KTW syndrome. Associated findings may include glaucoma, retinal vascular masses, cerebral aneurysm, polydactyly, syndactyly, lipomatosis, lymphedema, and ipsilateral hypertrichosis or hyperhidrosis. In these vascular malformations, dysplastic vessels *without* cellular proliferation are seen, in contrast to hemangiomas *with* endothelial cell proliferation.

The *differential diagnosis* includes extensive pure limb venous malformations (slow-flow, hemodynamically inactive lesions, called cavernous hemangiomas in the past, in which the overlying skin is blue, muscles and joints may be involved, and a coagulopathy may be present); Maffucci's syndrome (vascular malformations, usually venous or venous combined with lymphatic) in association with bony abnormalities (dyschondroplasia, enchondromas, and multiple fractures); Proteus syndrome (hemihypertrophy, macrodactyly, exostoses, epidermal nevi, lipomas and complex combined vascular malformations of the limb); CHILD syndrome (congenital hemidysplasia with ichthyosiform erythroderma [or nevus] and limb defects);

and phakomatosis pigmentovascularis, which includes extensive port-wine stains plus either melanocytic (aberrant Mongolian spots or speckled lentiginous nevi) or epidermal nevi.

The inheritance of KTW syndrome typically is sporadic. However, recent reports have suggested autosomal dominant inheritance. Evidence for localization of the KTW gene to the long arm of chromosome 5 or to the short arm of chromosome 11 has been reported.

A well-recognized complication in patients with lymphatic malformations in KTW syndrome is recurrent bacteremia, as occurred in the present patient. The fragile vesicles of lymphangioma circumscriptum are easily traumatized and provide portals of entry for bacteria. Management of these patients, therefore, requires prompt diagnosis and treatment of any febrile illness. Management of the hypertrophy or gigantism of the limb includes compression elastic stockings, intermittent pneumatic compression devices, and shoe lifts to prevent scoliosis. Orthopedic surgical repair should be delayed and conservative. Surgical removal of arteriovenous malformations and cosmetic corrections of other vascular abnormalities should be undertaken only when absolutely necessary. Overly aggressive and early surgical repair has led to disastrous results.

Additional potential complications in KTW syndrome include stasis dermatitis, skin ulcers, cellulitis, intestinal involvement with GI bleeding and anemia, phlebitis, and thrombosis.

In the present patient, treatment included antibiotics for septic episodes and compression elastic stockings. By the age of 18 months, she was running and walking despite a greatly enlarged right leg. At the age of 3, she is being considered for some conservative orthopedic and vascular surgical procedures.

Clinical Pearls

1. The nomenclature of complex vascular malformations is in flux. Klippel-Trénaunay-Weber syndrome is entrenched in the literature and refers to a combination of capillary, lymphatic, venous, and arteriovenous malformations with limb hypertrophy.

2. The differential diagnosis of complex combined vascular malformations with limb involvement includes Klippel-Trénaunay, Parks-Weber, Proteus, and CHILD syndromes, as well as extensive pure limb venous malformations.

3. Treatment of children with complex combined vascular malformations and limb hypertrophy should be conservative. Aggressive, early surgical intervention has resulted in poor outcomes.

REFERENCES

1. Enjolras O, Mulliken JB: The current management of vascular birthmarks. Pediatr Dermatol 10:311–333, 1993.
2. Whelan AJ, Watson MS, Porter FD, et al: Klippel-Trénaunay-Weber syndrome associated with a 5:11 balanced translocation. Am J Med Genet 59:492–494, 1995.
3. Bird LM, Jones MC, Kuppermann N, et al: Gram-negative bacteremia in four patients with Klippel-Trénaunay-Weber syndrome. Pediatrics 97:739–741, 1996.
4. Ceballos-Quintal JM, Pinto-Escalante D, Castilla-Zaparata I: A new case of Klippel-Trénaunay Weber (KTW) syndrome: Evidence of autosomal dominant inheritance. Am J Med Genet 663:426–427, 1996.
5. Teekhasaenee C, Ritch R: Glaucoma in phakomatosis pigmentovascularis. Ophthalmology 104:150–157, 1997.
6. Enjolras O, Ciabrini D, Mazoyer E, et al: Extensive pure venous malformations in the upper and lower limb: A review of 27 cases. J Am Acad Dermatol 36:219–225, 1997.

PATIENT 15

A 6-year-old boy with patchy alopecia

A 6-year-old boy demonstrated asymptomatic, round patches of scalp alopecia that had progressively worsened over 6 months. Past history revealed atopic dermatitis since the age of 3 years. He was otherwise in good health, and there was no family history of alopecia.

Physical Examination: Scalp: several round areas of smooth alopecia with no evidence of scarring or scale; mild erythema at margins of some of these patches, with short, broken-off hairs (see figure). Nails: normal. Remainder of physical examination: normal.

Laboratory Findings: CBC with differential, blood glucose, and thyroid function tests: normal. Fungal culture of hair: negative. Microscopic examination of peripheral broken-off hair: "exclamation-point" hair.

Question: What is your diagnosis?

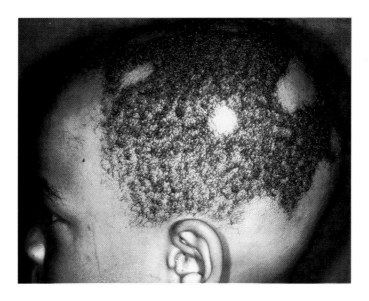

Diagnosis: Alopecia areata

Discussion: Alopecia areata is an autoimmune disorder characterized by the sudden appearance of sharply defined, round or oval patches of complete hair loss, most commonly located on the frontal or parietal scalp. The incidence is 17 per 100,000 individuals per year; therefore, approximately 1% of the population is affected by the age of 50. The clinical picture varies from a single, small, round scalp patch of alopecia, to total scalp involvement, to involvement of total body hair (eyelashes, eyebrows, beard, pubic hair, and skin). Systemic involvement is illustrated by frequent nail changes (10–44%) and occasional eye involvement (most often lens opacities, seen in alopecia universalis).

Alopecia areata has been associated with various autoimmune or endocrine diseases, including vitiligo, thyroid disease, diabetes mellitus, pernicious anemia, ulcerative colitis, Addison's disease, lupus erythematosus, and trisomy 21. Therefore, in addition to a thorough history and physical examination, screening blood work such as CBC with differential, thyroid function tests, and blood glucose should be performed.

The characteristic histopathologic picture of alopecia areata is a lymphocytic peribulbar infiltrate composed mostly of T-helper cells ("swarm of bees"). It appears that antibodies in patients with alopecia areata target structures of the hair follicle, most commonly the outer and inner root sheaths, the matrix, and the hair shaft. Current investigations are attempting to identify other hair follicle antigens that are increased in patients with alopecia areata.

The natural history of alopecia areata includes **frequent spontaneous remissions** and exacerbations. The overall frequency of spontaneous remission after 1 year is estimated at 60%. The clinician should be cognizant of the remission rate when considering treatment options. Patients with atopic dermatitis, a longer course of alopecia at diagnosis, and more widespread hair loss, such as the ophiasis pattern (posterior occiput and temporal band of alopecia) have a worse prognosis. The aforementioned prognostic factors need to be considered when developing a therapeutic plan.

Therapy of alopecia areata depends on the age of the patient, extent and duration of the hair loss, and associated factors such as atopy or immunologic dysfunction. If the prognosis is poor at the outset, any therapy is likely to fail. Because of the high spontaneous remission rate, not treating is a viable option. Psychological and cosmetic support always is appropriate. Topical corticosteroid therapy coupled with the contact irritant anthralin is used frequently in limited disease. Intralesional corticosteroids may be helpful in older, highly motivated children and adults. Minoxidil, psoralen plus UVA (PUVA), and systemic steroids occasionally are prescribed. Currently the most promising therapy is topical immunotherapy using contact allergens. Dinitrochlorobenzene is no longer used because it is mutagenic. Squaric acid dibutyl ester is nonmutagenic but unstable, and results have been disappointing. Diphenylcyclopropenone (diphencyprone, DPCP) is both nonmutagenic and stable. It is under study, and positive results are being reported, even in children. However, DPCP typically is not used in children under 12 years of age.

The present patient was treated with high-potency topical corticosteriods applied twice daily and anthralin 0.25% cream applied for 4 hours at night and washed off. The scalp hairs began to regrow after 2 months, and the topical steroids were decreased to once daily. At the end of 1 year, the child's hair had regrown completely. Whether this was due to the medical intervention as requested by the parents or a spontaneous remission remained unclear.

Clinical Pearls

1. Alopecia areata has a high rate of spontaneous remission within the first year; therefore, observation is a viable recommendation to patients or their parents.

2. Antibodies directed against structures of anagen hair follicles are increased in patients with alopecia areata, and the expression of hair follicle antigen may determine the localization and severity of the disease process.

3. In severe, nonresponsive, and nonremitting alopecia areata, alopecia totalis, or alopecia universalis, topical immunotherapy with DPCP is a valid treatment option.

REFERENCES

1. Sahn EE: Alopecia areata in childhood. Semin Derm 14:9–14, 1995.
2. Gordon PM, Aldrige RD, McVittie E, et al: Topical diphencyprone for alopecia areata: Evaluation of 48 cases after 30 months' follow-up. Br J Dermatol 134:869–871, 1996.
3. Schuttelaar ML, Hamstra JJ, Plinck EP, et al: Alopecia areata in children: Treatment with diphencyprone. Br J Dermatol 135:581–585, 1996.
4. Tosti A, Guidetti MS, Bardazzi F, et al: Long-term results of topical immunotherapy in children with alopecia totalis or alopecia universalis. J Am Acad Dermatol 35:199–201, 1996.
5. Lebwohl M: New treatments for alopecia areata. Lancet 349:222–223, 1997.
6. Tobin DJ, Hann SK, Song MS, et al: Hair follicle structures targeted by antibodies in patients with alopecia areata. Arch Dermatol 133:57–61, 1997.

PATIENT 16

A newborn with erythematous, linear streaks and vesicles

A 4-week-old girl had been born with linear, erythematous streaks on the legs, buttocks, and trunk. Some vesicles ruptured, producing yellow crusts. The infant was treated with systemic antibiotics for 4 weeks without improvement.

Physical Examination: General: healthy and active. Vital signs: normal. Skin: linear, erythematous streaks and vesicles, some with hemorrhagic crusts (see figure), on legs and buttocks.

Laboratory Findings: Cultures and scrapings of vesicles: negative for bacteria and fungi. Tzanck preparation: no multinucleated giant cells; sheets of eosinophils. Blood cultures: no growth. CBC: mild eosinophilia. Skin biopsy: pending.

Question: What is the diagnosis and the appropriate work-up of this infant?

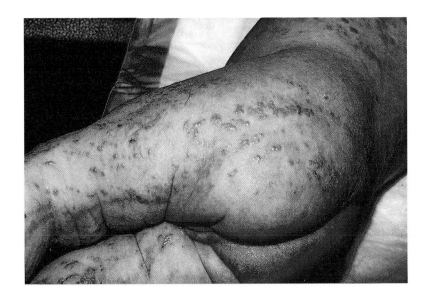

Diagnosis: Incontinentia pigmenti

Discussion: Incontinentia pigmenti (IP) is a rare genodermatosis characterized by four overlapping cutaneous stages and frequent neuroectodermal defects, most commonly central nervous system, ocular, and dental anomalies. IP most often is an X-linked dominant trait with in utero male lethality. The hereditary form is linked to Xq28, and the sporadic form is linked to Xp11.21. There have been a few reports of IP in males, most with Klinefelter syndrome (47,XXY karyotype). A recent case of transmission from a normal father to his two daughters suggested that the father was a gonadal mosaic for the IP mutation.

The clinical stages begin at birth, first with linear erythema and vesicles that follow Blaschko's developmental lines. Thus, the streaks are linear on the extremities, swirling on the trunk, and V-shaped over the spine. The second stage consists of verrucous papules, also predominantly located on the extremities in a linear pattern. The third stage consists of hyperpigmented macules and patches on the trunk again following Blaschko's lines, although not usually occurring in the same locations as previous erythematous or vesicular lesions. The fourth stage, if present, consists of streaky hypopigmentation and atrophy on the lower extremities.

Systemic involvement in IP is common. Central nervous system involvement occurs in a third of patients, typically presenting as seizures, mental retardation, paralysis, microcephaly, or motor retardation. Eye anomalies occur in a third, with strabismus, keratitis, and retinal detachment reported. Dental abnormalities most commonly reported are partial anodontia and pegged teeth. Hair and nail abnormalities also have been described.

The *differential diagnosis* of vesicles in infants is extensive and includes infectious (bacterial, fungal, and viral) and noninfectious etiologies. Management of IP includes thorough evaluation by a pediatric ophthalmologist, a pediatric neurologist, and a pediatric dentist. Mothers and sisters of patients with IP should be examined for cutaneous stigmata as well as ophthalmologic and dental abnormalities.

In the present patient, the biopsy specimen revealed eosinophilic spongiosis with spongiotic microvesicles in the epidermis and a mixed dermal infiltrate containing numerous eosinophils. Individual necrotic or dyskeratotic keratinocytes were present in the epidermis. Eosinophils were noted on the Tzanck preparation. The only therapy instituted was topical tap water compresses and topical antibiotics. All erythematous streaks and blisters resolved within 3 months. At the age of 2 years, white, verrucous papules developed on the dorsum of the patient's fingers, but these resolved 6 months later. At the age of 4, swirly, hyperpigmented streaks developed on her abdomen and buttocks. The only extracutaneous involvement to date is two pegged teeth.

Clinical Pearls

1. Incontinentia pigmenti typically is an X-linked dominant trait with in utero male lethality. However, IP in males has been reported in association with Klinefelter syndrome or genetic mosaicism.

2. An unaffected father may transmit IP to his daughters through the mechanism of gonadal mosaicism.

3. An infant with the diagnosis of IP requires evaluation for associated anomalies of the central nervous system, eyes, and teeth.

REFERENCES

1. Sahn EE, Davidson LS: Incontinentia pigmenti: Three cases with unusual features. J Am Acad Dermatol 31:852–857, 1994.
2. Sahn EE: Vesiculopustular diseases of neonates and infants. Pediatrics 6:442–446, 1994.
3. Kirchman TT, Levy ML, Lewis RA, et al: Gonadal mosaicism for incontinentia pigmenti in a healthy male. J Med Genet 32:887–890, 1995.
4. Ferreira RC, Ferreira LC, Forstot L, et al: Corneal abnormalities associated with incontinentia pigmenti. Am J Ophthalmol 123:549–551, 1997.

PATIENT 17

A 2-year-old boy with photosensitivity, freckling, and hypopigmentation

A 2-year-old boy suffered a severe, blistering sunburn with photophobia and conjunctivitis at the age of 6 months. He remained extremely photosensitive and subsequently developed freckling and hypopigmented macules on the face, dorsum of the hands, and V of the neck. He is the first child of parents who are first cousins. There is no family history of skin disease, and he is not receiving medications.

Physical Examination: Vital signs and development: normal for age. Skin: erythema, scaling, and hyperpigmented macules over face, dorsum of hands, forearms, and anterior neck; white atrophic plaques and telangiectasia scattered on face (see figures).

Laboratory Findings: CBC and chemistry profile: normal. Antinuclear antibody: negative. Skin biopsy specimen from forearm: pending.

Questions: What is the differential diagnosis? What is the most likely diagnosis? What is the optimum management for this child?

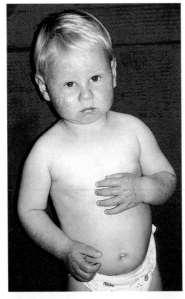

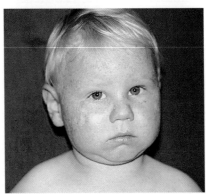

Diagnosis: Xeroderma pigmentosa

Discussion: Xeroderma pigmentosa (XP) comprises a rare, heterogeneous group of genetic diseases that prevent repair of DNA excisions occurring in cells exposed to UV radiation. The inability to repair is due to deficient endonuclease activity. This defect in nucleotide excision repair produces a multitude of physical findings. The incidence of XP ranges from 1:40,000–1:250,000 and is autosomal recessive. Parental consanguinity may be present. There are eight complementation groups that are identified based on in vitro cell-fusion studies. Gene locus depends on complementation type.

Clinical findings include **early photosensitivity** with **photophobia** and conjunctivitis and/or severe sunburn reactions, usually in the first few months of life. Erythema and scaling persist, with hyperpigmented macules developing thereafter. There may be crusts on the palpebral margins with squinting. Atrophic, hypopigmented plaques with numerous telangiectasias develop. Actinic keratoses and keratoacanthomas may follow. By the age of 6 years, most children will have a malignancy in a sun-exposed area.

In addition to premalignant lesions, complications include squamous cell carcinoma of the anterior third of the tongue and a greater than 1000-fold increase in the incidence of basal cell carcinoma, squamous cell carcinoma, or malignant melanoma. The eyes are involved in up to 80% of cases, with photophobia, conjunctivitis, telangiectasias, ectropion, symblepharon, ankyloblepharon, corneal vascularization or ulcers, cataracts, and carcinomas. Neurologic abnormalities occur in 20%, mostly in complementation groups A and D. The neurologic changes are progressive and may include sensorineural deafness.

The diagnosis is confirmed by unscheduled DNA synthesis (UDS) assay. Prenatal diagnosis of XP also is possible with the UDS assay, but 4–5 weeks are required for results. A new test, the single cell gel electrophoresis assay (comet assay) appears to be as accurate as the UDS assay in identification of nucleotide excision repair–deficient phenotypes, with results available within 24 hours.

The *differential diagnosis* of an infant with severe photosensitivity includes severe sunburn, drug-induced phototoxic eruption, polymorphous light eruption, neonatal lupus erythematosus, erythropoietic protoporphyria, congenital erythropoietic porphyria, Bloom syndrome, Rothmund-Thomson syndrome, Hartnup disease, and Cockayne syndrome. Hyperpigmentation similar to that seen in XP also occurs in radiodermatitis, dyskeratosis congenita, multiple lentigines syndrome, scleroderma, and urticaria pigmentosa. Early skin cancers in children also are seen in the basal cell nevus syndrome. Early melanoma occurs in familial atypical mole and melanoma syndrome.

The management of patients with XP begins with strict sun avoidance. Ultraviolet (UV)-blocking sunglasses with side shields should be worn at all times. These children also should avoid exposure to dental UV light. Sunscreen containing physical blockers is to be worn indoors and out, and strict photoprotection via clothing, hats, and avoidance must be practiced. Genetic counseling, ophthalmologic consultation, and neurologic consultation are all appropriate. Automobile windows should be fitted with UV-blocking film.

Prompt and complete treatment of precancers and cancers is imperative. Dermabrasion has been tried in children under general anesthesia to reduce new tumor formation. Oral isotretinoin or low-dose etretinate may decrease tumor formation, as well. As the deficient enzymes are identified, enzyme therapy is being attempted. Testing is ongoing using liposome delivery to the skin via a lotion of prokaryotic DNA repair enzymes specific for UV-induced DNA damage.

The diagnosis was confirmed in the present patient by a UDS assay performed on his cultured skin fibroblasts. Results showed a markedly decreased unscheduled DNA synthesis, at 10% of normal. Photoprotection, sun avoidance, and home schooling were recommended. Despite strict adherence to this medical advice, several actinic keratoses developed at the age of 4, and at the age of 6 a squamous cell carcinoma developed on his lower lip.

Clinical Pearls

1. Early severe sunburn reaction is a clue to the diagnosis of xeroderma pigmentosa.

2. Prenatal diagnosis of XP may become practical with the use of the single cell gel electrophoresis assay (comet assay).

3. Liposome lotion to deliver the missing enzyme to the skin may provide a viable therapeutic option for XP in the near future.

4. Strict sun avoidance from an early age decreases the incidence of malignancy and early death in XP. Avoidance of dental UV light exposure also is recommended.

REFERENCES

1. Finkelstein E, Lazarov A, Halevy S: Treatment of xeroderma pigmentosum variant with low-dose etretinate. Br J Dermatol 134:815–816, 1996.
2. Ocampo-Candiani J, Silva-Siwady G, Fernandez-Gutierrez L, et al: Dermabrasion in xeroderma pigmentosum. Dermatol Surg 22:575–577, 1996.
3. Yarosh D, Klein J, Kibitel J, et al: Enzyme therapy of xeroderma pigmentosum: Safety and efficacy testing of T4N5 liposome lotion containing a prokaryotic DNA repair enzyme. Photodermatol Photoimmunol Photomed 12:122–130, 1996.
4. Alapetite C, Benoit A, Moustacchi E, et al: The comet assay as a repair test for prenatal diagnosis of xeroderma pigmentosum and trichothiodystrophy. J Invest Dermatol 108:154–159, 1997.

PATIENT 18

A 7-year-old boy with diffuse nail changes

A 7-year-old boy experienced gradual changes of all his toenails and fingernails over the previous year. The changes included roughness, longitudinal striations, pits, and an opaque whiteness. He was otherwise in excellent health.

Physical Examination: Nails: white opaque discoloration, roughness, numerous tiny pits, onychorrhexis, thinning of nail plate (see figure). Remainder of physical examination: normal.

Laboratory Findings: Fungal culture of nail clippings: no growth. Punch biopsy specimen (3 mm) of one toenail bed: pending.

Question: What is the most likely diagnosis?

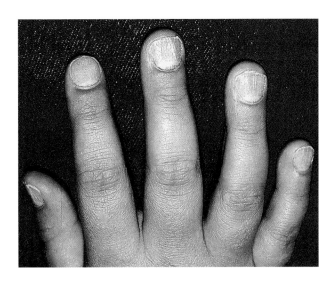

Diagnosis: Twenty-nail dystrophy

Discussion: Twenty-nail dystrophy of childhood was described in 1977 as the gradual appearance of the following nail plate changes: longitudinal grooves and furrows, onychorrhexis (longitudinal striations or splits), thinning of the nail plate, and trachyonychia (rough, sandpaper texture). These changes often result in distal chipping and splitting, with subsequent snagging and tearing of the nails. There often is a whitish, opaque appearance to the nail plates.

The *differential diagnosis* of twenty-nail dystrophy includes lichen planus, which usually causes changes in the skin, scalp, and buccal mucosa as well; psoriasis, usually with other changes present, but two types may show nail changes only (acrodermatitis continua of Hallopeau and dermatitis repens of Crocker); chronic eczema, usually with additional changes; dermatophyte infection, differentiated by the results of fungal culture; alopecia areata; and dyskeratosis congenita. The latter two may show trachyonychia for several years prior to the other classic findings. The classic nail change in lichen planus is pterygium caused by attachment of the proximal nail fold to the underlying nail bed, with destruction of the nail. The histopathologic findings on a small punch biopsy specimen of the nail bed or matrix will reveal the underlying disease.

Some authors believe that twenty-nail dystrophy of childhood is not a specific entity, but rather is a clinical sign of one of the above disease processes, most likely lichen planus. Reported associations include ichthyosis vulgaris and hypogammaglobulinemia. Congenital, hereditary, and adult-onset twenty-nail dystrophy also have been recognized.

Management of twenty-nail dystrophy begins with observation for several months, since associated diseases may appear after the nail changes occur. A fungal culture is done first, to exclude dermatophyte infection. If no additional treatable disease can be diagnosed, consider intervention. Strong topical steroids or steroids injected into the nail matrix generally have not produced good results in twenty-nail dystrophy. There is one report in the literature of success with topical soak psoralen plus UVA (PUVA). The use of nail hardeners may decrease the roughness and splitting and, therefore, decrease symptoms. Occasionally, systemic steroids or systemic retinoids have been used successfully in lichen planus of the nail to prevent complete nail loss. Whether or not a nail bed or matrix biopsy is performed depends upon the clinical situation.

In the present patient, the punch biopsy specimen demonstrated lichen planus. Since he was asymptomatic, the parents declined intervention. He will be followed clinically.

Clinical Pearls

1. Twenty-nail dystrophy of childhood may be seen in adults and may affect any number of nails.

2. Twenty-nail dystrophy may be caused by lichen planus, psoriasis, eczema, dermatophyte infection, alopecia areata, or dyskeratosis congenita.

3. The management of twenty-nail dystrophy should be conservative. Some cases improve spontaneously over months to years. Intralesional steroids in children are painful and may produce severe atrophy.

REFERENCES
1. Silverman RA: Pediatric disease. In Scher RK, Daniel CR (eds): Nails. Therapy, Diagnosis, Surgery. Philadelphia, WB Saunders, 1990, pp 82–105.
2. Taniguchi S, Kutsuna H, Tani Y, et al: Twenty-nail dystrophy (trachyonychia) caused by lichen planus in a patient with alopecia universalis and ichthyosis vulgaris. J Am Acad Dermatol 33:903–905, 1995.
3. Ohta Y, Katsuoka K: A case report of twenty-nail dystrophy. J Dermatol 24:60–62, 1997.

PATIENT 19

An 8-month-old girl with fever and multiple, erythematous, tender nodules

A previously healthy 8-month-old girl suffered pustules on the chin that rapidly enlarged into erythematous, tender nodules. The nodules subsequently developed central necrosis with the formation of a black eschar. Over the next 2 days, a fever developed, and 16 similar lesions arose on her extremities.

Physical Examination: Temperature: 39.1°C; pulse 110. Skin: 16 erythematous, firm, tender nodules 1–3 cm in diameter over arms, thighs, chin, and trunk; thick, black, adherent eschar in center of older lesions; hemorrhagic central bulla in new lesions (see figure). Lymph nodes: 1–2 cm and movable in inguinal and axillary areas.

Laboratory Findings: Hct normal; WBC 2500/μl with 50% bands; platelets normal. Blood culture: no growth. Nitroblue tetrazolium (NBT) reduction studies and integrin levels: pending. Trephine punch skin biopsies: pending.

Question: What is the differential diagnosis of this clinical presentation?

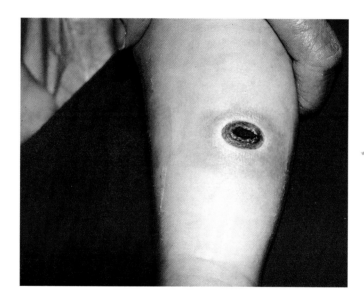

Diagnosis: Septic panniculitis due to acquired idiopathic neutropenia

Discussion: Panniculitis is inflammation of the subcutaneous fat and has numerous possible causes. In childhood, erythema nodosum is the most common cause, but other possible entities include: alpha-1 antitrypsin deficiency, the common cold, connective tissue disease, factitial disorder, sclerema neonatorum, subcutaneous fat necrosis of the newborn, drugs, granuloma annulare, sarcoidosis, and infections.

Fever with tender, red nodules, bullae, necrosis, and black eschar formation strongly suggests an infectious etiology, including deep fungal, atypical mycobacterial, and bacterial infections. A single lesion is highly suggestive of ecthyma gangrenosum secondary to pseudomonas sepsis; occasionally the lesions are multiple. Bullous Sweet's syndrome associated with leukemia may present similarly. Bullous pyoderma gangrenosum and vasculitis (with or without connective tissue disease) also are possibilities. Lymphomatoid papulosis and Mucha-Habermann disease usually feature smaller lesions.

Chronic idiopathic neutropenia (CIN) is thought to be antibody-mediated, with an onset early in infancy and up to 3 years of age. It typically eventuates in spontaneous remission. Most children with CIN do not need specific treatment unless they become symptomatic with frequent or severe infections. Infections that may be seen include recurrent upper respiratory infections, pneumonia, chronic otitis media, cellulitis, gingivitis, bacteremia, perirectal abscesses, and septic panniculitis. Febrile seizures may occur with fevers of unknown origin.

In those children with CIN who need treatment, management includes prompt and thorough treatment of acute infections with systemic antibiotics. Prophylactic antibiotics, glucocorticoids, and IV immunoglobulin also have been used successfully. Recombinant human granulocyte colony–stimulating factor (G-CSF) has been effective, with recent reports of promising results with low-dose G-CSF. In a single report, a dose < 5mcg/kg subcutaneously every 2 to 7 days kept the absolute neutrophil count > 1000/µl. Recombinant human G-CSF is thought to work in childhood CIN by overcoming the effects of the antibody or by decreasing the expression of the offending leukocyte antigen. It may improve neutrophil function, which has been depressed due to circulating antineutrophil antibodies.

In the present patient, a trephine punch was used to obtain a deep core of subcutaneous tissue. The skin biopsy revealed a superficial and deep neutrophilic infiltrate with lobular panniculitis and small vessel thrombosis consistent with either sepsis or alpha-1 antitrypsin deficiency. The alpha-1 antitrypsin level was normal in this child. The tissue culture revealed a pure growth of *Pseudomonas aeruginosa*. The NBT reduction was normal, as were integrins CD 11/18. After vigorous and prolonged treatment with high-dose intravenous antibiotics and topical care, the lesions began to heal, but her absolute neutrophil count remained extremely low. A bone marrow biopsy showed reactive hyperplasia with no evidence of leukemia or other myeloproliferative diseases. The diagnosis of autoimmune neutropenia (CIN) was made. Other causes of neutropenia in this child, such as cyclic neutropenia, connective tissue disease, and malignancy, were excluded.

Many months of intravenous antibiotics as well as recombinant G-CSF were necessary to completely heal the lesions. The adherent eschars were removed after treatment with warm, 40% urea soaks 4–6 hours per day for 8 weeks. Two years later, the child continues to require treatment with G-CSF to maintain an absolute neutrophil count above 1500/µl and to prevent recurrent infections. The areas of panniculitis have healed, leaving depressed scars.

Clinical Pearls

1. Septic panniculitis is a medical emergency that requires immediate treatment of the infection as well as a search for an underlying cause such as connective tissue disease, malignancy, or idiopathic neutropenia.

2. Recurrent infections and poor healing in children can be the result of chronic autoimmune neutropenia.

3. Recombinant human G-CSF, in low doses, is effective in the treatment of symptomatic children with chronic, idiopathic, autoimmune neutropenia.

REFERENCES

1. Adame J, Cohen PR: Eosinophilic panniculitis: Diagnostic considerations and evaluation. J Am Acad Dermatol 34:229–234, 1996.
2. Bernini JC, Wooley R, Buchanan GR: Low-dose recombinant human granulocyte colony-stimulating factor therapy in children with symptomatic chronic idiopathic neutropenia. J Pediatr 129:551–558, 1996.
3. Guynes RD, Huey RL, McMullan MR, et al: Case records of the Department of Medicine University of Mississippi Medical Center. Acute panniculitis secondary to fungal infection, most likely Aspergillus species. J Miss State Med Assoc 37:610–615, 1996.
4. Tok J, Abrahams I, Ravits MA, et al: Surgical pearl: The trephine punch for diagnosing panniculitis. J Am Acad Dermatol 35: 980–981, 1996.
5. Matsumura Y, Tanabe H, Wada Y, et al: Neutrophilic panniculitis associated with myelodysplastic syndromes. Br J Dermatol 136:142–144, 1997.

PATIENT 20

A 28-year-old man with a pruritic, generalized, erythematous eruption

A healthy 28-year-old man cut his foot on a glass fragment in his yard. He was treated with cephalexin. Six days later he awoke with fever, malaise, and a pruritic, generalized, erythematous eruption. The following day, numerous minute pustules appeared on the extremities. He had no personal or family history of psoriasis and was not receiving other medications.

Physical Examination: Temperature 40.3°C; pulse 110; respirations 34; blood pressure 120/82. Skin: symmetric, erythematous, edematous plaques over trunk and extremities, many with numerous 0.5-mm pustules in a nonfollicular distribution (see figure); mucous membranes, palms, and soles spared.

Laboratory Findings: WBC 18,300/μl; ESR 35 mm/hr. KOH: no fungal hyphae. Gram stain of pustule: no bacteria; numerous neutrophils. Cultures of blood and pustules: sterile. Skin biopsy: pending.

Question: What is the most likely underlying diagnosis? How can it be confirmed?

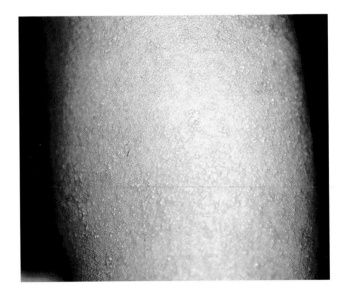

Diagnosis: Acute generalized exanthematous pustulosis induced by cephalexin

Discussion: Acute generalized exanthematous pustulosis (AGEP) is a rare reaction pattern first described in 1980. It most often is caused by drugs, and eruptions in the drug-induced reaction typically are morbilliform (macular and papular), urticarial, or fixed. Other reported causes of AGEP are viruses, such as enterovirus and cytomegalovirus, and mercury hypersensitivity. Drugs implicated in AGEP include amoxicillin, ampicillin, erythromycin, cyclin, nadoxolol, carbamazepine, nifedipine, cephalexin, cephradine, cefazolin, diltiazem, naproxen, norfloxacin, trimethoprim-sulfamethoxazole, itraconazole, hydroxychloroquine, terbinafine, and dexamethasone.

The predominant clinical feature is widely distributed, symmetrical, nonfollicular pustules on an erythematous base affecting the extensor surfaces and trunk. There is fever, leukocytosis, and prompt resolution over 2 weeks when the offending drug is withdrawn.

The *differential diagnosis* of AGEP includes pustular psoriasis, subcorneal pustular dermatosis of Sneddon-Wilkinson, and fungal or bacterial infection. Infection is excluded by gram stain, KOH, and appropriate cultures. A patient with acute generalized pustular psoriasis often has a previous history of psoriasis. Subcorneal pustular dermatosis is usually localized to flexural areas, especially the groin, axilla, and submammary areas.

The histopathologic examination of AGEP helps to confirm the diagnosis. Occasionally, systemic steroids are used in the treatment of more severe cases.

In the present patient, the skin biopsy revealed subcorneal pustules filled with neutrophils, a perivascular, mixed infiltrate in the papillary dermis, and no evidence of vasculitis. The eruption totally resolved at 1 month after withdrawal of cephalexin, and a patch test was performed. The cephalexin patch test results were positive, with minute pustules on an erythematous base, which on biopsy revealed the identical histologic picture as in the previous skin biopsy. The positive patch test confirmed the diagnosis of AGEP secondary to cephalexin.

Clinical Pearls

1. Acute generalized exanthematous pustulosis, most often caused by antibiotic or other drug use, is being reported more frequently.

2. The treatment of AGEP is withdrawal of the offending drug.

3. Corticosteroids have been reported to cause AGEP.

4. The diagnosis of AGEP can be confirmed by patch testing with the offending drug, which should reproduce the original clinical and histopathologic picture. There is one report of patch testing resulting in a recurrent generalized eruption.

REFERENCES

1. Assier-Bonnet H, Saada V, Bernier M, et al: Acute generalized exanthematous pustulosis induced by hydroxychloroquine. Dermatology 193:70–71, 1996.
2. Demitsu T, Kosuge A, Yamada T, et al: Acute generalized exanthematous pustulosis induced by dexamethasone injection. Dermatology 193:56–58, 1996.
3. Sawhney RA, Dubin DB, Otley CC, et al: Generalized exanthematous pustulosis induced by medications. Int J Dermatol 35: 826–827, 1996.
4. Park YM, Kim JW, Kim CW: Acute generalized exanthematous pustulosis induced by itraconazole. J Am Acad Dermatol 36: 794–796, 1997.

PATIENT 21

A 10-year-old boy with enlarging white patches on his chest

A 10-year-old African-American boy noticed a white spot on his right upper chest. The patch extended in a linear and segmental fashion over the next 6 months. There was no family history of depigmentation. The child was in excellent health, and there was no history of atopic dermatitis.

Physical Examination: Skin (Wood's light examination): several large, depigmented patches on right upper chest and back; multiple smaller macules and patches extending down right shoulder and arm (see figure); no evidence of follicular repigmentation. Ophthalmologic examination: normal.

Laboratory Findings: CBC, fasting blood glucose, and thyroid function tests: normal. Biopsy specimen from center of a white patch: pending.

Questions: What is the most likely diagnosis? What is the prognosis for this patient?

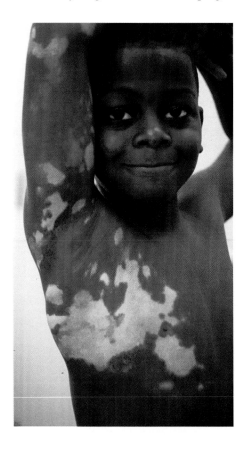

Diagnosis: Vitiligo, segmental type

Discussion: Vitiligo is a depigmenting disorder of the skin produced by destruction of melanocytes. It affects approximately 1% of the population, and there are no racial, sexual, or regional differences in incidence. Family history is positive for vitiligo in approximately a third of cases. Onset occurs prior to the age of 18 in 50% of patients.

In the **generalized type** of vitiligo, there are symmetrical, acral, and periorificial depigmented patches. In the **localized type**, a single patch, halo nevus, or segmental, zosteriform, or dermatomal involvement is present. In segmental vitiligo, a single or several contiguous dermatomes are involved, with onset tending to be at an earlier age and progression more rapid. The most common dermatome involved in segmental or zosteriform vitiligo is the trigeminal area. Vitiligo demonstrates Koebnerization, with appearance or worsening following trauma or sunburn.

The eyes are affected in up to 40% of patients. Uveitis, choreoretinal scars, and melanocytic destruction in the pigment epithelium of the retina may occur. Most of these changes affect the periphery of the retina, so that vision is not impaired. Autoimmune diseases reported to be associated with vitiligo include alopecia areata, insulin-dependent diabetes mellitus, hypoadrenalism, hypoparathyroidism, thyroid disease, pernicious anemia, mucocutaneous candidiasis, and scleroderma. However, segmental vitiligo is infrequently associated with autoimmune diseases.

Skin biopsy of *early* lesions of vitiligo reveals an inflammatory infiltrate in the upper dermis, and the melanocyte density is decreased, with degenerative changes. There also are degenerative changes seen in keratinocytes, which suggests that vitiligo is not a disease of melanocytes alone.

The *differential diagnosis* of segmental vitiligo includes nevus depigmentosus (achromic nevus or hypomelanosis of Ito), which is present at birth and remains stable; tinea versicolor with postinflammatory hypopigmentation (not depigmentation), which shows scale; and postinflammatory hypopigmentation such as pityriasis alba (also not depigmented). Wood's light examination is helpful in differentiating hypopigmentation and depigmentation.

Management of the patient with vitiligo involves psychological counseling, particularly in children, sunscreens and sun avoidance, and cosmetic masking agents or stains such as black walnut stain or self-tanning creams containing dihydroxyacetone. Moderate- to high-potency steroids sometimes are effective. Psoralen plus UVA (PUVA) produces a response in 50–70% of patients, but 20 to 25 treatments are required before any change is seen, and a good response often requires 100 to 200 treatments. Many physicians do not use PUVA in children under 12 because of the risk of severe burns as well as the unknown long-term risks of skin cancer and lentigines. Surgical procedures, which have produced variable results, include epidermal grafts using suction blisters and mini-grafting from skin that has been stimulated with PUVA. In the most severe, cosmetically debilitating cases of vitiligo, total body pigmentation may be obtained with monobenzyl ether of hydroquinone.

In the present patient, skin biopsy showed absence of melanocytes and no inflammatory infiltrate. The diagnosis was discussed in detail with the parents. Sunscreen was prescribed for the involved area, and the patient was directed to apply moderately strong topical corticosteroids twice daily. There was no further progression over the ensuing 2 years, but normal pigmentation did not return.

Clinical Pearls

1. Because eye abnormalities are common in vitiligo, an ophthalmologic examination is indicated in newly diagnosed patients.

2. Segmental vitiligo tends to have an earlier onset than generalized vitiligo; however, the segmental type is more easily treated, particularly in children.

3. New surgical procedures involving melanocytic transplants have shown promising cosmetic results in vitiligo.

REFERENCES

1. Drake LA, Dinehart SM, Farmer ER, et al: Guidelines of care for vitiligo. J Am Acad Dermatol 35:620–626, 1996.
2. Hann SK, Lee HJ: Segmental vitiligo: Clinical findings in 208 patients. J Am Acad Dermatol 35:671–674, 1996.
3. Suga Y, Butt KI, Takimoto R, et al: Successful treatment of vitiligo with PUVA-pigmented autologous epidermal grafting. Int J Dermatol 35:518–522, 1996.
4. Nordlund JJ, Majumder PP: Recent investigations on vitiligo vulgaris. Dermatol Clin 15:69–78, 1997.

PATIENT 22

A 75-year-old man with a plaque on the buttock

A 75-year-old Caucasian man presented with a mildly pruritic plaque on the buttock, which appeared 10 years previously. Gradual enlargement and central clearing of the plaque had produced a C-shape. The patient had mild hypertension treated with hydrodiuril for the past 20 years. He had adult-onset diabetes mellitus, controlled with an oral hypoglycemic agent. He was otherwise in excellent health.

Physical Examination: Blood pressure 140/90. Skin: large, red-brown, scaly plaque, C-shaped and sharply demarcated with central clearing, on left buttock (see figure). Lymph nodes: no lymphadenopathy. Abdomen: no hepatosplenomegaly or abdominal masses.

Laboratory Findings: CBC and chest radiograph: normal. Skin biopsy specimen from plaque: pending.

Questions: What is the most likely diagnosis? What additional tests are required?

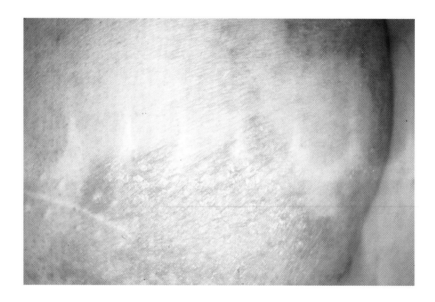

Diagnosis: Cutaneous T-cell lymphoma, plaque stage

Discussion: Cutaneous T-cell lymphoma (CTCL) refers to a heterogenous group of lymphoproliferative diseases with specific characteristics. Malignant clonal T-lymphocytes demonstrate epidermotropism, or localization to the skin. Once this occurs, the malignant T-cells grow locally or spread hematogenously. Local growth may be contained by host immunologic factors (as in the present patient) so that 10 or more years may elapse without any noticeable affect on the host. Hematogenous spread initially can be controlled by lymph nodes and the reticuloendothelial system. When a plaque of CTCL no longer is controlled by local host factors, progression to the tumor stage occurs. The cells in the tumor stage are more aggressive histopathologically as well as clinically.

The incidence of CTCL in the United States is about 0.3 per 100,000 individuals per year. It is more common in men, African-Americans, and the elderly. Variants of CTCL include plaque-stage mycosis fungoides, tumor-stage mycosis fungoides, Sezary syndrome (erythroderma), alopecia mucinosa, granulomatous slack skin, and Ki-1+ lymphoma.

Clinical characteristics of cutaneous T-cell lymphoma depend upon the stage. Plaque-stage CTCL shows sharply demarcated plaques with a geographic appearance due to central clearing and coalescence of adjacent areas. These features produce island sparing, a finding that also is seen in pityriasis rubra pilaris. Symptoms that may or may not be present include scaling, pruritus, and hypopigmentation. The *differential diagnosis* of plaque-stage CTCL includes pagetoid reticulosis (Woringer-Kolopp disease, a localized variant of CTCL), Bowen's disease, tinea corporis, and contact dermatitis.

The work-up of CTCL in early stages includes a thorough physical examination, chest radiograph, CBC and smear, Sezary preparation, blood chemistries, and skin biopsy examination. An abdominal computed tomography scan also is useful in the identification of intra-abdominal lymphadenopathy or hepatosplenomegaly. The following examinations are *not* helpful in early CTCL, unless there is a specific indication: liver-spleen scan, gallium scan, lymph node biopsy, and bone marrow biopsy. Southern blotting of the T-cell receptor (TCR) gene is extremely useful in confirming the diagnosis. In a normal individual, there are millions of different T-cell clones present, and it is impossible to detect one particular gene rearrangement on Southern blot examination. In cutaneous T-cell lymphoma, the expansion of a single T-cell clone in skin, blood, or lymph node is presumed evidence of malignancy. In the appropriate clinical setting, the identification of TCR gene rearrangement supports the diagnosis of CTCL.

The most important prognostic factor in CTCL of the mycosis fungoides or Sezary syndrome type is the extent and type of skin involvement. Staging evaluations for CTCL measure involvement of skin (T stage), lymph nodes (LN stage), and viscera (V stage).

Management of CTCL includes topical or intralesional corticosteroids, topical nitrogen mustard (mechlorethamine) or carmustine, psoralen plus UVA, narrow band UVB, interferon, photopheresis, electron beam therapy, retinoids, and systemic chemotherapy.

In the present patient, skin biopsy revealed a polymorphous, band-like infiltrate in the upper dermis, with eosinophils, normal lymphocytes, and atypical lymphocytes (Lutzner cells, with characteristic cerebriform nuclei and scant cytoplasm). These cells individually infiltrated the epidermis without spongiosis (epidermotropism). There were several intraepidermal collections of atypical lymphocytes (Pautrier's microabscesses). A KOH examination was negative for hyphal elements. TCR gene rearrangement studies showed a clonal proliferation. Abdominal CT scan was negative. Because there was no evidence of systemic involvement, symptoms were mild, and the patient was 75 years old, he was treated for the local pruritus with topical steroids, and he is being followed closely.

Clinical Pearls

1. A solitary plaque of cutaneous T-cell lymphoma can remain stable for years, probably due to local host factors.

2. An extensive and costly evaluation of the patient with early CTCL is not indicated.

3. Liver-spleen scan, gallium scan, lymph node biopsy, and bone marrow biopsy have not been found useful in the evaluation of early CTCL unless there is a specific indication on history, physical examination, chest radiograph, screening blood work, or abdominal computed tomography scan.

4. Southern blotting of the T-cell receptor gene may identify an expanded T-cell clone, which is supportive evidence of a malignant process.

REFERENCES

1. Duvic M, Hester JP, Lemak NA: Photopheresis therapy for cutaneous T-cell lymphoma. J Am Acad Dermatol 35:573–579, 1996.
2. Whittaker S: T-cell receptor gene analysis in cutaneous T-cell lymphomas. Clin Exp Dermatol 21:81–87, 1996.
3. Demierre MF, Foss FM, Koh HK: Proceedings of the International Consensus Conference on Cutaneous T-cell Lymphoma: Treatment Recommendations. Boston, Massachusetts, October 1994. J Am Acad Dermatol 36:460–466, 1997.
4. Herrick C, Heald P: The dynamic interplay of malignant and benign T cells in cutaneous T-cell lymphoma. Dermatol Clin 15:149–157, 1997.
5. Toro JR, Stoll HL, Stomper PC, et al: Prognostic factors and evaluation of mycosis fungoides and Sezary syndrome. J Am Acad Dermatol 37:58–67, 1997.

PATIENT 23

A 2-year-old girl with a facial eruption

A 2-year-old child was diagnosed with acute lymphoblastic leukemia at the age of 1 year and underwent successful chemotherapy. Following remission, she received monthly maintenance chemotherapy. A mildly pruritic facial eruption was noted on one of her monthly chemotherapy visits.

Physical Examination: Skin: many intact and excoriated 1- to 3-mm erythematous papules and pustules on face (see figure).

Laboratory Findings: Hct 30%, WBC 1500/µl with normal differential. Gram stain of pustule: numerous neutrophils, no organisms. Potassium hydroxide (KOH) stain: no yeast or fungal elements; numerous *Demodex folliculorum* mites.

Question: What is your diagnosis?

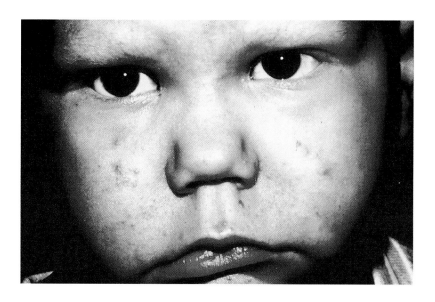

Diagnosis: Demodicidosis in an immunosuppressed child

Discussion: Demodicidosis is a pustular and papular eruption caused by proliferation of the normally commensal hair follicle mites, *Demodex folliculorum* and *Demodex brevis*. These mites are permanent ectoparasites in humans, but they are never found in neonates and rarely found in children. The mites increase in prevalence with age. Healthy populations show 10–13% incidence of Demodex organisms on skin scrapings or cutaneous biopsy specimens. Demodex mites live in follicles from areas with the greatest concentration of sebaceous glands, including the nasolabial folds, nose, and eyelids. This may explain the low prevalence in children, in whom sebum production is low.

It is not uncommon for unusual facial eruptions to develop in immunosuppressed children. Children with leukemia, those receiving chemotherapy, and children with AIDS or congenital immunodeficiencies may present with unusual facial eruptions. The *differential diagnosis* of demodicidosis includes dermatophyte infection, candidiasis, drug eruption, impetigo, folliculitis, and acneiform eruptions such as acne rosacea, granulomatous rosacea, and perioral dermatitis.

The diagnosis is readily established on KOH preparation, which reveals numerous *D. folliculorum* mites with no fungal hyphae present. Gram stain and culture are negative.

Treatment with permethrin 5% cream overnight clears the eruption rapidly and provides confirmation of the diagnosis. Other treatments include topical metronidazole cream, lindane lotion, and oral erythromycin.

In the present patient, KOH stain revealed *D. folliculorum* mites. Immunosuppression set the stage for the facial eruption. The patient was treated with permethrin, and her skin condition resolved within 4 days.

Clinical Pearls

1. *Demodex folliculorum* and *Demodex brevis* mites are normal inhabitants of the pilosebaceous follicle, but may be pathogenic under certain conditions.

2. Demodicidosis, a pustular eruption of the face, may result from the immunosuppression of chemotherapy, malignancy, AIDS, or congenital immunodeficiencies.

3. Demodicidosis can be treated successfully with either topical permethrin 5% cream or topical lindane 1% lotion.

REFERENCES

1. Sahn EE, Sheridan DM: Demodicidosis in a child with leukemia. J Am Acad Dermatol 27:799–801, 1992.
2. Ivy SP, Mackall CL, Gore L, et al: Demodicidosis in childhood acute lymphoblastic leukemia: An opportunistic infection occurring with immunosuppression. J Pediatr 127:751–754, 1995.
3. Barrio J, Lecona M, Hernanz JM, et al: Rosacea-like demodicidosis in an HIV-positive child. Dermatology 192:143–145, 1996.
4. Nakagawa T, Sasaki M, Fujita K, et al: *Demodex* folliculitis on the trunk of a patient with mycosis fungoides. Clin Exp Dermatol 21:148–150, 1996.
5. Castanet J, Monpoux F, Mariani R, et al: Demodicidosis in an immunodeficient child. Pediatr Dermatol 3:219–220, 1997.

PATIENT 24

A 10-year-old boy with a hypopigmented patch and erythematous papules

A 10-year-old boy in excellent health noticed an enlarging white patch on his abdomen 2 years previously. The lesion was treated intermittently with emollients and mild topical corticosteroids. One year later, erythematous papules appeared within the plaque.

Physical Examination: Skin: a 9-cm hypopigmented patch containing scattered 2- to 10-mm erythematous papules and nodules on left lateral abdomen (see figure). Remainder of examination: normal. Lymph nodes: no lymphadenopathy. Abdomen: no hepatosplenomegaly.

Laboratory Findings: CBC with peripheral smear, blood chemistries, chest radiograph, and CT of the abdomen: normal. Biopsy from largest erythematous nodule: pending.

Question: What are the diagnosis and prognosis in this child?

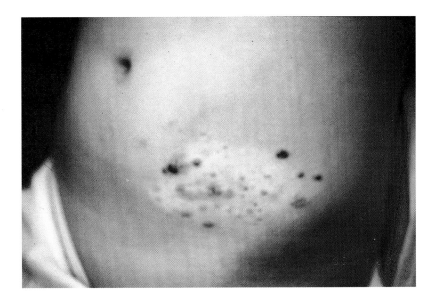

Diagnosis: Cutaneous T-cell lymphoma, localized

Discussion: Cutaneous T-cell lymphoma (CTCL) is a T-helper cell lymphoma characterized by epidermotropism early, and lymph node, viscera, and bone marrow involvement later. About 75% of patients are diagnosed after the age of 50. Onset is rare in patients under 20 years of age, but CTCL has been documented in a 22-month-old infant.

In one large study, the incidence of malignant skin tumors in children was 1.4% of all superficial skin tumors biopsied. Of these, two-thirds were primary malignancy and one-third were metastatic. Tumor types and relative frequencies were as follows: rhabdomyosarcoma 25%, lymphoma 19%, basal cell carcinoma 13%, leukemia 13%, neuroblastoma 10%, malignant melanoma 6%, squamous cell carcinoma 6%, sarcoma 4%, schwannoma 2%, and ependymoma 2%. In another study, 20% of non-Hodgkin's lymphomas in childhood were of the peripheral T-cell type. Most common was the Ki-1+ large cell lymphoma. Less common peripheral large T-cell lymphomas included pleomorphic T-cell lymphoma, angiocentric immunoproliferative lymphoma, angioimmunoblastic lymphadenopathy–like T-cell lymphoma, and cutaneous T-cell lymphoma.

The *differential diagnosis* of a patch containing erythematous papules and nodules includes other malignant cutaneous tumors; unusual localized inflammatory conditions, such as psoriasis or lichen planus; pityriasis lichenoides et varioliformis acuta; and lymphomatoid papulosis. A hypopigmented patch is more frequently found in childhood CTCL than in adult-onset CTCL.

Treatment of childhood CTCL often is appropriately conservative. Topical carmustine (BCNU) or mechlorethamine (nitrogen mustard) and topical corticosteroids frequently are used. Other therapies that have been successful in children include tar or anthralin, ultraviolet B or psoralen plus ultraviolet A (PUVA), and electron beam or x-ray therapy. A combination of PUVA plus interferon-alpha 2a resulted in successful treatment of an 8-year-old child with plaque-stage mycosis fungoides, stage IIa. Systemic chemotherapy is appropriate for later stages of disease. The prognosis in children with early-onset CTCL is not worse than in adult-onset CTCL.

The present patient's skin biopsy revealed a band-like mixed infiltrate in the dermis with cerebriform lymphocytes scattered throughout the epidermis, some in collections (Pautrier's microabscesses). There was no spongiosis in the epidermis. Since the work-up of this child was entirely negative, and he was asymptomatic, strong topical corticosteroids were applied twice daily to the localized plaque, with resolution of the erythematous papules and nodules over 2 months. The corticosteroid therapy then was tapered and discontinued. Six months later, the erythematous papules and nodules recurred. Again, therapy with strong class I corticosteroids resulted in resolution of the nodules. The patient continues to be closely followed.

Clinical Pearls

1. Cutaneous T-cell lymphoma is rare in children but does occur, and even has been reported in infancy.
2. CTCL should be included in the differential diagnosis of nonresponsive chronic dermatoses in childhood.
3. CTCL occurring in childhood does not have a more aggressive course than that presenting in adults.
4. Hypopigmentation in association with CTCL occurs more frequently in young patients.

REFERENCES

1. Orozco-Covarrubias de la L, Tamayo-Sanchez L, Duran-McKinster C, et al: Malignant cutaneous tumors in children. J Am Acad Dermatol 30:243–249, 1994.
2. Agnarsson BA, Kadin ME: Peripheral T-cell lymphomas in children. Semin Diagn Pathol 12:314–324, 1995.
3. Tay YK, Weston WL, Aeling JL: Treatment of childhood cutaneous T-cell lymphoma with alpha-interferon plus PUVA. Pediatr Dermatol 13:496–500, 1996.
4. Zackheim HS, McCalmont TH, Deanovic FW: Mycosis fungoides with onset before 20 years of age. J Am Acad Dermatol 36:557–562, 1997.

PATIENT 25

A 4-month-old girl with unilateral, hyperpigmented papules on the trunk and leg

A 4-month-old girl was noted at birth to have hyperpigmented papules arranged in streaks on the leg and swirls on the abdomen. She was otherwise in good health, and there was no family history of similar skin findings, inherited disease, or ichthyosis.

Physical Examination: General: developmentally normal. Skin: verrucous hyperpigmented papules in a swirled pattern on right side of abdomen (see figure, *left*); similar verrucous hyperpigmented papules in a linear distribution down posterior right thigh and leg (see figure, *right*). Remainder of physical exam: normal.

Laboratory Findings: Chest radiograph, electrocardiogram, electroencephalogram, and brain MRI: normal. Skin biopsy specimen: pending. Consultation was requested from pediatric neurology and pediatric ophthalmology.

Questions: What is the most likely diagnosis? What are your treatment options?

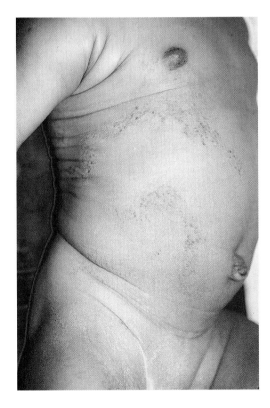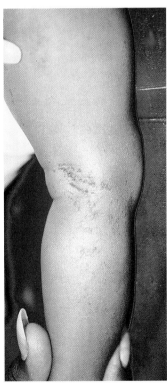

Diagnosis: Epidermal nevus of the nevus unius lateris type

Discussion: Epidermal nevi are hamartomas or overgrowths of normal components of skin or adnexal structures. They usually present at birth or shortly thereafter, and extension may continue for several years. The following terms have been used to describe variants of epidermal nevi: nevus verrucosus, the most common type being a solitary warty lesion; nevus unius lateris, in which unilateral, verrucous, linear papules are seen on the extremities and swirls or whorls are seen on the trunk; ichthyosis histrix, which refers to generalization of the epidermal nevus with bilateral, usually symmetric, distribution on the trunk and limbs; nevus comedonicus, which is characterized by keratin plugs and dilated hair follicles; and inflammatory linear verrucous epidermal nevus (ILVEN), which is erythematous and psoriasiform. Some authors include nevus sebaceus of Jadassohn as a subtype of epidermal nevus. Ichthyosis histrix also is referred to as systematized epidermal nevus.

The *differential diagnosis* of a linear epidermal nevus includes linear psoriasis, linear porokeratosis, linear lichen planus, and linear Darier's disease. Epidermal nevi can resemble acanthosis nigricans, eczema, or the verrucous (second) stage of incontinentia pigmenti.

Epidermal nevi are distributed along developmental lines (lines of Blaschko) and are thought to result from somatic mosaicism. The pattern, therefore, in **systematized epidermal nevus** is that of linear lesions on the limbs; swirls, whorls, and a marbleized pattern on the abdomen; and a V-shape over the spine.

An epidermal nevus with epidermolytic hyperkeratosis is thought to represent a mosaic genetic disorder of suprabasal keratin. Patients with this type of epidermal nevus can produce children with widely disseminated epidermolytic hyperkeratosis (bullous congenital ichthyosiform erythroderma). Therefore, genetic counseling will be necessary at the appropriate time for this patient.

The epidermal nevus syndrome refers to the association of epidermal nevi with systemic abnormalities, most commonly neurologic, ophthalmologic, or skeletal. Central nervous system abnormalities include mental retardation, seizures, deafness, hydrocephalus, porencephaly, and cerebrovascular malformations. Ocular abnormalities include lid involvement, colibomas, cysts, microphthalmia, and corneal opacities. Skeletal problems include kyphosis, scoliosis, short limbs, hemihypertrophy, and syndactyly. Rarely, cardiac, renal, or endocrine abnormalities may occur. Although the syndrome usually occurs with widespread epidermal nevi, there can be internal involvement with small epidermal nevi, particularly when located on the head. Late complications include the development of skin cancer within the epidermal nevus, but this is rare compared to the development of cancers in nevus sebaceus of Jadassohn.

Management of epidermal nevi is symptomatic and cosmetic. Topical or intralesional corticosteroids may relieve pruritus. Anthralin and liquid nitrogen have been used in ILVEN. The combination of 5-fluorouracil and tretinoin as well as the recent use of calcipotriol have produced some good results in epidermal nevi. Electrocautery, cryotherapy, dermabrasion, surgical excision, and shave excision followed by phenol peel each have produced variable results. There are recent reports of success using the pulsed ruby laser or CO_2 laser.

In the present patient, the histopathologic examination revealed compact hyperkeratosis, moderate acanthosis, and papillomatosis. Epidermolytic hyperkeratosis, frequently seen in systematized epidermal nevi, also was demonstrated. The neurologic and ophthalmologic evaluations revealed no abnormalities. Because her skin biopsy showed evidence of epidermolytic hyperkeratosis, she will be at risk for producing a child with generalized epidermolytic hyperkeratosis and, therefore, will require genetic counseling. She has been followed for 1 year without requiring treatment.

Clinical Pearls

1. The epidermal nevus syndrome is rare, but may be seen with small as well as systematized epidermal nevi.

2. A biopsy of an epidermal nevus should be done to exclude epidermolytic hyperkeratosis.

3. Patients with epidermolytic hyperkeratosis have an increased risk of producing a child with generalized epidermolytic hyperkeratosis (bullous congenital ichthyosiform erythroderma).

4. There are several cosmetic treatment options for epidermal nevi. Any surgical procedure should be delayed until growth has ceased, to minimize the likelihood of scarring.

REFERENCES

1. Paller AS, Syder AJ, Chan YM, et al: Genetic and clinical mosaicism in a type of epidermal nevus. N Engl J Med 331:1408–1415, 1994.
2. Baba T, Narumi H, Hanada K, et al: Successful treatment of dark-colored epidermal nevus with ruby laser. J Dermatol 22:567–570, 1995.
3. Hohenleutner U, Wlotzke U, Konz B, et al: Carbon dioxide laser therapy of a widespread epidermal nevus. Lasers Surg Med 16:288–291, 1995.
4. Gurecki PJ, Holden KR, Sahn EE et al: Developmental neural abnormalities and seizures in epidermal nevus syndrome. Develop Med Child Neuro 38:716–723, 1996.
5. Tay YK, Weston WL, Ganong CA, et al: Epidermal nevus syndrome: association with central precocious puberty and wooly hair nevus. J Am Acad Dermatol 35:839–842, 1996.

PATIENT 26

A 70-year-old, obese man with bullae on his extremities

A 70-year-old, obese man was taking a thiazide diuretic and propranolol for 20 years for hypertension. Two weeks prior to admission, large, tense, and flaccid bullae developed on his legs and spread to involve his arms and palms. He was otherwise well. He denied any change in topical or systemic medications.

Physical Examination: Weight 335 pounds. Skin: numerous 3- to 13-mm tense and flaccid bullae, some on skin-colored and others on erythematous base, scattered over forearms, thighs, legs, and palms (see figure); several ulcers or crusts from ruptured bullae; blister fluid clear; mucous membranes spared. Lymph nodes: normal. Abdomen: normal.

Laboratory Findings: CBC, chest radiograph: normal. Serum chemistries: normal, except blood glucose 205 mg/dl. Skin biopsy specimen: pending. Indirect immunofluorescent study: pending.

Questions: What is the probable diagnosis? What is your immediate course of treatment?

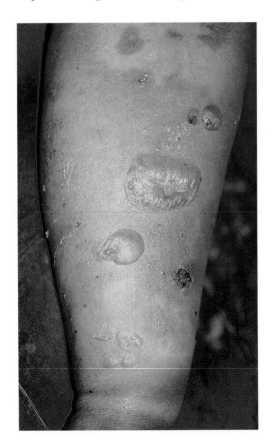

Diagnosis: Bullous pemphigoid

Discussion: Bullous pemphigoid is the most common of the autoimmune blistering diseases. It is seen in all ages, especially in the elderly. Autoantibodies are formed against proteins that are part of the hemidesmosomes and that have molecular weights of 230 and 180 kDa. Histopathologic examination reveals a subepidermal blister with eosinophils in both the upper papillary dermis and the blister cavity. Eosinophils typically are found lined up at the dermoepidermal junction. Direct immunofluorescence of perilesional skin reveals linear IgG, C3, or both at the dermoepidermal junction. Indirect immunofluorescence shows a circulating antibasement-membrane antibody.

Many drugs have been implicated as causes of bullous pemphigoid, including penicillamine, furosemide, penicillin, 5-fluorouracil, psoralen, amiodarone, and sulfonamides. One study found more frequent use of neuroleptics and diuretics, specifically aldosterone antagonists such as spironolactone, in patients with bullous pemphigoid.

There have been rare reports of malignancy in association with bullous pemphigoid. A recent study demonstrated that the serum of patients with bullous pemphigoid and malignancies reacted only to the bullous pemphigoid antigen with a molecular weight of 180 kDa. This is the minor bullous pemphigoid antigen, also called BPAg2.

Indirect immunofluorescence on salt-split skin currently is considered to be a sensitive and reliable assay for bullous pemphigoid screening. Immunoblot assay may reveal additional circulating antibodies to BPAg2 in those patients who show a negative indirect immunofluorescence.

The minor bullous pemphigoid antigen (180 kDa) has been studied intensively. It is a hemidesmosomal transmembrane glycoprotein that appears to have a collagen-like triple helix portion with a globule on one end and a variable portion on the other. This portion is thought to represent one of the major components of the anchoring filaments of the basement membrane zone.

The *differential diagnosis* of a patient with large blisters on the extremities (as in the present case) includes epidermolysis bullosa acquisita, bullous eruption of systemic lupus erythematosus, linear IgA disease, bullous disease of dialysis, bullous impetigo, bullosus diabeticorum, vasculitis, erythema multiforme, allergic contact dermatitis, bullous fixed drug eruption, arthropod bites, and trauma or burns. In different clinical settings, herpes gestationis, cicatricial or localized bullous pemphigoid, and chronic bullous dermatosis of childhood also should be considered.

Treatment usually involves systemic corticosteroids, often in association with a steroid-sparing immunosuppressant such as azathioprine, cyclophosphamide, or dapsone. Topical potent corticosteroids frequently are helpful. In severe cases, pulse intravenous cyclophosphamide has produced good results. In individuals who cannot tolerate systemic corticosteroids, such as the elderly, good results have been obtained with oral tetracycline and niacinamide.

In the present patient, who was obese, hypertensive, hyperglycemic, and elderly, systemic steroids were considered undesirable. Therefore, he received a trial of oral tetracycline and niacinamide, along with strong topical corticosteroids twice daily. On this regimen, the blistering decreased over the ensuing months, so that he could be maintained on this regimen with only two or three new blisters per month.

Clinical Pearls

1. Bullous pemphigoid is an autoimmune blistering disease that may be associated with drugs or malignancy.

2. Successful treatment most often requires systemic steroids combined with an additional immunosuppressive medication, or tetracycline combined with niacinamide.

3. Recent research on the 180 kDa bullous pemphigoid antigen suggests that it may represent one of the major components of the anchoring filaments of the basement membrane zone.

REFERENCES

1. Bustuji-Garin S, Joly P, Picard-Dahan C, et al: Drugs associated with bullous pemphigoid: A case-control study. Arch Dermatol 132:272–276, 1996.
2. Ghohestani R, Kanitakis J, Nicolas JF, et al: Comparative sensitivity of indirect immunofluorescence to immunoblot assay for the detection of circulating antibodies to bullous pemphigoid antigens 1 and 2. Br J Dermatol 135:74–79, 1996.
3. Hirako Y, Usukura J, Nishizawa Y, et al: Demonstration of the molecular shape of BP180, a 180-kDa bullous pemphigoid antigen and its potential for trimer formation. J Biol Chem 271:13739–13745, 1996.
4. Muramatsu T, Iida T, Tada H, et al: Bullous pemphigoid associated with internal malignancies: Identification of 180-kDa antigen by Western immunoblotting. Br J Dermatol 135:782–784, 1996.
5. Hornschuh B, Hamm H, Wever S, et al: Treatment of 16 patients with bullous pemphigoid with oral tetracycline and niacinamide and topical clobetasol. J Am Acad Dermatol 36:101–103, 1997.

PATIENT 27

**An 11-year-old boy with recurrent, spontaneously healing papules and
nodules on the face and extremities**

An 11-year-old boy sustained scattered erythematous papules and nodules, which developed ulcerated, necrotic centers and spontaneously healed. Other than minimal tenderness, these were asymptomatic, and the child remained in good health. The ulcerated lesions healed leaving small scars.

Physical Examination: Vital signs: normal. Skin: scattered erythematous papules and nodules over the face, arms, and legs (see figures), 3–12 mm in diameter, some central ulceration or necrotic crusts; mucous membranes, palms, and soles spared; lesions rare on trunk. Lymph nodes: not enlarged. Abdomen: no hepatosplenomegaly.

Laboratory Findings: CBC with peripheral smear, serum chemistries, and chest radiograph: normal. Skin biopsy: pending.

Questions: What is your diagnosis? What are your therapeutic recommendations?

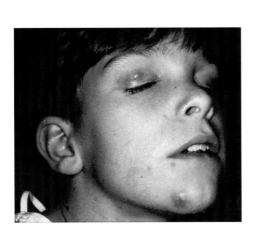

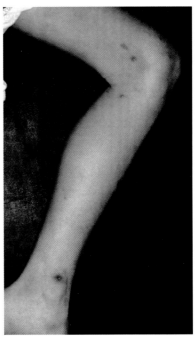

Diagnosis: Lymphomatoid papulosis

Discussion: Lymphomatoid papulosis (LP) is a chronic, self-healing, lymphoproliferative disease of the skin that usually is clinically benign but histologically malignant. It is characterized by crops of erythematous papules and nodules that either ulcerate or crust and eventually heal with scarring. In some patients LP appears to be a reactive skin condition, while in others it is most consistent with a localized lymphoid malignancy. Approximately 10–20% of patients with LP have an associated lymphoma, which may be discovered before or at diagnosis or may develop later. LP may show T-cell receptor (TCR) gene rearrangement on Southern blot analysis, despite benign clinical behavior. One study found that neither DNA flow cytometry nor TCR gene rearrangement studies could accurately predict which patients with LP would develop lymphoma.

Two types of activated T-cell can be seen in LP: type A, which is characterized by the **Reed-Sternberg type of activated T-cell**, and type B, the **Sezary cell type**, which has a cerebriform nucleus.

Childhood LP usually follows a similar clinical course as adult LP, with a few exceptions. First, in childhood LP the initial outbreak may be followed by decreasing frequency and numbers of lesions, until the disease ceases completely. Second, children can have a localized area of LP that remains stable for many years before generalizing. Third, children occasionally present with hundreds of lesions.

The diagnostic evaluation of a child with lymphomatoid papulosis includes a careful physical examination, CBC, serum chemistries, and a chest radiograph. In addition to the initial diagnostic biopsy, any lesion that becomes suspicious for lymphoma (enlarging or persistent skin lesion) should be biopsied. Other studies, such as bone marrow examination, CT scans, and TCR gene rearrangement studies, are indicated if evidence of lymphoma (e.g., atypical skin lesions, lymphadenopathy, or circulating atypical lymphocytes) develops. Because of the 10–20% risk of lymphoma, which may occur many years later, all patients with LP should be examined carefully every 6–12 months for the rest of their lives.

Treatments successfully used in LP include: systemic antibodies, potent topical corticosteroids, psoralen plus ultraviolet A, ultraviolet B, low-dose methotrexate, and systemic corticosteroids. The prognosis of LP in children is thought to be better than that in adults, with a spontaneous resolution more likely. However, lifetime follow-up still is necessary. Of those who do experience lymphoma, the types seen include cutaneous T-cell lymphoma (mycosis fungoides), Hodgkin's disease, and large cell lymphoma (CD30+). The prognosis of these lymphomas remains good if they are limited to the skin. The risk of systemic lymphoma developing in a patient with LP is less than 5%.

In the present patient, the skin biopsy showed a superficial and deep infiltrate of atypical-appearing lymphocytes with hyperchromatic, pleomorphic nuclei. In this child, the atypical lymphocytes were Ki-1+ (CD30+), consistent with type A lymphomatoid papulosis. Potent topical steroids were applied to individual lesions, and he was placed on oral erythromycin. His lesions cleared over the ensuing 3 months. The antibiotic was then stopped, but 3 months later a new outbreak occurred. A 3-month course of oral tetracycline produced resolution, and he has had no new lesions in 3 years.

Clinical Pearls

1. Lymphomatoid papulosis is rare in childhood and may be more likely to resolve spontaneously than in adulthood.
2. The risk of lymphoma in association with lymphomatoid papulosis is approximately 10–20%, and lymphoma may occur years after the original diagnosis.
3. TCR gene rearrangement studies and DNA flow cytometry cannot predict which patients with LP will develop lymphoma. Therefore, lifetime clinical follow-up is required.

REFERENCES

1. Beljaards RC, Willemze R: The prognosis of patients with lymphomatoid papulosis associated with malignant lymphomas. Br J Dermatol 126:596–602, 1992.
2. El-Azhary RA, Gibson LE, Kurtin PJ, et al: Lymphomatoid papulosis: A clinical and histopathologic review of 53 cases with leukocyte immunophenotyping, DNA flow cytometry, and T-cell receptor gene rearrangement studies. J Am Acad Dermatol 30:210–218, 1994.
3. Zirbel GM, Gellis SE, Kadin ME, et al: Lymphomatoid papulosis in children. J Am Acad Dermatol 33:741–748, 1995.
4. Orchard GE: Lymphomatoid papulosis: A low-grade T-cell lymphoma? Br J Biomed Sci 53:162–169, 1996.
5. Paul MA, Krowchuk DP, Hitchcock MG, et al: Lymphomatoid papulosis: Successful weekly pulse superpotent topical corticosteroid therapy in three pediatric patients. Pediatr Dermatol 13:501–506, 1996.
6. Towyama K, Tokura Y, Yagi H, et al: Lymphomatoid papulosis in children. Eur J Dermatol 7:291–294, 1997.

PATIENT 28

A 76-year-old man with an erythematous, pruritic plaque on the arm

A 76-year-old man underwent a successful, triple vessel, coronary artery bypass graft procedure. Two days later, he noted an erythematous, pruritic plaque on his left arm. The patient stated that the lesion had a "burning" sensation. He denied previous skin disease.

Physical Examination: Temperature 37°C. Skin: erythematous, edematous, sharply demarcated plaque on dorsum of forearm, measuring 15 × 5 cm (see figure); white scale and excoriations present; warmth over area, without erythematous streaks. Lymph nodes: no lymphadenopathy. Chest: sternotomy scar with skin staples in place.

Laboratory Findings: KOH examination of scale: negative for fungal hyphae. CBC and differential: normal.

Questions: What is the diagnosis? How would you confirm it?

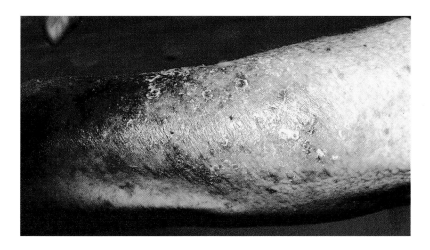

Diagnosis: Contact dermatitis, irritant type

Discussion: Contact dermatitis is the most common of all eczemas and is classified into two types: irritant (occurs more frequently) and allergic. The key to making the diagnosis of a contact dermatitis is recognition of the geometric, nonanatomic shape of the lesion, which means that the cause is exogenous.

The most common causes of irritant contact dermatitis are solvents, detergents, petroleum products, cutting fluids, foods, plants, and certain types of dust. However, many other chemicals and substances can produce an irritant contact dermatitis if contributing factors are present, such as a long exposure time, occlusion, humidity, and trauma.

A biopsy may be done to exclude other conditions. Contact dermatitis often shows nonspecific changes, such as intercellular edema, a superficial perivascular infiltrate, vasodilatation, acanthosis, parakeratosis, exocytosis, and spongiotic vesicles. An irritant contact dermatitis also may lead to epidermal necrosis.

Treatment of irritant contact dermatitis primarily involves elimination of the cause. Topical corticosteroids and moisturizers are helpful. If there is severe itching in an acute contact dermatitis, an ice pack or ice water compresses will provide immediate relief from pruritus.

Patch testing to exclude allergic contact dermatitis may be considered after the reaction has completely subsided. Patch tests must be evaluated carefully. False positive patch tests are frequent due to the "angry back" phenomenon, in which an active dermatitis in one area produces an excited skin state elsewhere (on the back under the patches). If one patch test is strongly positive, it may produce other positives which require further evaluation. Exogenous substances can produce an irritant reaction. Patch testing may be falsely negative if all the conditions producing the original reaction, such as sweating or occlusion, are not present.

In the present patient, a biopsy was not indicated. Additional history obtained from an operating room nurse revealed that chlorhexidine gluconate surgical scrub had spilled during preparation for the bypass procedure and had leaked under the patient's left arm. His arm rested in the pool of chlorhexidine gluconate throughout the surgical procedure and was discovered only when he was moved. His current condition was treated with cool compresses and a moderate-strength topical corticosteroid, with resolution of the plaque over the subsequent 3 weeks.

Clinical Pearls

1. A dermatitis with a geometric shape that does not correspond to any anatomic pattern strongly suggests that the cause is exogenous (contact dermatitis).

2. Severe pruritus in acute contact dermatitis can be relieved immediately by the application of ice packs or ice water compresses.

3. Patch testing to exclude or confirm an allergic contact dermatitis is easily performed, but interpretation may be problematic. Both false positive and false negative results can occur.

REFERENCES
1. Fisher AA: Contact Dermatitis, 3rd ed. Philadelphia, Lea and Febiger, 1986.
2. Stingeni L, Lapomarda V, Lisi P: Occupational hand dermatitis in hospital environments. Cont Derm 33:172–176, 1995.
3. Lee JY, Wang BJ: Contact dermatitis caused by cetrimide in antiseptics. Cont Derm 33:168–171, 1995.

PATIENT 29

A 61-year-old woman with burning, red feet

A 61-year-old woman sustained cold injury to her feet 20 years previously while on a ski trip. Since that time she noted intermittent burning, warmth, and redness of the feet. Her symptoms have gradually worsened so that an episode only ends after emersion of her feet in ice water. She is not taking any medicines, does not smoke, and is in good health otherwise.

Physical Examination: Blood pressure 125/85. Skin: sharply demarcated, erythematous, symmetrical plaques on forefeet and toes (see figure),which resolved with elevation and cold compresses. Remainder of physical examination: normal.

Laboratory Findings: CBC, platelet count, and blood smear: normal. Serum chemistries: normal. ANA and chest radiograph: negative. Skin biopsy: pending.

Question: What are the probable diagnosis, the differential diagnosis, and management options in this patient?

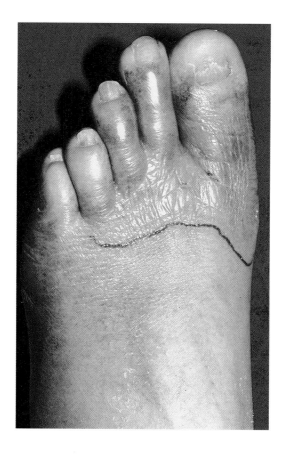

Diagnosis: Erythromelalgia, primary or idiopathic

Discussion: Erythromelalgia is a condition characterized by episodes of erythema, pain, and warmth in the skin of the feet and/or hands. Attacks are brought on by heat, exercise, or dependency of the limb and typically last 2–3 hours. Most often the forefeet, soles, or toes are involved. Erythromelalgia can be classified into three types: (1) early onset; (2) adult-onset, aspirin-responsive; and (3) adult-onset, aspirin-nonresponsive.

Primary or idiopathic erythromelalgia occurs at any age and usually is symmetrical. Secondary erythromelalgia most often is seen with polycythemia vera or thrombocythemia. Other associations that should be considered include connective tissue disease, myeloproliferative malignancy, hypertension, diabetes mellitus, gout, and calcium channel blocker use (verapamil or nifedipine). Causalgia and reflex sympathetic dystrophy also can produce similar burning pain in the extremities; however, these disorders are not relieved by ice water emersion, which promptly relieves erythromelalgia.

The pathogenesis of erythromelalgia is unknown but is related to abnormal platelet aggregation, aggravated by blood hyperviscosity or vessel wall damage. Prostaglandin disturbances also may play a role. Increased tone in precapillary arterioles may divert blood to the deep dermis and subcutaneous tissues, producing tissue hypoxia, heat, and erythema. Serotonin is thought to be involved in some cases.

In primary erythromelalgia, histologic examination demonstrates a mild perivascular infiltrate with mild endothelial swelling and thickened blood vessel basement membranes. This is a nonspecific finding, different from that reported in erythromelalgia associated with thrombocythemia. In the latter disease, there is fibromuscular intimal proliferation of arterioles with arteriolar and endarteriolar capillary thrombi. Venules and other capillaries usually are spared. Leukocytoclastic vasculitis usually is absent.

Thrombin generation does not occur in erythromelalgia associated with essential thrombocythemia. Therefore, intravascular activation and aggregation of platelets produce the microvascular sludging and occlusion in erythromelalgia. This explains why coumadin and heparin may not prevent attacks of erythromelalgia in thrombocythemia.

Management begins with excluding underlying diseases or drug causes. Acute episodes often are managed only with ice water compresses, elevation, and nonsteroidal anti-inflammatory drugs. Daily aspirin therapy often ameliorates both early-onset and aspirin-responsive adult-onset erythromelalgia. When aspirin is used to treat erythromelalgia associated with primary thrombocythemia or polycythemia vera, there is an increased risk of serious bleeding. Other medications that have been tried include heparin, propranolol, cyproheptadine (serotonin antagonist), and the platelet inhibitors dipyridamole, pentoxifylline, and ticlopidine. Successful treatment of three patients with the serotonin reuptake inhibitors venlafaxine and sertraline was recently reported.

In the present patient, histologic examination of the skin revealed features consistent with primary erythromelalgia. She was treated with daily aspirin therapy and heat avoidance, with marked improvement of symptoms.

Clinical Pearls

1. A history of pain relief with ice water emersion is typical of erythromelalgia and differentiates it from the pain of causalgia and reflex sympathetic dystrophy.
2. A biopsy of the skin in erythromelalgia often is useful, as it helps to exclude other associated diseases.
3. When aspirin therapy is used in erythromelalgia associated with primary thrombocythemia or polycythemia vera, there is an increased risk of serious bleeding.

REFERENCES

1. Drenth JP, Vuzevski V, Van Joost T, et al: Cutaneous pathology in primary erythromelalgia. Am J Dermatopathol 18:30–34, 1996.
2. Michiels JJ, van Genderen PJ, Lindemans J, et al: Erythromelalgic, thrombotic and hemorrhagic manifestations in 50 cases of thrombocythemia. Leuk Lymphoma 22(S):47–56, 1996.
3. Sakakibara R, Fukutake T, Kita K, et al: Treatment of primary erythromelalgia with cyproheptadine. J Auton Nerv Syst 58:121–122, 1996.
4. Van Genderen PJ, Lucas IS, van Strik R, et al: Erythromelalgia in essential thrombocythemia is characterized by platelet activation and endothelial cell damage but not by thrombin generation. Thromb Haemost 76:333–338, 1996.
5. Rudikoff D, Jaffe IA: Erythromelalgia: Response to serotonin reuptake inhibitors. J Am Acad Dermatol 37:281–283, 1997.

PATIENT 30

A 65-year-old man with pruritic plaques on his feet

A 65-year-old man complained of pruritic, scaly plaques on the soles and dorsum of his forefeet and toes. The plaques had been present for 5 years and were both hypopigmented and hyperpigmented. He used over-the-counter antifungal agents intermittently for 2 years, with no improvement. During the past year he changed his shoes twice, also with no improvement. There was no family history of psoriasis or atopic dermatitis.

Physical Examination: Skin: sharply demarcated, scaly, lichenified plaques—both hypopigmented and hyperpigmented—located symmetrically on soles, dorsum of toes, and dorsum of forefeet (see figure); interdigital toe webs, toenails, and hands uninvolved. Remainder of physical examination: normal.

Laboratory Findings: Two KOH examinations (feet and dorsum of toes): negative for hyphal elements. Skin biopsy: pending.

Questions: What is the differential diagnosis of this presentation? What additional history is necessary?

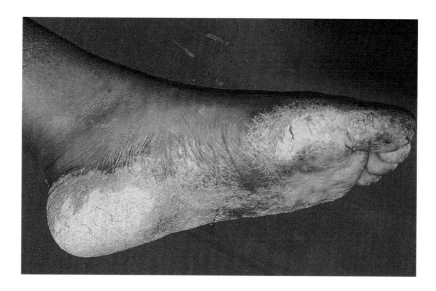

Diagnosis: Contact dermatitis, allergic

Discussion: Contact dermatitis is the most common of the eczematous conditions. Allergic contact dermatitis occurs less frequently than the irritant type. In an unsensitized person, approximately 5–10 days are required after first exposure to an allergen for the appearance of clinical allergy. In a sensitized person histopathologic changes are seen in the skin within 3 hours, and clinical allergy is present in 12–24 hours. A recent study of patients with allergic contact dermatitis demonstrated that their keratinocytes produce interferon-gamma in response to challenge with relevant antigens, but not irrelevant antigens. This **keratinocyte amplification** of the allergic response could explain the rapidity of the clinical response seen in allergic contact dermatitis.

The *differential diagnosis* includes tinea pedis, which always involves the plantar surface of the foot; occasionally, both feet and one hand are involved. Psoriasis can produce this picture, but typically with additional changes in the skin and nails. Atopic dermatitis also can mimic allergic contact dermatitis. In the correct clinical setting, pityriasis rubra pilaris, Reiter's syndrome, keratodermas, dyskeratosis congenita, ectodermal dysplasia, ichthyosis, and Sezary syndrome should be considered.

An eruption on the dorsum of the toes, the forefoot, and soles, in a symmetric distribution with sparing of the interdigital web spaces, is highly suggestive of a shoe dermatitis. The most frequent cause of shoe dermatitis is the additives to the rubber and rubber-based adhesives, including accelerators, stabilizers, vulcanizers, and antioxidants. Of these, the most frequent sensitizers are tetramethylthiuram (TMT) and mercaptobenzothiazole (MBT). Both are included in standard patch test kits. However, many other rubber additives are not included; therefore, patch testing with a piece of the suspected shoe is recommended. Even this method can result in false negatives, because the allergen concentration is too low when placed on normal back skin.

In addition to the numerous known chemicals and drugs that can produce an allergic contact dermatitis in susceptible individuals, recent reports have implicated corticosteroids, mupirocin, and calcipotriol as contact allergens.

In the present patient, histopathologic examination was consistent with a chronic contact dermatitis, showing a mixed perivascular infiltrate, acanthosis, hyperkeratosis, spongiosis, and—most helpfully—an absence of psoriasis, pityriasis rubra pilaris, and tinea pedis. Additional history finally extracted from this patient revealed that he wore 5-year-old slippers 8–12 hours per day. He underwent standard patch testing as well as patch testing with a piece of material from the inner sole of his slipper. Positive reactions to TMT, MBT, and to the piece of slipper resulted. He switched to 100% cotton slippers without rubber adhesive or rubber components and was prescribed topical steroid ointment. The patient gradually improved over the ensuing 3 months.

Clinical Pearls

1. In an unsensitized person, allergic contact dermatitis takes approximately 5–10 days to develop after the first exposure. In a sensitized person, however, changes may be noted within hours.

2. The most frequent causes of shoe dermatitis are the rubber additives tetramethylthiuram and mercaptobenzothiazole.

3. In shoe dermatitis, patch testing with a piece of the shoe may give a false negative result because the allergen concentration may be too low when placed on normal back skin.

REFERENCES

1. Garcia-Bravo B, Camacho F: Two cases of contact dermatitis caused by calcipotriol cream. Am J Contact Dermat 7:118–119, 1996.
2. Howie SE, Aldridge RD, McVittie E, et al: Epidermal keratinocyte production of interferon-gamma immunoreactive protein and mRNA is an early event in allergic contact dermatitis. J Invest Dermatol 106:1218–1223, 1996.
3. Roul S, Ducombs G, Leaute-Labreze C, et al: Footwear contact dermatitis in children. Contact Dermatitis 35:334–336,1996.
4. Beltrani VS, Beltrani VP: Contact dermatitis. Ann Allergy Asthma Immunol 78:160–173, 1997.
5. Cohen DE, Brancaccio RR: What is new in clinical research in contact dermatitis. Dermatol Clin 15:137–148, 1997.
6. Zappi EG, Brancaccio RR: Allergic contact dermatitis from muciprocin ointment. J Am Acad Dermatol 36:266, 1997.

PATIENT 31

A 24-year-old man with edema and erythema of the penis and scrotum

A healthy, 24-year-old man complained of edema, erythema, and tenderness of the penile and scrotal skin. He denied trauma, fever, and chills. Past history revealed several months of intermittent abdominal cramping and diarrhea 5 years previously, which was successfully treated with sulfasalazine and prednisone without recurrence.

Physical Examination: Temperature: 37.1°C. Skin: sharply demarcated, erythematous, and tender plaques on the scrotum and penis (see figure); no ulcerations or abnormalities of the perirectal area. Lymph nodes: no lymphadenopathy. Mouth: normal. Abdomen: normal.

Laboratory Findings: CBC: normal. Screening chemistries: negative. Chest radiograph: negative. Tuberculosis skin test: negative. Skin biopsy for routine examination, stains for organisms, cultures for mycobacterium, fungi, and bacteria, and polarizing microscopy: pending.

Questions: What is the differential diagnosis in this patient? What further tests are necessary to arrive at a precise diagnosis?

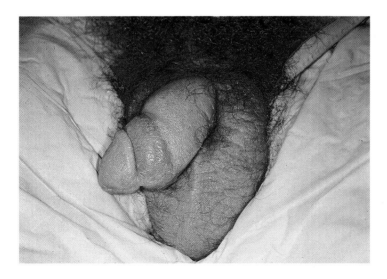

Diagnosis: Metastatic Crohn's disease

Discussion: Crohn's disease is a chronic, relapsing, inflammatory bowel disease that may involve any segment of the gastrointestinal (GI) tract. The skin is affected in 22–44% of patients, with several types of disorder. Direct extension is the most common cutaneous manifestation, with lesions (e.g., nodules, ulcers, fissures) located in a perianal, perifistular, or peristomal location. Nonspecific cutaneous reactions seen with Crohn's disease include erythema nodosum, pyoderma gangrenosum, erythema multiforme, and oral aphthae. Skin signs of malabsorption or malnutrition may occur, and intraoral manifestations include pyostomatitis vegetans, cobblestoning, ulcers, and angular cheilitis. Metastatic Crohn's disease (MCD) refers to skin involvement that is noncontiguous with GI tract lesions and is separated from these abnormalities by normal skin. It was first described by Parks, et al. in 1965, and as of 1997 the literature contained reports of 80 cases.

MCD is seen most often when the large intestine is involved, although Crohn's disease itself is more common in the small bowel. MCD may or may not parallel the severity of the intestinal disease. The diagnosis can be problematic when there is not a previous diagnosis of Crohn's disease. MCD most commonly affects the lower legs, but also can be seen on the trunk, groin, axillae, and, rarely, the face.

In children, the cutaneous lesions of MCD commonly precede the GI manifestations, which contrasts with the course in adults. In addition, genital involvement occurs more frequently in children.

Histopathologic examination of skin involved in MCD shows noncaseating granulomas with epithelioid cells and a variable number of Langhans multinucleated giant cells throughout the dermis. The granulomas are surrounded by lymphocytes and plasma cells. A recent report on MCD noted necrobiotic granulomas, similar to those seen in granuloma annulare, necrobiosis lipoidica diabeticorum, and rheumatoid nodules in a perivascular location.

The *different diagnosis* includes cellulitis and early necrotizing fasciitis of the scrotum (Fournier's gangrene). The latter disorder is a polymicrobial infection also known as bacterial synergistic gangrene. Other infections that can present with a similar picture include histoplasmosis, filariasis, lymphogranuloma venereum, herpes simplex virus, tuberculosis, actinomycosis, and mumps. Also in the differential diagnosis are cutaneous polyarteritis nodosa, sarcoidosis, severe seborrheic dermatitis, and sclerosing lipogranuloma (reaction to injection with oil or paraffin, iatrogenic or factitial). The scrotum rarely is involved with a primary, sexually transmitted disease or tinea. When the scrotum alone is involved with erythema and scale, lichen simplex chronicus or mite infestation is suggested. Patients with MCD may have a positive C-ANCA.

Treatments that have been used in MCD include oral, topical, and intravenous antibiotics (in particular sulfasalazine), metronidazole, cytotoxic agents (6-mercaptopurine and azathioprine), and surgical excision, including excision of the entire scrotal and penile skin with skin grafting.

In the present patient, the skin biopsy showed chronic edema with lymphangiectasis, chronic inflammation, and many noncaseating granulomas with Langhans giant cells. Stains for bacteria, acid-fast organisms, and fungus were negative. Tissue cultures likewise were negative for *Mycobacterium tuberculosis*, fungus, and bacteria. The polarizing microscopic examination revealed no evidence of oil or foreign material. Although the patient had no current symptoms of GI disease, he was referred for a colonoscopy, which revealed loss of vascularity, friability, and linear ulcerations with cobblestone appearance. A colon biopsy revealed acute and chronic inflammation of the colonic mucosa and submucosa consistent with Crohn's disease. He was treated with metronidazole, systemic corticosteroids, and strong topical corticosteroids, with gradual resolution of the scrotal and penile erythema and edema. A repeat colonoscopy 2 months later showed partial resolution of the abnormal findings.

Clinical Pearls

1. Metastatic Crohn's disease (noncontiguous, cutaneous) is rare, and in adults the underlying gastrointestinal disease usually is manifest.
2. In children, cutaneous lesions generally precede the gastrointestinal disease.
3. Genital disease is more common in children than adults.
4. Patients with MCD may have a positive C-ANCA.
5. Although gastrointestinal Crohn's disease typically involves the small bowel, when cutaneous Crohn's disease is present, it is more commonly associated with colorectal disease.

REFERENCES

1. Parks AG, Moroson BC, Pegum JS: Crohn's disease with cutaneous involvement. Proc R Soc Med 58:241, 1965.
2. Cockburn AG, Krolikowski J, Balogh K, et al: Crohn's disease of penile and scrotal skin. Urology 15:596–598, 1980.
3. Neri I, Bardazzi F, Fanti PA, et al: Penile Crohn's disease: A case report. Genitourin Med 71:45–46, 1995.
4. Chen W, Blume-Peytavi U, Goerdt S, et al: Metastatic Crohn's disease of the face. J Am Acad Dermatol 35:986–988, 1996.
5. Hackzell-Bradley M, Hedblad MA, Stephansson EA: Metastatic Crohn's disease. Arch Dermatol 132:928–932, 1996.
6. Phillips SS, Baird DB, Joshi VV, et al: Crohn's disease of the prepuce in a 12-year-old boy: A case report and review of the literature. Pediatr Pathol Lab Med 17:497–502, 1997.
7. Polysangam T, Heubi JE, Eisen D, et al: Cutaneous Crohn's disease in children. J Am Acad Dermatol 36:697–704, 1997.
8. Sangueza OP, Davis LS, Gourdin FW: Metastatic Crohn's disease. South Med J 90:897–900, 1997.

PATIENT 32

A 3-month-old boy with a scalp plaque and cervical lymphadenopathy

A 3-month-old infant sustained a pustule on the left parietal scalp, which gradually enlarged into a plaque over the following month despite two courses of systemic antibiotics. Pronounced cervical lymphadenopathy and torticollis developed, necessitating hospital admission.

Physical Examination: Vital signs: normal. Neck: torticollis with left cervical lymphadenopathy measuring 3 × 5 cm. Skin: 2-cm, crusted, eroded plaque on left parietal scalp (see figure). Abdomen: no hepatosplenomegaly.

Laboratory Findings: CBC, differential, and Westergren ESR: normal. Chest radiograph: normal, with the exception of left neck mass. Skin biopsy from scalp nodule: suppurative and granulomatous dermatitis. Stains and cultures: pending.

Questions: What is the most likely diagnosis? How would you confirm the diagnosis?

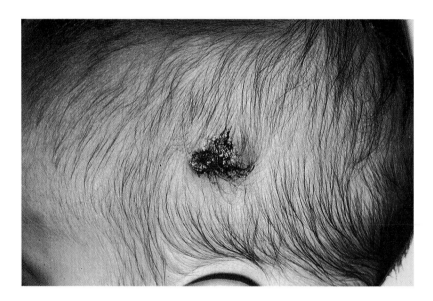

Diagnosis: Chronic granulomatous disease

Discussion: Chronic granulomatous disease (CGD) represents a group of rare genetic diseases characterized by dermatitis, recurrent furuncles and pyodermas, and skin abscesses. The incidence of CGD is 1 in 500,000, and 90% of patients are male. The classic X-linked recessive inheritance pattern is seen in 60–65% of all patients. Onset usually is in early childhood, but the diagnosis may be delayed. In one recent study of 11 patients with CGD, the median age at diagnosis was 22 years, and symptoms began at 3.6 years. The diagnosis of CGD must be considered in adolescents and adults with unexplained infections or granulomas.

In CGD, there is disordered bacterial and fungal killing by phagocytic leukocytes due to a defect in one of the membrane or cytosolic components of the nicotinamide adenine dinucleotide phosphate (NADPH)-oxidase system. This system generates the toxic oxygen metabolites necessary for microbicidal activity; if one of these components is missing, intracellular bacterial and fungal killing cannot occur. To date, four components of the NADPH-oxidase complex have been identified, sequenced, cloned, and characterized. Genes that code for these polypeptides are located on chromosomes X (Xp21.1), 1 (1q25), 7 (7q.11.23) and 16 (16p24). The subunits of the NADPH-oxidase complex are gp91phox, p47phox, p67phox, and p22phox.

Skin manifestations occur in 60–70% of CGD patients. Dermatitis is present in a third and resembles an infectious periorificial type rather than typical atopic or seborrheic dermatitis of childhood. Other dermatologic manifestations include miliaria pustulosa, cutaneous granulomas, dermal fixed plaques, chronic paronychia, perirectal abscesses and fistulae, and acne-like furuncles or severe acne vulgaris.

Recurrent and chronic infections are the hallmark of CGD. Most commonly seen are pneumonia; pyodermas and draining furuncles, especially of the axillae and groin; and lymphadenopathy with draining lymph nodes. Also seen are hepatic abscesses, osteomyelitis, septicemia, otitis media, pyelonephritis, conjunctivitis, and sinusitis. Rarely (less than 5%) brain abscess, pericarditis, and meningitis may occur. These chronic infections may result in anemia of chronic disease, short stature, hypergammaglobulinemia, hepatomegaly, splenomegaly, and chronic diarrhea.

The most commonly seen infectious organisms are *Staphylococcus aureus, Aspergillus* species,
Escherichia coli, Klebsiella, Proteus, Pseudomonas, Salmonella, *Serratia marcescens*, Nocardia, and Candida. Catalase-positive organisms are most common because catalase-negative organisms, such as *Enterococcus fecalis* and *Streptococcus viridans*, produce H_2O_2, which the CGD phagocyte can use for its killing reactions. The nitroblue tetrazolium (NBT) test is based on the observation that normal leukocytes phagocytose and reduce NBT dye, producing a change in color from colorless to dark blue. In patients with CGD, there is no color change. The chemiluminescence test is more specific, and molecular genetic subtyping is done in specialized laboratories. Prenatal diagnosis is available.

The histologic pattern is a suppurative and granulomatous dermatitis in involved internal organs as well as the skin. A characteristic golden-yellow granular pigment is seen in histiocytes, both in the skin and visceral granulomas, probably representing lipofuscin bodies derived from lysosomes.

The treatment of CGD starts with treatment of infection, often with prolonged intravenous antibiotics and surgical debridement or drainage, if appropriate. Prophylactic antibiotics on a daily basis, especially with trimethoprim-sulfamethoxazole (TMP/SMX), has improved the prognosis in these children. It appears that TMP/SMX has the ability to directly stimulate bacteriocidal activity. Interferon-gamma, a major activator of macrophages through its ability to induce cytochrome b-588 synthesis, has been used on a tri-weekly basis with good results. Since prophylactic antibiotic use has increased, there has been a concomitant emergence of aspergillus infection. It is now one of the greatest risks of CGD, and therefore it is imperative that patients be instructed to avoid sources of aspergillus. These sources include wet barns, hay, fresh-cut grass, wood shavings, and hospitals undergoing renovation. Itraconazole is prescribed when aspergillus infection develops. Bone marrow transplantation is controversial. When there is a matched sibling donor or an allergy to TMP/SMX, bone marrow transplant has proved lifesaving. Gene therapy currently is being developed. There are early successful reports of reconstitution of the NADPH-oxidase complex by retrovirus-mediated gene transfer.

In the present patient, the histologic pattern was consistent with CGD. Stains and cultures revealed *S. marcescens* sensitive to TMP/SMX. The infection responded to systemic TMP/SMX, which later was adjusted to a daily prophylactic regimen.

Clinical Pearls

1. Female carriers of X-linked CGD as well as patients with autosomal recessive CGD have shown discoid lupus erythematosus–like skin changes. These patients may show photosensitivity, aphthous stomatitis, and Raynaud's phenomenon.

2. The effectiveness of prophylactic TMP/SMX appears to be due to its ability to directly stimulate bacteriocidal activity in addition to its antimicrobial action.

3. Aspergillus infection has emerged as a major threat to children with CGD; therefore, they must be instructed to avoid sources of this fungus.

REFERENCES

1. Sahn EE, Migliardi RT: Crusted scalp nodule in an infant: Chronic granulomatous disease of childhood. Arch Dermatol 130:105–108, 1994.
2. Liese JG, Jendrossek V, Jansson A, et al: Chronic granulomatous disease in adults. Lancet 346:220–223, 1995.
3. Calvino MC, Maldonado MS, Otheo E, et al: Bone marrow transplantation in chronic granulomatous disease. Eur J Pediatr 155:877–899, 1996.
4. Segal AW: The NADPH oxidase and chronic granulomatous disease. Mol Med Today 2:129–135, 1996.
5. Dohil M, Prendiville JS, Crawford RI, et al: Cutaneous manifestations of chronic granulomatous disease. J Am Acad Dermatol 36:899–907, 1997.
6. Zicha D, Dunn GA, Segal AW: Deficiency of p67phox, p47phox or gp91phox in chronic granulomatous disease does not impair leucocyte chemotaxis or motility. Br J Haematol 96:543–550, 1997.

PATIENT 33

A 70-year-old man with a pruritic, spreading eruption

A 70-year-old man complained of a severely pruritic eruption which began on his mid-chest and spread over 5 years to involve his trunk, upper arms, groin, buttocks, and upper thighs. He had no fever, weight loss, or arthritis and was in reasonably good health. Mild hypertension had been controlled with a thiazide diuretic for the past 10 years.

Physical Examination: Vital signs: normal. Skin: diffuse poikiloderma on the chest, upper arms, back, buttocks, groin, and proximal thighs (see figure); atrophic patches with hyperpigmented and hypopigmented areas, telangiectasia, and scale. Lymph nodes: normal. Abdomen: no hepatosplenomegaly or masses.

Laboratory Findings: CBC, peripheral smear, serum chemistries, and chest radiograph: normal. Skin biopsy: pending.

Questions: What is the diagnosis for this constellation of skin findings? What are the possible underlying associations?

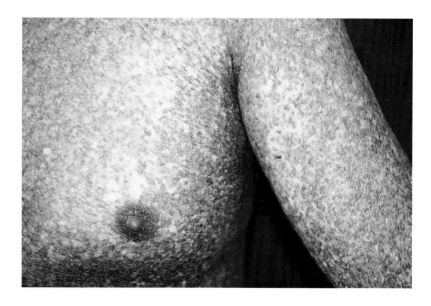

Diagnosis: Poikiloderma atrophicans vasculare associated with T-cell lymphoma

Discussion: Poikiloderma refers to skin changes of diffuse atrophy, often with "cigarette paper–like wrinkling," telangiectasia, hyperpigmentation, and hypopigmentation. Localized poikiloderma occurs in poikiloderma of Civatte or in chronic radiation injury. Poikiloderma atrophicans vasculare (PAV) is a chronic, scaly dermatitis characterized by poikiloderma. It most often is seen in middle-aged or older individuals and is frequently symmetrical, involving the chest, buttocks, breasts, and flexures.

PAV is classified into four types: idiopathic; associated with connective tissue disease (lupus erythematosus, dermatomyositis, or scleroderma); associated with malignancy (cutaneous T-cell lymphoma [CTCL]) or Hodgkin's disease; and associated with genetic disease. The following syndromes can show poikilodermatous changes, but appear in early childhood: Weary syndrome (hereditary acrokeratotic poikiloderma), also known as Grither syndrome (poikiloderma, palmoplantar keratoderma, acrokeratotic papules); Kindler syndrome (poikiloderma, bullae, proximal webbing of digits); Rothmund-Thomson syndrome (poikiloderma congenitale); focal dermal hypoplasia (Goltz syndrome); dyskeratosis congenita; xeroderma pigmentosa; ataxia telangiectasia; hereditary sclerosing poikiloderma (sclerotic bands in the flexures, palms, soles, and fingers); Bloom syndrome; Cockayne syndrome; and Werner syndrome. In addition, chronic graft versus host disease may present as PAV.

Histopathologic examination of idiopathic PAV or of that associated with connective tissue disease shows epidermal atrophy, vacuolar changes in the basement membrane, and a dense, band-like infiltrate in the upper dermis. PAV associated with lymphoma often demonstrates the changes of patch-stage mycosis fungoides, with abnormal cerebriform lymphocytes and epidermotropism.

PAV associated with genetic disease presents at an early age, and other features of the syndrome are detectable to help make the diagnosis. However, PAV in association with CTCL has occurred in childhood, so this possibility must be kept in mind. PAV associated with connective tissue disease usually occurs late in the course of the underlying disease, so that the diagnosis is known. Usually the patches occur on both exposed and covered areas and are relatively asymptomatic. In contrast, PAV associated with malignancy tends to be extremely pruritic, often precedes or heralds the malignancy, and typically occurs in covered areas.

In the present patient, the skin biopsy revealed the typical findings of patch-stage mycosis fungoides. An MRI of the abdomen revealed no abnormalities. Since his only complaint was itching, he was treated conservatively with topical steroid cream and topical nitrogen mustard ointment. The pruritus resolved within 3 months, but the eruption remained unchanged. He is being followed closely for return of symptoms or spread of disease.

Clinical Pearls

1. Poikiloderma occurring in a child may represent a genodermatosis, connective tissue disease, or early cutaneous T-cell lymphoma.
2. Poikiloderma atrophicans vasculare most often is associated with lymphoma.
3. Localized poikiloderma may be seen in poikiloderma of Civatte (neck) and chronic radiation injury (at site of previous irradiation).

REFERENCES
1. Fortson JS, Schroeter AL, Esterly NB: Cutaneous T-cell lymphoma (parapsoriasis en plaque): An association with pityriasis lichenoides et varioliformis acuta in young children. Arch Dermatol 126:1449–1453, 1990.
2. Wakelin SH, Stewart EJ, Emmerson RW: Poikilodermatous and verrucous mycosis fungoides. Clin Exp Dermatol 21:205–208, 1996.

PATIENT 34

A 1-month-old boy with dark brown plaques on his arm

A 1-month-old infant was born with a large, dark brown plaque on his right forearm and hand and three smaller similar plaques located proximally on his arm. Pregnancy, delivery, and health of the infant were entirely normal.

Physical Examination: Vital signs: normal. Neurologic examination: normal. Skin: dark brown plaque in a "glove distribution" extending from tips of fingers to middle of forearm, encircling wrist and involving palm; three similar but smaller, dark brown, round plaques noted on proximal arm (see figure). Lymph nodes: normal.

Laboratory Findings: Skin biopsy from dorsum of wrist: pending.

Questions: What is the most likely diagnosis? How would you counsel the parents?

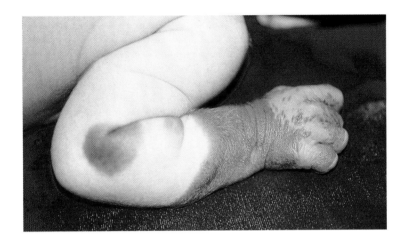

Diagnosis: Congenital melanocytic nevus

Discussion: Congenital melanocytic nevi (CMN) are nevi with specific histologic features that are present at birth or slightly thereafter. They are classified into three types based on size: the giant CMN is > 20 cm in diameter and occurs in 1:20,000 births; the intermediate CMN is 2–20 cm and occurs in 0.6% of births; the small CMN is < 2 cm and occurs in 1% of newborns.

The *differential diagnosis* of a CMN at birth includes café au lait macule, Mongolian spot (usually more blue in color), nevus of Ota or Ito (characteristic location and color), epidermal nevus, early-onset lentigo (often linear), and postinflammatory hyperpigmentation (as is seen in transient neonatal pustular melanosis or acropustulosis infantum).

The most important complication of CMN is **malignant melanoma**. Giant CMN carry a lifetime risk of melanoma of 5–15%, with the risk much greater in children under 10 years old. The lifetime risk of a malignant melanoma developing in a small CMN has been estimated at 0.8–4.9%, with the risk greatest after puberty. The risk of development of malignant melanoma in a giant CMN appears related to location. The risk is much higher in giant CMN in an axial location, whereas large CMN on an extremity almost never develop melanoma. The satellite nevi that frequently accompany giant CMN have never been reported to degenerate into malignant melanoma. Another complication of giant CMN is involvement of underlying tissue and bone. **Cosmetic problems** can be of major importance.

Neurocutaneous melanosis is defined as the association of a large CMN with leptomeningeal melanocytosis. There may or may not be central nervous system (CNS) melanoma or CNS symptoms. If CNS symptoms do develop, the prognosis is extremely poor even if no melanoma is present. There is an increased risk of neurocutaneous melanosis if the giant CMN is located in a posterior-axial site (head, neck, back, or buttocks), or if satellite melanocytic nevi are present. Symptoms in neurocutaneous melanosis are due to intracranial compression and obstruction, and seizures, spina bifida, or meningomyelocele may be present.

On histologic examination, features that suggest CMN include infiltration of nevus cells between collagen bundles in single file fashion and into nerves, blood vessels, and appendages. There also may be deep infiltration of nevus cells in the dermis.

Management of CMN is controversial. Because of the high risk of malignant melanoma, excision of posterior-axial giant or large CMNs should be undertaken if feasible. Tissue expanders and staged excisions often are required. Continued surveillance of all CMNs is necessary, with prompt biopsy of any areas suggestive of melanoma. If a giant CMN is located in a posterior-axial location, MRI should be done to evaluate the possibility of CNS melanosis. Although there is no current treatment for CNS melanosis, knowledge of its presence may help in management decisions. Cosmetic benefit has been obtained with dermabrasion or curettage, but some clinicians point out that melanoma may still develop in the melanocytes remaining in the deep dermis, and it could be obscured by the scarring that follows both procedures.

The present patient exhibited a "glove distribution" of intermediate-sized CMN; therefore, he was at low risk of malignant melanoma developing over his lifetime. The cosmetic deformity of the lesion was the parents' biggest concern; however, aggressive surgical procedures might functionally impair the child's dominant hand. Dermabrasion, laser therapy, and curettage were discussed but not encouraged. The child will be closely followed, and plastic surgery using tissue expansion is a future option.

Clinical Pearls

1. The risk of malignant melanoma developing in a giant melanocytic nevus is greatest in patients under the age of 10; in small congenital nevi, risk is greatest post-puberty.

2. Malignant melanoma almost never develops in a giant CMN on an extremity and reportedly has never developed in a satellite nevus associated with a giant CMN.

3. A giant CMN in the posterior-axial location has a high risk of neurocutaneous melanosis, and an MRI should be performed.

REFERENCES

1. De David M, Orlow SJ, Provost N, et al: Neurocutaneous melanosis: Clinical features of large congenital melanocytic nevi in patients with manifest central nervous system melanosis. J Am Acad Dermatol 35:529–538, 1996.
2. Marghoob AA, Schoenbach SP, Kopf AW, et al: Large congenital melanocytic nevi and the risk for the development of malignant melanoma: A prospective study. Arch Dermatol 132:170–175, 1996.
3. De David M, Orlow SJ, Provost N, et al: A study of large congenital melanocytic nevi and associated malignant melanomas: A review of cases in the New York University Registry and the world literature. J Am Acad Dermatol 36:409–416, 1997.
4. Ruiz-Maldonado R, Orozco-Covarrubias M: Malignant melanoma in children. Arch Dermatol 133:363–371, 1997.

PATIENT 35

A 9-year-old girl with red plaques on the extremities and trunk

A previously healthy 9-year-old girl noticed pruritic, erythematous, scaly plaques on her extremities and trunk 4 weeks previously. She had no family history of skin disease, no history of drug intake, and no preceding illness.

Physical Examination:　Vital signs: normal. Skin: sharply demarcated, erythematous plaques with silver-white scale symmetrically distributed over extensor surfaces of extremities (see figure) and trunk; scattered guttate papules on trunk. Throat: no erythema. Perirectal area: erythema and mild scale.

Laboratory Findings:　CBC and ESR: normal. Throat and perirectal cultures for group A β-hemolytic streptococcus: pending. Skin biopsy from an erythematous plaque on leg: pending.

Question:　What is the probable diagnosis in this child?

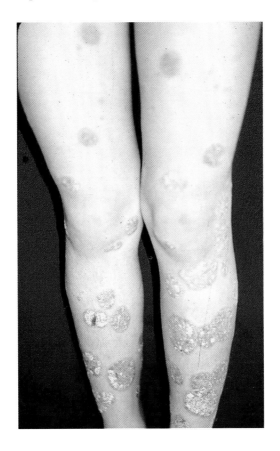

Diagnosis: Psoriasis vulgaris

Discussion: Psoriasis (vulgaris) is a papulo-squamous skin disorder affecting approximately 1–3% of the population. Although there are many ways to classify psoriasis, five common forms include: plaque-type, guttate (drop-like), pustular, erythrodermic, and arthritic (seen in 7% of hospitalized psoriatic patients). In childhood psoriasis, plaque-type is seen in 53%, and guttate psoriasis is seen in 34% of cases.

Psoriasis usually is asymptomatic, but may be pruritic, causing confusion with atopic dermatitis. The silvery-white scale may be thick or micaceous. Distribution often is symmetrical on the extensor surfaces, but may be flexural, and often involves the palms, soles, and scalp. Nails are involved in 25–50% of patients, and the most common findings are pitting, onycholysis, subungual hyperkeratosis, subungual "oil spotting," and koilonychia. Scalp involvement occurs in up to 80%. If the scale on the scalp is firm, adherent, and asbestos-like, it is referred to as tinea amiantacea. Geographic tongue may be present and is characterized by serpiginous, annular, white patches on the dorsum of the tongue. The Koebner or isomorphic phenomenon, in which new disease appears at sites of skin injury, is characteristic of psoriasis. This injury may include trauma or minor irritation, for example from clothing, sunburn, or irradiation.

The *differential diagnosis* includes other papulosquamous diseases, particularly lichen planus, tinea corporis, seborrheic dermatitis, and pityriasis rosea. In the pruritic variety of psoriasis, atopic dermatitis also must be considered. Scalp psoriasis can be confused with tinea capitis, and nail psoriasis can resemble onychomycosis.

A **drug history** is extremely important, as many agents can precipitate or exacerbate psoriasis. Among these are lithium, beta blockers, antimalarials, iodide, progesterone, salicylate, penicillin, nystatin, and discontinuation of systemic steroids. Alcohol also can exacerbate psoriasis.

In children, guttate psoriasis frequently is associated with a preceding **streptococcal pharyngitis** or **perianal dermatitis**. Therefore, when guttate lesions are seen in children it is important to obtain swabs from both the posterior pharynx and perianal area to exclude group A β-hemolytic streptococcal infection.

The histopathology of a psoriatic plaque reflects increased epidermal cell proliferation or turnover in addition to dermal alterations. The following was found on the skin biopsy of this child: acanthosis with elongation of the rete ridges and parakeratosis of the epidermis, neutrophilic microabscesses in the epidermis (Kogoj spongioform pustules and Monro microabscesses), a decreased granular layer, elongation of the dermal papillae with dilated capillary loops, and a moderate dermal infiltrate of lymphocytes and monocytes.

Treatment of psoriasis begins with topical corticosteroids. In children with guttate psoriasis and an associated infection, antibiotic treatment often produces a remission. Intralesional steroids and steroids under occlusion are used less commonly. Tar, either alone or in association with natural sunlight, or UVB irradiation can be helpful in children. Anthralin creams, particularly applied with the short-contact method, are effective and well-tolerated in childhood psoriasis; however, irritation and staining of skin and clothing may occur. Topical calcipotriol also has been used safely in children according to a recent study, which found no calcium or bone abnormalities in the study subjects. Systemic therapy for psoriasis in children is used only with severe recalcitrant psoriasis, pustular psoriasis, psoriatic erythroderma, or psoriatic arthritis. Methotrexate, either intramuscular or by mouth, has been prescribed in these circumstances. Systemic corticosteroids are not recommended because of the rapid flare that follows their discontinuation. Psoralen plus UVA (PUVA) has been used in children, but one recent study reported the development of two basal cell carcinomas before the age of 21 in a child who had been treated with PUVA for 6 years. Additional risks include cataracts, actinic damage, and other skin cancers. Oral retinoids, sulfasalazine, and cyclosporine A are not recommended for use in childhood psoriasis, but have proved useful in difficult cases of adult psoriasis.

In the present patient, the pharyngeal culture was negative, but the perianal swab showed group A β-hemolytic streptococcus. She was treated for 1 month with oral erythromycin and moderately strong topical corticosteroids. At her 6 week checkup, she was 90% cleared. The plan at that point was to add natural sunlight to her regimen and taper her off the topical corticosteroids.

Clinical Pearls

1. The Koebner or isomorphic phenomenon, in which psoriasis is exacerbated in sites of skin injury, can be seen following mild irritation from clothing, sunburn, irradiation, accidental trauma, and surgery.

2. Flares of guttate psoriasis in children frequently are associated with streptococcal pharyngitis or perianal streptococcal dermatitis. These infections are easily treated with oral antibiotics, which often leads to a remission.

3. In any new case of psoriasis, precipitating or exacerbating factors (especially lithium, beta-blockers, and antimalarials) must be excluded.

REFERENCES

1. Kumar B, Dhar S, Handa S, et al: Methotrexate in childhood psoriasis. Pediatr Dermatol 11:271–273, 1994.
2. Zvulunov A, Anisfeld A, Metzker A: Efficacy of short-contact therapy with dithranol in childhood psoriasis. Int J Dermatol 33:808–810, 1994.
3. Stern RS, Nichols KT: Therapy with orally administered methoxsalen and ultraviolet A radiation during childhood increases the risk of basal cell carcinoma: The PUVA Follow-up Study. J Pediatr 129:915–917, 1996.
4. Oranje AP, Marcoux D, Svensson A, et al: Topical calcipotriol in childhood psoriasis. J Am Acad Dermatol 36:203–208, 1997.

PATIENT 36

A newborn boy with hyperpigmented, linear streaks

A newborn was noted to have hyperpigmented, linear streaks on his left leg, thigh, buttock, and trunk. There was no family history of similar hyperpigmentation or neurologic disease.

Physical Examination: General: healthy-appearing. Skin: hyperpigmented, linear streaks distributed over left trunk, buttock, thigh, and leg (see figure); sparing of the face, mucous membranes, palms, and soles. Remainder of physical examination: normal.

Laboratory Findings: Skin biopsy of normal and hyperpigmented skin: pending.

Question: What is the most likely diagnosis?

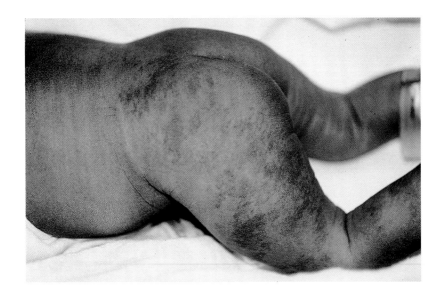

Diagnosis: Linear and whorled nevoid hypermelanosis

Discussion: Linear and whorled hyper-melanosis (LWNH) was first described in 1988 by Kalter, et al. Onset is at birth or within the first few weeks of life, with whorls, streaks, and patches of hyperpigmentation that follow Blaschko's developmental lines. The distribution is asymmetric and spares the palms and soles as well as the mucous membranes. A second type of presentation which occurs during the second decade and shows unilateral involvement of one quadrant only has been described. There appears to be a spectrum between these two presentations.

Similar clinical presentations noted prior to 1988 were given various names, such as zosteriform reticulate hyperpigmentation, zosteriform lentiginous nevus, and reticulate hyperpigmentation of Ijima. LWNH appears to represent a heterogeneous collection of disorders with underlying **somatic mosaicism**.

The *differential diagnosis* includes the third stage of incontinentia pigmenti, which demonstrates preceding vesicles or hyperkeratotic lesions and occurs in girls; skin biopsy provides differentiation. An early epidermal nevus may present with streaks following Blaschko's lines but later becomes palpable. Hypomelanosis of Ito presents with the same pattern and distribution, but the lesions are hypopigmented rather than hyperpigmented. However, it frequently is difficult to determine the normal skin color when the pigmentary abnormalities are widespread. Naegeli-Franceschetti-Jadassohn syndrome can present with a reticular hyperpigmentation, but begins in adolescence and includes other findings as well. Rarely reported associated problems in patients with LWNH include mental retardation, cerebral palsy, unspecified congenital and neurologic defects, and family history.

Histologic examination of the abnormally pigmented skin reveals increased melanin pigment in the basal layer, with prominence or vacuolization of basal melanocytes. However, there is no vacuolization of basal keratinocytes, no pigment incontinence, and no dermal melanophages as may be seen in incontinentia pigmenti.

In the present patient, the histopathologic examination was consistent with LWNH. Cultured fibroblasts from normal and hyperpigmented dermis, as well as peripheral blood lymphocytes, revealed a normal XY karyotype without evidence of chimerism or mosaicism. A thorough neurologic examination by the pediatric neurologist was normal. The child will be followed on a regular basis.

Clinical Pearls

1. Linear and whorled nevoid hypermelanosis probably is a heterogeneous collection of disorders with underlying somatic mosaicism.

2. LWNH must be differentiated from the third stage of incontinentia pigmenti, which occurs only rarely in boys.

3. LWNH may be associated with neurologic or other congenital defects, although rarely.

REFERENCES

1. Kalter DC, Griffiths WA, Atherton DJ: Linear and whorled nevoid hypermelanosis. J Am Acad Dermatol 19:1037–1044, 1988.
2. Akiyama M, Aranami A, Sasaki Y, et al: Familial linear and whorled nevoid hypermelanosis. J Am Acad Dermatol 30:831–833, 1994.
3. Nehal KS, Pe Bonito R, Orlow SJ: Analysis of 54 cases of hypopigmentation and hyperpigmentation along the lines of Blaschko. Arch Dermatol 132:1167–1170, 1996.
4. Quecedo E, Febrer I, Aliaga A: Linear and whorled nevoid hypermelanosis: A spectrum of pigmentary disorders. Pediatr Dermatol 14:247–248, 1997.

PATIENT 37

A 17-old-year girl with facial lesions and seizure disorder

A 17-year-old mentally retarded girl was brought by her mother for treatment of worsening "acne" lesions on the face. She had used topical benzoyl peroxide for several years without benefit. The seizure disorder began in infancy and was partially controlled with oral phenytoin. There was no family history of a seizure disorder, similar facial lesions, or mental retardation.

Physical Examination: Mental age: approximately 7 years. Skin: multiple 1- to 8-mm, hyper-pigmented, dome-shaped papules symmetrically located over cheeks and forehead; hypopigmented macule on left upper lip; large, rectangular, hypopigmented macule on arm; pink-yellow plaque consisting of small papules with an "orange peel" appearance on back (see figures). Fundoscopic, nail, and cardiac examinations: normal. Woods light examination: multiple, "confetti-sized," white macules on shins. Dental examination: tiny pits in tooth enamel.

Laboratory Findings: Brain MRI: calcified cortical tubers. Renal ultrasound: polycystic kidneys.

Questions: What is this syndrome? Should further work-up be done? What treatment options are available for the facial lesions?

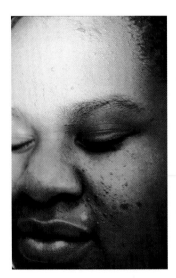
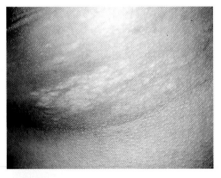
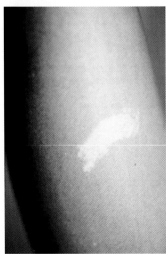

Diagnosis: Tuberous sclerosis

Discussion: Tuberous sclerosis (TS) is a geno-dermatosis characterized by multiple hamartomas of the skin, eyes, central nervous system, heart, kidneys, lungs, and bones. The classic triad described in 1908 consisted of angiofibromas of the face (originally misnamed adenoma sebaceum), mental retardation, and seizures. There is a direct relationship between seizures and mental retardation: the younger the age at onset of seizures, the more severe the mental retardation. However, 40% of patients with TS have normal intelligence.

The incidence of TS is reported to be 1:10,000, but may be as high 1:6000. Inheritance is autosomal dominant, but the spontaneous mutation rate is high, estimated at 66–75%. Locus heterogeneity is established: one gene is located on chromosome 9q34 (TSC1), and the other gene is located on chromosome 16p13 (TSC2). The protein product of the TSC2 gene is tuberin, a polypeptide with a role in growth suppression. High levels of tuberin are present in cortical neurons and in the blood vessels of many organs, including kidney and skin, which typically are affected by TS. Therefore, partial inactivation of the TSC2 tumor suppressor gene results in tumors as well as focal dysplasias.

Clinical findings of tuberous sclerosis are numerous. Angiofibromas of the face usually begin between the ages of 2 and 6 years and increase in number. They are symmetrical and usually involve the nasolabial fold. The differential diagnosis of facial angiofibromas includes trichoepitheliomas, syringomas, tricholemmomas (as seen in Cowden's disease), milia, xanthomas, verrucae, and acne vulgaris. **Hypopigmented macules** are the earliest cutaneous marker of TS. There are four types, of which the most common is the polygonal macule, as seen on the present patient's arm. The most characteristic is the ash-leaf macule, which has a lance-ovate shape. The third type is the confetti macule, which is seen in the pretibial areas. The fourth type is the dermatomal hypopigmented macule. The **shagreen patch** is a connective tissue nevus most commonly seen over the sacrum, but in our patient was on the back. Fibrous plaques may be present on the face or forehead and are thought by some investigators to be a poor prognostic sign. Periungal fibromas ("garlic clove tumors") appear after puberty and, therefore, are not helpful in making the diagnosis in infancy. These also are called Koenen's tumors. Café au lait macules are increased in individuals with TS. Diffuse skin bronzing occasionally is seen.

Oral findings include gingival fibromas and enamel pits in the teeth. Kidney lesions include angiomyolipomas and renal cysts, which occur in 15% of patients, but are not found in the neonatal period. One study found that renal disease in TS tends to be associated with increased retinal hamartomas, cardiac rhabdomyomas, and skin lesions. Cardiac rhabdomyomas may be seen in infancy in TS and regress with age; however, they can cause sudden death in the first year of life. Fifty percent of all cardiac rhabdomyomas occur in patients with TS. Eye findings include retinal gliomas and other hamartomas, papilledema, and optic atrophy. A fully dilated, indirect ophthalmoscopy is necessary to reveal diagnostic retinal hamartomas in infants. The two characteristic types are the "mulberry" or "frog's egg" tumor and pale, flat lesions.

In addition to an ophthalmologic examination, the work-up of a child suspected of having TS includes a brain MRI to exclude the presence of cortical tubers (when calcified these appear as brain stones on radiograph or CT scan), subependymal hamartomas, astrocytomas, periventricular calcification (curvilinear shape), and dilated lateral ventricles. Positron emission tomography (PET) brain scans, which measure glucose metabolism in the brain, have been studied recently in patients with TS. They probably are useful only when brain surgery is contemplated, or when the EEG, CT, and MRI show unifocal or unilateral abnormalities. The PET scan provides information about overall brain integrity, and may help identify contralateral tubers. A renal ultrasound can identify cysts and tumors. It is imperative to examine first-degree relatives, since there have been recent reports of asymptomatic parents of a TS child who themselves show brain CT scan findings compatible with TS. Parents and siblings probably should have a CT or MRI of the brain prior to genetic counseling.

The incidence of hypopigmented macules in the general population was thought to be about 0.3%, but recent studies have shown a much higher incidence, with 4.7% of a healthy population having at least one white spot. These findings imply that the incidence of white spots in the normal population has been underestimated and that white spots occurring in an otherwise healthy individual without a family history of TS does not necessitate an extensive work-up. The differential diagnosis of calcified brain lesions includes Sturge-Weber syndrome, congenital toxoplasmosis, lipoid proteinosis, basal cell nevus syndrome, and calcified neoplasms.

The management of tuberous sclerosis begins with seizure control at an early age, since this may lead to improved mental development. Evaluation and close follow-up for the appearance of tumors or malformations in organ systems is necessary.

Intractable epilepsy may be seen in TS and can be successfully treated with surgical removal of the epileptogenic focus, if clearly identified. Treatment of the angiofibromas of the face is cosmetic and not entirely satisfactory. Often, simple tangential shave excision is sufficient. Dermabrasion, electrodesiccation, and cryotherapy also are used. More recently the CO_2 laser and the copper vapor laser have produced good results.

In the present patient, the extent of her disease was limited to brain, skin, and kidney. There was no evidence of brain malignancy or functional renal disease. Since evaluation of her siblings and parents revealed no evidence of TS, she was classified as a sporadic case. She will be followed closely in neurology, dermatology, and renal clinics, and is in an appropriate learning environment at her school. Cosmetic improvement in the angiofibromas of the face was obtained with simple shave excisions and the use of Monsel's solution for hemostasis, which provided a darker scar compatible with her natural complexion.

Clinical Pearls

1. Hypopigmented macules are the earliest cutaneous marker of tuberous sclerosis. The most characteristic is the ash-leaf or lance-ovate macule.

2. The most common white spot in TS is the polygonal macule. The incidence of white spots in a normal, healthy population without TS may be as high as 4.7%.

3. A Woods lamp should be used when examining the skin for white spots.

4. Seizures plus white spots in infancy necessitates an evaluation for TS.

5. Fully dilated, indirect ophthalmoscopy must be performed to diagnose retinal hamartomas in infancy.

REFERENCES

1. Curatolo P: Neurological manifestations of tuberous sclerosis complex. Childs Nerv Syst 12:515–521, 1996.
2. Halley DJ: Tuberous sclerosis: Between genetic and physical analysis. Acta Genet Med Gemellol 45:63–75, 1996.
3. O'Hagan AR, Ellsworth R, Secic M, et al: Renal manifestations of tuberous sclerosis complex. Clin Pediatr 35:483–489, 1996.
4. Vanderhooft SL, Francis JS, Pagon RA, et al: Prevalence of hypopigmented macules in a healthy population. J Pediatr 129:355–661, 1996.
5. Rintahaka PJ, Chugani HT: Clinical role of positron emission tomography in children with tuberous sclerosis complex. J Child Neurol 12:42–52, 1997.
6. Wienecke R, Maize JC Jr, Reed JA, et al: Expression of the TSC2 product tuberin and its target Rap 1 in normal human tissues. Am J Pathol 150:43–50, 1997.

PATIENT 38

A 3-month-old infant with white spots on the face and diaper area

A 3-month-old boy experienced asymptomatic, erythematous, scaly plaques on the face and diaper area at the age of 1 month. The redness resolved with the use of petrolatum and cocoa butter, but white patches remained. There was no family history of skin disease, and the child was otherwise in excellent health.

Physical Examination: Skin: hypopigmented macules and patches with scale over face, accentuated in nasolabial folds and eyebrows (see figure); similar lesions in deep folds of neck, behind ears, in axillae, and in diaper area; yellowish, thick, scaly plaques adhered to scalp. Nails: no pitting.

Laboratory Findings: Potassium hydroxide examination: no hyphae. Fungal culture of scalp plaques: no growth.

Question: What is the most likely diagnosis and the most appropriate treatment?

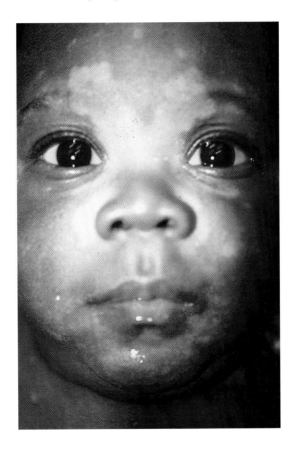

Diagnosis: Seborrheic dermatitis with postinflammatory hypopigmentation

Discussion: Seborrheic dermatitis is a common, chronic, papulosquamous dermatosis characterized by redness and scaling on the face, scalp, and intertriginous areas. Onset of infantile seborrheic dermatitis typically occurs between 2 and 10 weeks of age; otherwise, onset is during puberty or thereafter. In children, the thick scalp scale is called "**cradle cap**." Eyelid involvement can produce a seborrheic blepharitis.

The *differential diagnosis* of seborrheic dermatitis in infants primarily includes atopic dermatitis and psoriasis or sebopsoriasis. Scabies, contact dermatitis, and tinea capitis or corporis should be excluded. Less common entities that can produce a seborrheic picture include biotin deficiency, HIV infection, acrodermatitis enteropathica, Langerhans cell histiocytosis (Letterer-Siwe disease, which features petechiae), and Leiner's disease (C5 and/or C3 dysfunction, diarrhea, and failure to thrive).

Histologically, seborrheic dermatitis shows focal parakeratosis with pyknotic neutrophils in the horn, particularly concentrated around the follicular ostia. There is acanthosis and a superficial perivascular infiltrate, as well as spongiosis with neutrophils.

The etiology of seborrheic dermatitis is unclear, but several studies have supported a causative role for *Pityrosporon ovale* yeast. Seborrheic dermatitis improves with ketoconazole, and there is increased incidence in HIV infection due to depressed cell-mediated immunity. Some studies have found an increased number of *P. ovale* organisms in the skin of patients with seborrheic dermatitis. Also noted is an increased association between seborrheic dermatitis and tinea versicolor and an increased incidence of seborrheic dermatitis in certain neurologic abnormalities. One recent study found that *P. ovale* antigen produced peripheral blood monocyte (PBMC) proliferation in healthy volunteers, but not in patients with seborrheic dermatitis. Furthermore, PBMC from patients with seborrheic dermatitis showed a markedly depressed production of the cytokines Il-2 and IFN-γ, but increased production of IL-10 compared to normals when stimulated with *P. ovale* antigen. The authors concluded that heavy skin colonization with *P. ovale* and seborrheic dermatitis may be related to altered cytokine production as well as altered cell-mediated immunity.

Treatment of seborrheic dermatitis involves topical corticosteroid creams or solutions and ketoconazole cream or shampoo. Additional softening agents, such as tar shampoo, may be required for severe disease. Terbinafine solution recently has been shown to produce good results.

The prognosis in infants with seborrheic dermatitis usually is good, with clearing in 3–4 weeks; rarely, taking up to 6 months. A recent study revealed the following outcomes of infantile seborrheic dermatitis: psoriasis developed in 1/88 infants; atopic dermatitis developed in 4/88; and adult seborrheic dermatitis developed in 7/88. The authors concluded that infantile seborrheic dermatitis is a predictor of adult seborrheic dermatitis.

Mild topical corticosteroid cream was prescribed for the present patient, and the parents were reassured. Repigmentation eventually occurred after 9 months. The parents were cautioned that the child might develop seborrheic dermatitis as an adolescent or adult.

Clinical Pearls

1. *Pityrosporon ovale* appears to be involved in the etiology of seborrheic dermatitis according to studies of colonization, treatment with antifungals, cytokine production, and cell-mediated immunity alterations.

2. Infantile seborrheic dermatitis that shows petechiae or hemorrhagic crusts immediately raises the possibility of Langerhans cell histiocytosis.

3. Infantile seborrheic dermatitis may be a predictor of adolescent- or adult-onset seborrheic dermatitis, and parents of these patients should be so informed.

REFERENCES

1. Mimouni K, Mukamel M, Zeharia A, et al: Prognosis of infantile seborrheic dermatitis. J Pediatr 127:744–746, 1995.
2. Faergemann J, Jones JC, Hettler O, et al: *Pityrosporon ovale (Malassezia fufur)* as the causative agent of seborrheic dermatitis: New treatment options. Br J Dermatol 134:12–15, 1996.
3. Neuber K, Kroger S, Gruseck E, et al: Effects of *Pityrosporon ovale* on proliferation, immunoglobulin (IgA, G, M) synthesis, and cytokine (IL-2, IL-10, IFN gamma) production of peripheral blood mononuclear cells from patients with seborrheic dermatitis. Arch Dermatol Res 288:532–536, 1996.

PATIENT 39

A 43-year-old man with an enlarging plaque on the shin

A 43-year-old man noted an asymptomatic, scaly, red papule on his shin 2 years previously. The papule enlarged to form a plaque, which has continued to grow. He was diagnosed with insulin-dependent diabetes mellitus at the age of 11, and he has mild diabetic retinopathy.

Physical Examination: Skin: large, erythematous, sharply demarcated plaque in right anterior tibial area, with areas of atrophy, yellowish pigmentation, and hyperpigmentation (see figure). Remainder of skin exam: normal.

Laboratory Findings: Blood glucose: 150–400 mg/dl; hemoglobin A1C elevated at 9.8%. Skin biopsy of right leg plaque: pending.

Questions: What is the diagnosis? The differential diagnosis? What is the best course of treatment?

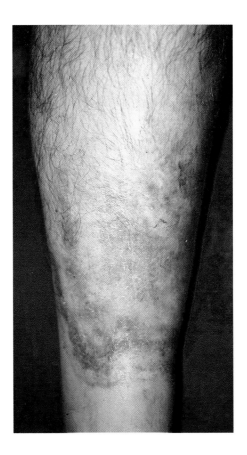

Diagnosis: Necrobiosis lipoidica diabeticorum

Discussion: Necrobiosis lipoidica (NL) is a granulomatous skin condition that is associated with insulin-dependent diabetes mellitus (IDDM) in about two-thirds of cases (necrobiosis lipoidica diabeticorum [NLD]). However, NLD develops in less than 1% of diabetic patients. An asymptomatic, scaly, red papule appears, most often on the anterior tibial area, and slowly enlarges. Later, atrophy with a waxy, translucent appearance may develop along with telangiectasias. Fat deposits produce a yellowish discoloration. Ulcerations in the atrophic center of these plaques occur in about a third of patients. Healing is accompanied by cribriform scarring. Unless there is ulceration, these plaques are asymptomatic. In 15% of cases, NL lesions are not confined to the legs; other locations include the face, scalp, hands, fingers, and forearms. However, only about 2% of patients experience lesion-free legs.

The *differential diagnosis* of pretibial plaques is extensive. Pruritic entities in that location include lichen amyloidosis (yellow, conical papules), hypertrophic lichen planus, lichen simplex chronicus (often linear), and Majocchi's *Trichophyton rubrum* folliculitis. Also in the differential are pretibial myxedema, Ehlers-Danlos type VIII (autosomal dominant with periodontitis), Meischer's granulomatosis, lichen planus-like drug eruption, deep fungal infection, squamous cell carcinoma, flat warts, scleromyxedema, morphia, and acrodermatitis chronica atrophicans (band-like).

The association between NL and IDDM has been studied extensively. Despite previous reports to the contrary, one recent study found evidence to support the conclusion that tight glucose control in IDDM can improve or prevent NLD. Another found that the presence of NLD in IDDM is associated with a significantly increased incidence of diabetic nephropathy and retinopathy. This association may be due to poorer glucose control in these patients.

Histologically, two patterns can be seen in NL. The first is the **necrobiotic pattern**, in which there are areas of degenerated collagen (necrobiosis) with increased mucin, a superficial and deep inflammatory infiltrate with histiocytes and epithelioid cells that palisade around the necrobiotic areas, thick-walled blood vessels, lipid deposits (foam cells), and, occasionally, foreign body giant cells. This was the pattern seen in the current patient. The second is the **granulomatous pattern**, in which there are granulomas composed of histiocytes, epithelioid cells, and giant cells containing asteroid bodies throughout the dermis. There also is an inflammatory infiltrate, but there may or may not be degenerated collagen or lipid deposits. Many patients fall in the middle of the spectrum. It is unknown why these reactions occur, but a recent study found that natural autoantibody activity against cytoskeleton proteins in sera was significantly increased in NL with or without IDDM, but not in IDDM alone or in healthy controls.

The treatment of NL often is unsatisfactory. Commonly, topical corticosteroids with or without occlusion are prescribed. Intralesional corticosteroids can produce good results, but they must be used cautiously since they can cause ulceration. Topical tretinoin has improved atrophy in a single case. Oral aspirin plus dipyridamole has proven helpful in the past. Pentoxiphylline, diaminodiphenylsulfone (Dapsone), and short courses of oral steriods also have been used. When ulcers have required grafting, NL frequently recurs around the edges of the graft.

In the present patient, control of his glucose level was not optimal. His insulin was increased with improvement in his hemoglobin A1C level. The leg plaque was treated with moderate-strength topical corticosteroids, with improved appearance.

Clinical Pearls

1. Necrobiosis lipoidica is associated with IDDM in about two-thirds of cases. However, less than 1% of diabetic patients have or will have necrobiosis lipoidica diabeticorum.

2. It is rare (about 2%) to see lesion-free legs in a patient with NL.

3. Contrary to previous reports, tight glucose control in IDDM may improve or prevent necrobiosis lipoidica diabeticorum.

REFERENCES

1. Haralambous S, Blackwell C, Mappouras DG, et al: Increased natural auotantibody activity to cytoskeleton proteins in sera from patients with necrobiosis lipoidica, with or without insulin-dependent diabetes mellitus. Autoimmunity 20:267–275, 1995.
2. Verotti A, Chiarelli F, Amerio P, et al: Necrobiosis lipoidica diabeticorum in children and adolescents: A clue for underlying renal and retinal disease. Pediatr Dermatol 12:220–223, 1995.
3. Cohen O, Yaniv R, Karasik A, et al: Necrobiosis lipoidica and diabetic control revisited. Med Hypotheses 46:348–350, 1996.
4. Heymann WR: Necrobiosis lipoidica treated with topical tretinoin. Cutis 58:53–54, 1996.

PATIENT 40

A 17-year-old girl with sudden growth in a congenital facial lesion

A 17-year-old Caucasian girl had been born with a yellowish plaque on her nose. At puberty, the plaque had thickened. Two months previously, a hyperpigmented papule began to enlarge at one end of the plaque.

Physical Examination: Skin: yellowish, waxy, 1 × 0.4 cm plaque with pebbly surface on nasal tip; hyperpigmented raised papule at one end of plaque (see figure). Lymph nodes: normal. Abdomen: no hepatosplenomegaly. Remainder of physical examination: normal.

Questions: What is the underlying congenital lesion? What is the most likely cause of the rapidly growing papule?

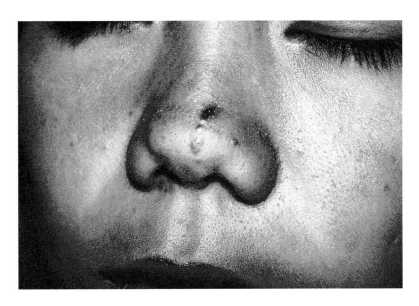

Diagnosis: Basal cell carcinoma developing in a nevus sebaceus of Jadassohn

Discussion: Nevus sebaceus of Jadassohn (NSJ) is a complex hamartoma typically affecting the scalp, face, or neck and usually present at birth. It presents as a pink or yellow, smooth plaque with alopecia. There are three clinical stages, each of which is related to the underlying histopathologic picture. At birth, there are hypoplastic sebaceous glands and hair follicles. There may be a pebbly, yellow surface secondary to the influence of maternal hormones on the sebaceous glands. At puberty, there is epidermal acanthosis, papillomatosis, and a marked increase in size and number of sebaceous, apocrine, and eccrine glands. However, hair follicles remain hypoplastic and incompletely developed. The third stage is the development of benign or malignant tumors, usually after puberty. Tumors develop in one-third of patients. Merkel cell hyperplasia has been noted in NSJ within lesions of trichoblastoma but not basal cell carcinoma. This suggests that Merkel cells may promote the growth of follicular germ structures and trichoblastomas.

An animal model of NSJ has been developed using the nude mouse grafting model. NSJ-like lesions with typical sebaceous gland hyperplasia, abortive hair follicles, and epidermal hyperplasia can develop in the presence of dermal cells only, with no epidermal components required.

Other than the cosmetic problem, a major consideration in the management of NSJ is the development of benign or malignant tumors. Aggressive malignant neoplasms are rare, developing in only about 1% of patients, and never in prepubertal children. Complete surgical excision prevents the development of tumors. Excision can be delayed until puberty so that the child's cooperation can be elicited in the surgical procedure. All children with a NSJ in a photoexposed area should use daily sunscreen and practice sun avoidance because of the increased risk of the development of malignancy.

The malignant neoplasm most commonly seen in NSJ is basal cell carcinoma, which develops in 5–7% of cases. Some reports have found an incidence as high as 50%, but these cases may represent benign trichoblastomas. Basal cell carcinomas almost always are small and do not show an aggressive growth pattern. The most common benign neoplasm is syringocystadenoma papilliforum, which occurs in 8–19% of patients with NSJ. Other benign and malignant neoplasms that have been reported include nodular hidradenoma, apocrine cystadenoma, keratoacanthoma, infundibulinoma, syringoma, tricholemmoma, proliferating trichilemmal cyst, squamous cell carcinoma, and apocrine carcinoma.

The linear sebaceus nevus syndrome is the occurrence of a linear NSJ with central nervous system involvement, most often mental retardation and seizures, but also including benign and malignant neoplasms. The syndrome is more frequent when the NSJ is on the midface. Involvement of other organ systems, such as the eye (optic glioma, conjunctival lipodermoids, and epibulbar complex choristoma of the sclera), liver (biliary tree adenoma), and skeletal system, have been reported. The linear sebaceus nevus syndrome is a variant of the epidermal nevus syndrome, which is discussed in more detail in Case 25.

In the present patient, a shave biopsy of the new growth revealed a nodular basal cell carcinoma in an underlying NSJ. A complete excision was undertaken, with plastic surgery repair and a good cosmetic outcome.

Clinical Pearls

1. In a newborn, the presence of a nevus sebaceous of Jadassohn raises three concerns: cosmesis, nevus sebaceus (epidermal nevus) syndrome, and neoplasm development.

2. Neoplasms arising in NSJ almost always are small, nonaggressive, and easily treated surgically. Observation and planned excision of small NSJ prior to puberty is a reasonable approach.

3. Since basal cell carcinoma is the most common neoplasm in NSJ, exposure of the nevus to sunlight should be avoided.

REFERENCES

1. Schulz T, Hartschuh W: Merkel cells in nevus sebaceous: An immunohistochemical study. Am J Dermatopathol 17:570–579, 1995.
2. Snow JL, Zalla MJ, Roenig KRK, et al: Sudden nodular growth in a congenital facial lesion: Squamous cell carcinoma arising in a nevus sebaceus of Jadassohn. Arch Dermatol 1341:1069–1072, 1995.
3. Prouty SM, Lawrence L, Stenn KS: Fibroblast-dependent induction of a murine skin lesion similar to human nevus sebaceus of Jadassohn. Lab Invest 76:179–189, 1997.

PATIENT 41

A 53-year-old man with pruritic, hyperpigmented papules on his legs

A 53-year-old man noted increasing and darkening papules over his anterior legs for the past 6 months. Pruritus was severe despite attempts to resolve the condition with numerous nonprescription topical preparations. He had no known medical illnesses and was not taking medications. He was otherwise in excellent health.

Physical Examination: Skin: hyperkeratotic, hyperpigmented, and scaly papules, nodules, and plaques distributed symmetrically over anterior legs; intraoral, nail, and remainder of skin examination normal. Abdomen: no hepatomegaly. Ophthalmologic: no icterus.

Laboratory Findings: Liver function tests and hepatitis screening examination: normal. Skin biopsy: pending.

Question: What is your diagnosis?

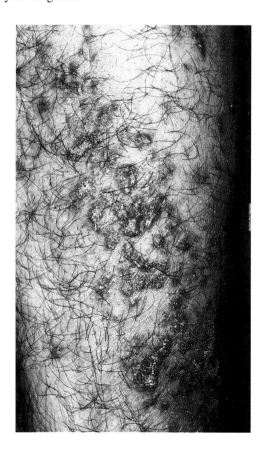

Diagnosis: Lichen planus, hypertrophic type

Discussion: Lichen planus is a chronic, papulosquamous dermatosis characterized by flat-topped, violaceous, polygonal papules with a faint lacy or shiny scale. It usually is pruritic and is located most commonly on the flexor forearms, legs, glans penis, and mouth. Worldwide incidence varies from about 0.3–1%. Mucous membranes are involved alone in 25% of patients and along with other areas in 40% of patients. Nail involvement is common and characteristically shows longitudinal ridging (onychorrhexis), roughening (trachyonychia), or pterygium formation.

Many different varieties of lichen planus have been described. Among these are vesiculobullous, hypertrophic, annular, linear, dermatomal, zosteriform, following lines of Blaschko, atrophic, lichen planus pemphigoides (bullae on normal as well as lichen planus–involved skin; not the coexistence of bullous pemphigoid and lichen planus), lichen planus/lupus erythematosus overlap, erosive or ulcerative (usually involving the feet), lichen planopilaris (follicular lichen planus of scalp which eventuates into pseudopelade of Brocq), and lichen planus actinicus (annular, on face).

Characteristic histologic findings of lichen planus include hyperkeratosis, focal hypergranulosis, acanthosis with irregular elongation and pointing of rete ridges (saw-tooth pattern), basal cell vacuolization, band-like dermal infiltrate near or obscuring the basal layer, and colloid (Civatte) bodies in the epidermis (degenerated keratinocytes). Colloid bodies are not specific to lichen planus; they also are seen in lupus erythematosus, lichen nitidus, graft-versus-host disease, lichenoid keratoses, and even normal skin. The damaged basal cells are unable to store melanin and "incontinence of pigment" occurs, with melanophages in the dermis and intense hyperpigmentation. **Wickham's striae** are the white, lacy and reticulated spots or lines seen on top of lichen planus papules. They represent focally increased thickness in the granular layer and epidermis.

The *differential diagnosis* of a patient with hypertrophic lichen planus is extensive and includes other papulosquamous diseases, such as psoriasis and tinea. Lichen simplex chronicus, granuloma annulare, lichen amyloidosis, and even Kaposi's sarcoma also should be considered. The complete differential for lesions on the anterior legs is listed in the discussion for Patient 39. Many drugs are associated with lichen planus–like eruptions, and these need to be considered. Heavy metals such as gold and photographic chemicals also can produce lichen planus–like drug eruptions. Several diseases associated with an increased incidence of lichen planus include graft-versus-host disease, autoimmune liver diseases (chronic active hepatitis and primary biliary cirrhosis), mysathenia gravis and thymoma, and ulcerative colitis. Several recent articles have supported the association between lichen planus and hepatitis C virus infection, and one study noted a strong association with erosive lichen planus.

Management of lichen planus includes antihistamines for itching and topical corticosteroids. Other treatments that have been used successfully include oral corticosteroids and psoralen plus UVA, diaminodiphenylsulfone (Dapsone), griseofulvin, topical and oral retinoids, topical cyclosporin A for intraoral lichen planus, and interferon-α-2a or 2b for generalized lichen planus that has failed other treatment. A recent study reported successful use of interferon-α-2a for chronic hepatitis C in a patient with mild hypertrophic lichen planus. Approximately two-thirds of patients with lichen planus have a spontaneous remission within 15 months. Those most likely to progress to chronic disease have the hypertrophic or lichen planopilaris varieties.

In the present patient, further history revealed that he had been consuming gold-containing liquor on a weekly basis for the past 6 months. This consumption was stopped, and he was placed on strong topical corticosteroids as well as oral antihistamines. Over the ensuing 6 months, his eruption gradually improved.

Clinical Pearls

1. Lichen planus (LP) may be triggered or aggravated by numerous substances or conditions, including medications, heavy metals, photographic chemicals, and diseases such as hepatitis C. Elimination of these factors may improve the LP.

2. Colloid or Civatte bodies representing degenerating keratinocytes are nonspecific and can be seen in LP as well as lupus erythematosus, lichen nitidus, graft-versus-host disease, lichenoid keratoses, and normal skin.

3. Approximately two-thirds of patients with LP experience spontaneous remission within 15 months. Hypertrophic LP and lichen planopilaris are the subtypes most likely to become chronic.

REFERENCES

1. Hildebrand A, Kolde G, Luger TA, et al: Successful treatment of generalized lichen planus with recombinant interferon-α-2b. J Am Acad Dermatol 33:880–883, 1995.
2. Areias J, Velho GC, Cerqueira R, et al: Lichen planus and chronic hepatitis C: Exacerbation of the lichen under interferon-α-2a therapy. Eur J. Gatroenterol Hepatol 8:825–828, 1996.
3. Ott F, Bollag W, Geiger JM: Efficacy of oral low-dose tretinoin (all-trans-retinoic acid) in lichen planus. Dermatology 102:334–336, 1996.
4. Sanchez-Perez J, De Castro M, Buezo GF, et al: Lichen planus and hepatitis C virus: Prevalence and clinical presentation of patients with lichen planus and hepatitis C virus infection. Br J Dermatol 134:715–719, 1996.
5. Schissel DJ, Elston DM: Lichen planus associated with hepatitis C. Cutis 61:90–92, 1998.

PATIENT 42

A 2½-year-old girl with face rash and muscle weakness

A 2½-year-old girl suffered an erythematous face rash following sun exposure. Her parents noted easy fatigability and muscle weakness increasing over the past 3 months.

Physical Examination: Temperature: 37.5°C. Skin: erythematous, slightly edematous patches over cheeks and eyelids; pink, scaly plaques over proximal interphalangeal, metacarpophalangeal, and distal interphalangeal joints of hands; telangiectasias visible on the upper eyelids and posterior nail folds (see figures). Musculoskeletal: proximal limb girdle weakness, with Gower's sign.

Laboratory Findings: CBC and differential: normal. Creatine phosphokinase, aspartate aminotransferase, and aldolase: mildly elevated. Skin biopsy: pending. Electromyogram (EMG): pending.

Question: What is the most likely diagnosis in this child?

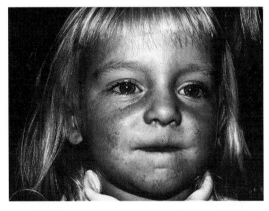

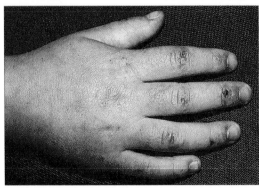

Diagnosis: Juvenile dermatomyositis

Discussion: Juvenile dermatomyositis (JDM) is characterized by symmetrical, proximal muscle weakness, skin rash of the hands and face, periorbital swelling, dysphagia, and photosensitivity. Onset is insidious in about half of affected children, and the skin rash predates other symptoms in 20%. A third of children experience a rapid onset of rash, usually after sun exposure, that is accompanied by weakness and muscle pain. Fever and easy fatigability may occur as well. The characteristic rash features erythema, sometimes in a purple-red heliotrope color, with or without edema of the eyelids. Gottron patches or papules—erythematous, scaly lesions—are located over the extensor surfaces of the skin on the joints of the hands, knees, and elbows. Capillaroscopy of the posterior nail folds often reveals capillary dilatation with loop drop-out.

Physical examination may reveal tenosynovitis of the hands and fingers, arthritis of the knees, and evidence of proximal muscle weakness in the limbs and neck as well as weakness in the pharynx or palate. Gower's sign refers to the attempts of the child to arise from the floor by pushing his hands against his shins, then knees, and then thighs to aid the weak proximal limb muscles.

The diagnosis is based on the classic distribution of the skin rash as well as proximal muscle weakness. Usually there is an increase in muscle enzymes such as creatine phosphokinase, aldolase, aspartate aminotransferase, and lactate dehydrogenase. An EMG confirms myositis with evidence of myopathy and denervation, with random fiber destruction and membrane instability. However, EMG may be painful for the child, and recent studies have suggested that muscle MRI provides ample information for diagnosis. Muscle biopsy also can be used to confirm the diagnosis but may miss areas of involvement, which can be spotty.

The *differential diagnosis* of JDM includes trichinosis, which produces myositis and eyelid changes; postviral myositis, which usually has no rash; other collagen vascular diseases; and primary myopathies, which also do not feature rash. The prognosis of JDM since the advent of oral corticosteroid use is much improved. More than 90% of children survive, and most recover after a single course of oral corticosteroids, which may need to be continued for up to 3 years. Unlike dermatomyositis in adults, JDM is not associated with malignancy. Calcinosis cutis is seen in up to 70% of patients with JDM as opposed to only about 5% in adult-onset dermatomyositis; it usually occurs later in JDM, from 6 months to 12 years after JDM onset, and may be associated with a worse prognosis. Involvement of gastrointestinal mucosa can result in ulcerations and perforations. Cardiac involvement can produce heart block or pericarditis. The retina and kidney rarely are affected. Localized lipodystrophy of connective tissue (panniculitis) occasionally is seen. Recent reports have noted partial lipodystrophy in association with JDM. A microvascular angiopathy with necrotizing vasculitis in the small blood vessels also is seen in JDM.

Treatment of JDM is primarily oral corticosteroids, which are effective in the majority of patients. Immunosuppressive agents such as azathioprine, cyclophosphamide, or methotrexate may need to be added. Hydroxychloroquine can be useful either as a steroid-sparing agent or as specific treatment for severe skin disease. High-dose, pulsed corticosteroids and cyclosporine A have produced good results. High-dose intravenous immunoglobulin has been used in children in whom all other therapies have failed and in those who experience severely adverse effects from steroids. The most common side effects from intravenous immunoglobulin are headache, nausea, and vomiting.

In the present patient, the histopathology revealed a superficial perivascular infiltrate with vacuolar changes of the basement membrane and mucin deposition in the dermis. Oral corticosteroids, sunscreen, and sun avoidance produced improvement in the face rash and muscle weakness within 4 weeks. Corticosteroid tapering was done gradually to prevent exacerbation. Over the course of 2 years, her disease remitted, and she was able to discontinue corticosteroids.

Clinical Pearls

1. Juvenile dermatomyositis is characterized by more frequent calcinosis cutis and more severe microvascular angiopathy than is adult-onset dermatomyositis.

2. Confirmation of myositis can be accomplished by measure of muscle enzymes, EMG, muscle biopsy, or MRI.

3. Children with JDM may arise from the floor by pressing their hands first against their shins, then against their knees, and then against their thighs—Gower's sign of proximal muscle weakness.

REFERENCES

1. Chung HT, Huang JL, Wang HS, et al: Dermatomyositis and polymyositis in childhood. Acta Paediatr Sin 35:407–414, 1994.
2. Sansome A, Dubowitz V: Intravenous immunoglobulin in juvenile dermatomyositis: Four-year review of nine cases. Arch Dis Child 72:25–28, 1995.
3. Vedanarayanan V, Subramony SH, Ray LI, et al: Treatment of childhood dermatomyositis with high-dose intravenous immunoglobulin. Pediatr Neurol 13:336–339, 1995.
4. Maugars YM, Berthelot JM, Abbas AA, et al: Long-term prognosis of 69 patients with dermatomyositis or polymyositis. Clin Exp Rheumatol 14:253–274, 1996.
5. Quecedo E, Febrer I, Serrano G, et al: Partial lipodystrophy associated with juvenile dermatomyositis: Report of two cases. Pediatr Dermatol 13:477–482, 1996.

PATIENT 43

A 4-year-old girl with a facial eruption

A 4-year-old African-American girl experienced a symmetrical, asymptomatic, papular eruption around the mouth and eyes. She was otherwise healthy, with no joint or eye complaints, fatigue, fever, or weight loss. The child had been prescribed a combination of high-potency corticosteroid and anti-fungal cream for chapped lips 3 months previously.

Physical Examination: Vital signs: normal. Skin: 1- to 2-mm, skin-colored papules around mouth and eyes; some hyperpigmentation around mouth (see figure); sparing of skin immediately adjacent to vermilion border. Lymph nodes: no lymphadenopathy. Joint and eye exam: normal.

Laboratory Findings: Potassium hydroxide (KOH) examination: negative for hyphal elements or Demodex mites. CBC, calcium, angiotensin converting enzyme, and liver profile: normal. Chest radiograph: normal. Ophthalmologic examination: normal. Small punch biopsy of skin: results pending.

Questions: What is the diagnosis? How would you treat this child?

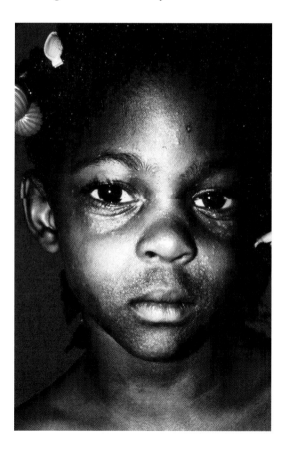

Diagnosis: Perioral dermatitis, granulomatous variant

Discussion: Perioral dermatitis (PD) is an inflammatory skin disease characterized by erythematous papules and pustules that was originally described in young women. Distribution is symmetrical around the mouth and chin, with a characteristic zone of sparing immediately adjacent to the vermilion border of the lips. The nose also is involved, specifically the nasolabial folds and the periocular area. The eyelids and glabella are involved in 20% of patients. The granulomatous form of perioral dermatitis (GPD) appears to be more frequent in children and is characterized by skin-colored papules in the same locations as just described, with characteristic findings on histopathologic examination.

Both PD and its variant GPD tend to be cyclical, and flares occur every few days to months. Most cases eventually resolve spontaneously, but this may take months to years. The only association consistent for both PD and GPD is the previous use of fluorinated corticosteroids on the face, often for a trivial dermatosis. Patients are unable to discontinue the fluorinated corticosteroid without experiencing a flare of the PD. The granulomatous variety has been reported to be more common in African-American children and clinically resembles sarcoidosis, but features less erythema, scale, and pustule formation than the nongranulomatous variety.

The *differential diagnosis* of GPD primarily includes sarcoidosis. Preschool sarcoidosis in young children involves the triad of skin lesions, uveitis, and arthritis. In older children, pulmonary symptoms also may be present; in all children, there is lymphadenopathy. Contact dermatitis can produce a similar picture, and reported causes include chewing gum, toothpaste, fingernail polish, and formaldehyde. However, contact dermatitis does not spare the area around the vermilion border. Tinea faciei and Demodex dermatitis, which can produce scaly, erythematous papules on children's faces, should be excluded with a KOH examination. Benign cephalic histiocytosis is characterized by brown-yellow to pink nodules on the face; a biopsy is diagnostic. Granulomatous acne rosacea may present with skin-colored facial papules, but is rare in children; usually flushing, telangiectasias, erythema, pustules, and cysts also are present. Granulosis rubra nasi, a familial condition seen in children, is characterized by hyperhidrosis; erythema, particularly of the nasal tip; and an absence of granulomas on biopsy. Lupus miliaris disseminatus faciei was originally described as a tuberculid, but may in fact represent granulomatous rosacea. Acne vulgaris is characterized by comedones, papules, pustules, and cysts, as well as involvement of the entire face.

Treatment can be problematic because discontinuation of fluorinated corticosteroids produces a flare. Some studies report spontaneous resolution over months to years without treatment. In children older than 8 years, oral tetracycline tapered over 2–3 months often produces clearing. In children younger than 8, metronidazole gel 0.75% b.i.d. over 2–3 months may be effective. Oral erythromycin also has produced good results in that age group. The use of a mild, nonfluorinated, topical corticosteroid ointment during treatment may help with irritation and dryness. Other topical agents that have been tried with variable success include sulfur preparations, topical erythromycin, and benzoyl peroxide. However, all three may cause irritation.

In the present patient, histopathologic examination of the skin revealed a lymphohistiocytic infiltrate with scattered multinucleated giant cells and spongiosis around hair follicles. There were numerous noncaseating granulomas, also in a perifollicular distribution. Polarization for foreign body presence was negative. Special stains for fungi and AFB were negative. The fluorinated corticosteroid preparation was immediately discontinued, and the child was begun on topical metronidazole gel and a low-potency, nonfluorinated corticosteroid ointment. She did not improve over the ensuing 4 weeks and therefore was placed on a course of oral erythromycin. Over the next 4 weeks, the eruption improved dramatically, and at the 6 month follow-up it was completely resolved.

Clinical Pearls

1. Granulomatous perioral dermatitis can mimic sarcoidosis, both clinically and histopathologically; therefore, sarcoidosis must be excluded whenever a diagnosis of GPD is made.

2. Both PD and its variant GPD are associated with previous fluorinated corticosteroid use on the face.

3. The primary treatment of perioral dermatitis is discontinuation of fluorinated corticosteroids, if present. Oral antibiotics and metronidazole gel may produce resolution.

REFERENCES

1. Frieden IJ, Prose NS, Fletcher V, et al: Granulomatous perioral dermatitis in children. Arch Dermatol 125:369–373, 1989.
2. Miller SR, Shalita AR: Topical metronidazole gel (0.75%) for the treatment of perioral dermatitis in children. J Am Acad Dermatol 31:847–848, 1994.
3. Hogan DJ: Perioral dermatitis. Curr Probl Dermatol 22:98–104, 1995.
4. Knautz MA, Lesher JL Jr: Childhood granulomatous periorificial dermatitis. Pediatr Dermatol 13:131–134, 1996.

PATIENT 44

A 2½-year-old boy with fever, erythema, and blisters

A previously healthy, 2½-year-old boy experienced fever and restlessness, followed 6 hours later by erythema with fragile blisters in the diaper area and around his mouth and nose. His parents had noticed a slight purulent drainage from one eye the day before. He was not taking medications.

Physical Examination: Temperature 38.5°C; pulse 120; respirations 42. Skin: macular erythema over neck, central face, ears, and groin, with superimposed crusted erosions and rare bullae (see figure); Nicholsky's sign positive; mucous membranes spared except for a small amount of purulent drainage in right medial palpebral fissure.

Laboratory Findings: WBC 16,000/μl with 40% bands. Gram stain of right eye drainage: groups of gram-positive cocci. Gram stain of blister fluid: sterile. Cultures from palpebral fissure drainage, nose, throat, groin, and blood: pending. Skin biopsy from perineal bulla edge: pending.

Question: What is your diagnosis?

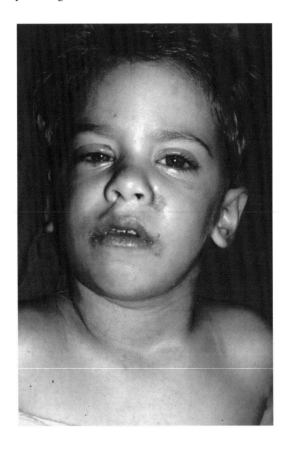

Diagnosis: Staphylococcal scalded skin syndrome

Discussion: Staphylococcal scalded skin syndrome (SSSS) is a toxin-mediated epidermolytic disease seen in neonates and children under the age of 5. It rarely is seen in adults because they have developed immunity to the organism producing the toxin and are better able to metabolize and excrete the toxin. Rare reports of SSSS in adults point to two major risk factors: immunocompromise and renal impairment. Recently, SSSS has been reported in an HIV-infected patient and in an immunocompetent adult. The mortality rate of SSSS in adults (approximately 50%) is much greater than in children (3–7%) due to underlying comorbidity.

The cause of SSSS is an exfoliative toxin, an exotoxin, that is produced by *Staphylococcal aureus* phage group II type 71 most commonly, but also by groups I and III. There are two serotypes of exotoxin, exfoliative toxin A (ETA) and exfoliative toxin B (ETB). Exfoliative toxin produces an intraepidermal separation leading to skin loosening and eventual peeling. A recent report on the x-ray crystal structure of ETA showed that it belongs to the chymotrypsin-like family of serine proteases.

Clinically, tender erythema around the lips and nose rapidly spreads to involve the upper body in infants and older children, and the entire body in neonates and immunocompromised adults. The tender, erythematous skin wrinkles and then rapidly exfoliates within 48 hours. Because the blisters are superficial, they are easily broken. Neck and axillae frequently are involved as well, but the mucosa is spared (unlike scarlet fever or Stevens-Johnson syndrome). After 48 hours, crusting, fissuring, and scaling occurs, with the characteristic "potato chip"

scale. Periorificial radial crusting and fissuring also may be seen. Fever is common.

The diagnosis is based on the clinical picture and the skin biopsy, which shows a split through the stratum granulosum. Cultures of distant sites may reveal a source of staphylococcal infection, most commonly in the nose, throat, ear, eye, wound site if present, umbilicus in neonate, vagina, and rectum. A new polymerase chain reaction test can detect ETA and ETB gene fragments in staphylococcal colonies isolated from patients with SSSS.

The *differential diagnosis* of SSSS includes scarlet fever and Kawasaki's disease, both of which feature mucosal involvement. Erythema multiforme demonstrates targetoid lesions. Toxic epidermal necrolysis is evident on skin biopsy in which full-thickness epidermal loss occurs. The differential also includes toxic shock syndrome, exfoliative erythroderma, burn, dermatitis herpetiformis, bullous pemphigoid, and sun burn.

Treatment mainly is supportive, with careful attention to fluid and electrolyte balance and prevention of infection. Penicillinase-resistant antibiotic is recommended, to decrease the incidence of sepsis and spread to other patients. Emollient creams may be used later in the course, if necessary.

In the present patient, the culture of the palpebral fissure drainage revealed *S. aureus* phage group II type 71, which produced ETA. The skin biopsy demonstrated the characteristic split through the stratum granulosum. He was treated with a penicillinase-resistant penicillin intravenously, and he recovered completely over 2 weeks with no scarring. The minor eye infection was thought to be the source of the staphylococcal infection.

Clinical Pearls

1. Staphylococcal scalded skin syndrome is common and has a low mortality rate in children under 5 years old . In adults, it is rare and severe, with a 50% mortality rate.

2. The cause of the stratum granulosum split in SSSS is one of two exotoxins, both of which appear to be proteases.

3. A new polymerase chain reaction test is sensitive and rapid in the detection of exotoxins A and B gene fragments in staphylococcal colonies isolated from patients with SSSS.

REFERENCES
1. Gemmell CG: Staphylococcal scalded skin syndrome. J Med Microbiol 43:318–327, 1995.
2. Sakurai S, Suzuki H, Machida K: Rapid identification by polymerase chain reaction of staphylococcal exfoliative toxin serotype A and B genes. Microbiol Immunol 39:379–386, 1995.
3. Farrell AM, Ross JS, Umasankar S, et al: Staphylococcal scalded skin syndrome in an HIV-1 seropositive man. Br J Dermatol 134:962–965, 1996.
4. Roeb E, Schonfelder T, Matern S, et al: Staphylococcal scalded skin syndrome in an immunocompromised adult. Eur J Clin Microbiol Infect Dis 15:499–503, 1996.
5. Vath GM, Earhart CA, Rago JV, et al: The structure of the superantigen exfoliative toxin A suggests a novel regulation as a serine protease. Biochemistry 36:1559–1566, 1997.

PATIENT 45

A 43-year-old woman with papules and plaques

A 43-year-old African-American woman noticed the appearance of skin-colored papules and plaques on her face during a 6-month period. She was otherwise in good health and was not taking medications.

Physical Examination: Skin: firm, skin-colored papules and plaques on eyelids and medial periocular skin; two reddish papules on left cheek (see figure). Lymph nodes: lymphadenopathy in anterior cervical and supraclavicular chains. Chest: normal. Abdomen: no hepatosplenomegaly. Remainder of physical examination: normal.

Laboratory Findings: CBC and serum chemistries: normal, except for elevated serum calcium. 24-hour urine: hypercalciuria. Angiotensin converting enzyme: elevated. Ophthalmologic examination including slit lamp: normal. Chest radiograph: bilateral symmetric hilar adenopathy. Skin tests for TB, candida, and mumps antigens: pending. Skin biopsy from face plaque: pending. Gallium scan: pending.

Question: What are the most likely diagnosis, prognosis, and treatment options?

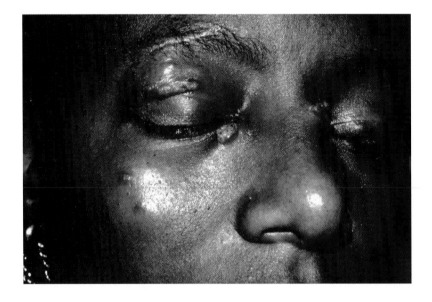

Diagnosis: Sarcoidosis

Discussion: Sarcoidosis is a multisystem disease of unknown etiology characterized by noncaseating granulomas occurring in any organ, but most often affecting the lungs, lymph nodes, skin, and eyes. It occurs most often in African-Americans, women, and individuals living in the Southeastern United States. The lungs are involved in 90% of patients, but only 30% have symptoms related to pulmonary fibrosis and adenopathy. The eyes are affected in 25–50%, frequently with conjunctival granulomas and lacrimal gland involvement. Up to 35% of patients experience skin disorder in sarcoidosis, most often at the beginning of the disease. Therefore, dermatologists frequently make the initial diagnosis.

Skin lesions in sarcoidosis have been classified as specific (those with noncaseating granulomas on biopsy) or nonspecific (those without granulomas on biopsy). The most common **specific skin lesions** are macular and papular eruptions, which are associated with acute forms of sarcoidosis and a good prognosis. Lupus pernio of Besnier affects the nose, cheeks, and ears, and has been associated with sarcoidosis of the upper respiratory tract as well as uveitis, bone cysts, and pulmonary fibrosis. Lupus pernio and the chronic plaque-like skin lesions are associated with a worse prognosis and more severe systemic involvement. Infiltrated plaques may be annular and also are associated with pulmonary fibrosis and a more severe chronic course. Other specific lesions of sarcoidosis include subcutaneous nodules and scar lesions. Rarely reported are erythrodermic infiltrated sarcoidosis lesions, usually of the lower extremities; ichthyosiform sarcoid, usually of the legs; hypopigmented macular lesions (more common in black patients); and ulcerative sarcoidosis (which appears in young women and blacks and typically involves the lower extremities).

The most common **nonspecific skin lesion** is erythema nodosum, which portends a good prognosis. Syndromes seen in sarcoidosis include: Löfgren's syndrome (uveitis, fever, and bilateral hilar adenopathy); a variant of Löfgren's syndrome (which also features inflammatory ankle swelling); Heerfordt's syndrome or uveoparotid fever (uveitis, facial nerve palsy, fever, and parotitis); and Jungling's disease or osteitis cystica tuberculisata (punched-out bone lesions seen around the nails and phalanges).

The *clinical differential diagnosis* includes granuloma annulare, histiocytoma, xanthoma, perioral dermatitis, urticaria pigmentosa, syringoma, syphilis, leprosy, and lymphoproliferative disease.

The histology of a specific skin lesion reveals noncaseating granulomas consisting of epithelioid (macrophage-derived) cells with giant cells, surrounded by a narrow zone of lymphocytes. Inclusion bodies that may be seen within the giant cells include the Schaumann body (calcium carbonate, phosphate, and iron), the asteroid body (lipoprotein), and the residual body (lipomucoprotein). The *histologic differential diagnosis* is broad and includes tuberculosis (caseating granulomas), atypical mycobacterium, deep fungal infections (histoplasmosis, cryptococcus, sporotrichosis), berylliosis, zirconiosis, tattoo dye, cutaneous leischmaniasis, tuberculoid leprosy, lymphoma, and syphilis. Therefore, it is necessary to perform special stains, cultures, and polarization.

The prognosis of sarcoidosis is good in younger patients with an acute onset. Skin findings that are associated with a worse prognosis include lupus pernio, chronic plaque-type skin lesions, and scar infiltrates. Treatment options for mild skin disease include topical and intralesional corticosteroids. The mainstay for disfiguring skin lesions or for severe systemic disease is oral corticosteroid therapy. Antimalarials can be helpful in skin disease alone. Other reported beneficial therapies include oral methotrexate, allopurinol, intralesional chloroquine, and thalidomide.

In the present patient, skin tests were negative, revealing cutaneous anergy. The skin biopsy showed noncaseating granulomas, with negative stains and cultures for acid-fast bacilli, fungus, and other organisms. Polarization revealed no foreign bodies. She was treated cautiously, with high-potency topical corticosteroids prescribed for the face plaques and close follow-up by her ophthalmologist to rule out glaucoma. The papules flattened significantly with this therapy, and she was pleased with the cosmetic result. Her pulmonary function tests, including diffusing capacity for carbon monoxide, were normal. The gallium scan showed a λ (lambda) pattern, indicating uptake in the right paratracheal and bilateral hilar modes, but no "panda face" pattern, which is produced by symmetrical lacrimal and parotid gland uptake. Her hypercalcemia and hypercalciuria were due to increased gastrointestinal absorption of calcium because of hypersensitivity to vitamin D.

Clinical Pearls

1. Specific skin lesions that correlate with a poorer prognosis in sarcoidosis include lupus pernio, plaque-type skin lesions, and scar infiltrates.

2. Inclusion bodies seen within giant cells in sarcoidosis are nonspecific: Schaumann bodies contain calcium; asteroid bodies contain collagen; and residual bodies contain lipo-mucoprotein granules.

3. Hypercalcemia in sarcoidosis is thought to be secondary to increased gastrointestinal absorption of calcium due to hypersensitivity to vitamin D. There also may be extrarenal production of 1, 25 dihydroxyvitamin D by some patients.

4. A gallium scan may provide useful information in sarcoidosis because it seems to correlate with the degree of lung parenchymal inflammation. When there is symmetrical uptake by lacrimal and parotid glands, a "panda face" image may be produced.

REFERENCES

1. Puryear DW, Fowler AA: Sarcoidosis: A clinical overview. Compr Ther 22:649–653, 1996.
2. Albertni JG, Tyler W, Miller OF: Ulcerative sarcoidosis: Case report and review of the literature. Arch Dermatol 133:215–219, 1997.
3. Fink CW, Cimaz R: Early onset sarcoidosis: Not a benign disease. J Rheumatol 24:174–177, 1997.
4. Mana J, Marcoval J, Graells J, et al: Cutaneous involvement in sarcoidosis. Arch Dermatol 133:882–888, 1997.
5. Newman LS, Rose CS, Maier LA: Sarcoidosis. N Engl J Med 335:1224–1234, 1997.

PATIENT 46

A 35-year-old woman with painful, blue papules on her hand

A 35-year-old woman noted the appearance of three blue papules on her lateral hand over a period of several months. The papules were intermittently painful, particularly with exposure to heat or cold. She had no gastrointestinal complaints, and there was no family history of similar lesions.

Physical Examination: Skin: blue, 5-mm nodule on right lateral hand at base of thumb; tender and compressible; two similar, but smaller, papules adjacent (see figure).

Laboratory Findings: CBC: normal. Stool hematest: negative for occult blood. Skin biopsy of larger nodule: pending.

Question: What is the differential diagnosis of this lesion?

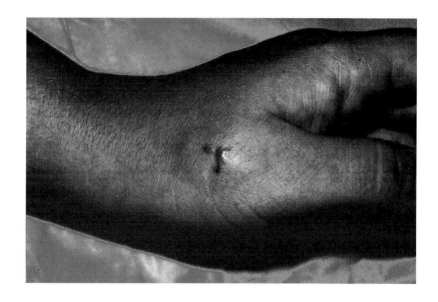

Diagnosis: Glomus tumor, multiple (glomangioma)

Discussion: Glomus tumors are benign neoplasms that arise from the glomus body and typically are solitary, but may be multiple (glomangiomas). The clinical and histopathologic characteristics of the two types differ. The solitary glomus tumor (SGT) is the most common type and is characterized by a small, blue-red papule or nodule that may be soft or firm, but usually is painful. Severe pain may occur, particularly in relation to temperature changes. These lesions usually are seen in adults and affect the extremities, most often the nail beds; however, they also can be seen on the neck, face, penis, and scrotum. Histopathologically, the SGT is circumscribed and encapsulated, with narrow vascular spaces surrounded by flattened endothelial cells. Collections of tightly packed glomus cells resemble epithelioid cells and contain clear to eosinophilic cytoplasm and large, pale nuclei.

Multiple glomus tumors (MGT) usually are asymptomatic, occasionally are painful, and typically are found in children. They may be localized but more commonly are widespread, and may be inherited in an autosomal dominant manner. A large GT may resemble a blue rubber bleb nevus. Rarely, a patient with generalized MGT shows Kasabach-Merritt syndrome (consumption coagulopathy). Histologically, these tumors are not encapsulated, and there are more, larger, and irregularly shaped vascular spaces. The vascular spaces are lined by a single layer of flattened endothelial cells as are the spaces in SGT, but in MGT there are few glomus cells.

The pathogenesis of both SGT and MGT is the same. The tumors arise from the Sucquet-Hoyer canal, which is the arterial segment of the cutaneous glomus body. The glomus body is an encapsulated structure that contains up to four direct connections between arterial and venous structures, thus permitting bypass of congested capillary beds. It is involved in temperature regulation, and when the shunts are open, blood flow into the area increases markedly. Glomus bodies are numerous in the palms and soles, especially around the fingernail beds and pads. They also are found in the skin of the ears and central face. Electron microscopy has shown that glomus cells are vascular smooth muscle cells in the Sucquet-Hoyer canal as well as in SGT amd MGT. In the glomus body, however, they are elongated; in the tumors, they are polyhedral. Glomus tumor cells react with desmin on immunostaining, which is consistent with a smooth muscle origin.

The *differential diagnosis* of SGT includes hemangiopericytoma (painless), eccrine spiradenoma, leiomyoma, malignant melanoma, blue nevus, and neurofibroma. The differential diagnosis of MGT includes blue rubber bleb nevus, cavernous hemangiomas, leiomyomas, venous malformations, lymphoma, leukemia cutis, angiosarcoma, Kaposi's sarcoma, metastatic carcinoma, dermatofibrosarcoma protuberans, and pseudolymphoma. Painful nodules on the skin include blue rubber bleb nevus, eccrine spiradenoma, neuroma, neurilemmoma, glomus tumor, angiolipoma, and leiomyoma (last two may be agminated or grouped).

Since glomus tumors are benign, simple excision is curative. Some clinicians have withheld excision when the lesion was asymptomatic; however, a biopsy should be performed if hemangiopericytoma or another lesion with malignant potential is in the differential diagnosis. In one report, the tunable, pulsed-dye laser was used for treatment of the superficial dermal component of MGT. Sclerotherapy also has been used.

In the present patient, the biopsy revealed the characteristic findings of MGT. Since she was asymptomatic, a simple excision was performed, with good cosmetic results.

Clinical Pearls

1. Glomus tumors are derived from smooth muscle cells of the Sucquet-Hoyer canal, the arterial segment of the arteriovenous shunts making up the glomus body.

2. The solitary glomus tumor may resemble a hemangiopericytoma, which has the potential to metastasize. A biopsy is required to differentiate the two lesions.

3. Multiple glomus tumors may resemble blue rubber bleb nevi and may produce (rarely) the Kasabach-Merritt syndrome (consumption coagulopathy) when generalized.

REFERENCES

1. Keefer CJ, Brantley B, De Lozier JB: Familial infiltrative glomangiomas: Diagnosis and treatment. J Craniofac Surg 7:145–147, 1996.
2. Miyano JA, Fitzgibbons TC: Glomangioma of the ankle simulating injury to the flexor hallucis longus: A case report. Foot Ankle Int 17:768–770, 1996.
3. Waguespack RL, Fair KP, Svetec DA, et al: Glomangioma of the penile and scrotal median raphe. J Urol 156:179, 1996.
4. Baselga E, Drolet BA, Fleming MS, et al: Multiple acquired vascular nodules. Pediatr Dermatol 14:327–329, 1997.

PATIENT 47

A 59-year-old liver transplant patient with enlarging, keratotic thigh lesions

A 59-year-old man underwent a cadaveric liver transplant 3 years previously to treat liver failure induced by hepatitis B virus. During the past 6 months, he noticed slowly enlarging, scaly, pruritic papules and plaques on his thighs. There was no family history of similar lesions. Medications included prednisone, azathioprine, and cyclosporin A.

Physical Examination: General: cushingoid appearance. Skin: acneiform eruption on face, upper chest, and upper back; several well-healed scars on abdomen; five brown, hyperkeratotic plaques measuring 4–14 mm scattered on anterior and posterior thighs, each with a raised border and central furrow (see figure). Lymph nodes: no adenopathy.

Laboratory Findings: CBC and screening chemistries: normal. HIV examination: negative. Skin biopsy from raised border of largest lesion: pending.

Question: What is your diagnosis?

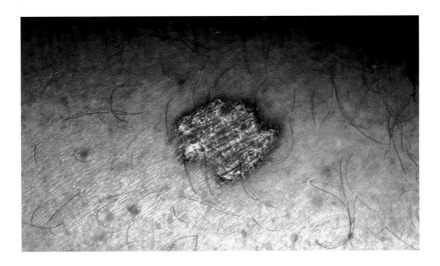

Diagnosis: Porokeratosis of Mibelli in an immunosuppressed patient

Discussion: Porokeratosis (PK) is a disorder of cornification characterized by a cornoid lamella. There are five types of PK, the first three of which can be inherited in an autosomal dominant fashion. Disseminated superficial actinic PK is the most common type, occurring on sun-exposed areas of women. Porokeratosis of Mibelli (PKM) usually arises in childhood, but may occur at any age. It most commonly is located on the extremities, but also can involve the face, trunk, or genitalia. PK palmaris plantaris et disseminata begins on the palms and soles and spreads to other areas. Linear PK can resemble linear verrucous nevus, linear psoriasis, linear lichen planus, or lichen striatus. Punctate PK involves only the palms and soles, with tiny lesions that resemble arsenical keratoses or punctate keratoderma. These five types do not appear to be genetically distinct, as several may occur together in one family.

The characteristic histologic finding in all types of PK is the **cornoid lamella**, a parakeratotic column within the keratin-filled furrow at the periphery of the hyperkeratotic plaque. Abnormal keratinocytes with pycnotic nuclei and perinuclear edema are located at the base of this parakeratotic column. Pathogenesis is related to proliferation of this abnormal clone of keratinocytes. The epidermis overlying the abnormal clone may be atrophic, normal, or (rarely) acanthotic.

Immunosuppression may exacerbate or initiate PK. Cancer chemotherapy, HIV infection, organ or bone marrow transplant, and certain drugs (e.g., high-dose corticosteroids) have been associated with the development or exacerbation of PK. In a single report, however, PK associated with liver failure improved after liver transplant despite immunosuppressive therapy. Trauma occasionally initiates the development of PK.

Because squamous cell carcinoma, Bowen's disease, and basal cell carcinoma have been reported in PK lesions, treatment and close follow-up are necessary. Malignant potential is evidenced by DNA polyploidy in 25% of PK lesions; an increased proportion of cells in PK lesions in S and G2/M phases; and p53 immunoperoxidase staining of lesional keratinocytes, normally not seen, which suggests mutant p53 in PKM as is known to occur in other keratinocyte neoplasms. (Normal, wild-type p53 is not detectable on this stain.)

Since the cornoid lamella is not specific, the histopathologic differential includes other entities, such as verruca vulgaris and actinic keratosis. The clinical differential of an annular plaque of PKM can include elastosis perforans serpiginosa, perforating granuloma annulare, annular elastolytic granuloma, annular tertiary syphilis, and lupus erythematosus.

Treatment options include topical 5-fluorouracil, topical retinoids, cryosurgery, surgical excision, electrosurgery, dermabrasion, and CO_2 laser ablation.

In the present patient, PKM was confirmed by the presence of a cornoid lamella on skin biopsy. Cryotherapy was attempted on two occasions with liquid nitrogen, but the lesions recurred rapidly. Topical 5-fluorouracil cream and tretinoin gel for 6 weeks resulted in complete resolution of all lesions but residual postinflammatory hyperpigmentation. He is being followed closely, since his immunosuppression will be life long.

Clinical Pearls

1. The characteristic histopathologic finding of the cornoid lamella in porokeratosis supports the diagnosis of PK, but may be seen in other clinical entities.

2. PK has been initiated or exacerbated by immunosuppression, including HIV infection, drugs, cancer, chemotherapy, or bone marrow transplantation.

3. The lesions of PK are premalignant and require treatment and close follow-up.

4. There are many treatment options for PK, none of which is superior. Topical 5-fluorouracil and tretinoin gel may be effective in combination.

REFERENCES

1. Dippel E, Haas N, Czarnetzki BM: Porokeratosis of Mibelli associated with active chronic hepatitis and vitiligo. Acta Derm Venereol 74:463–464, 1994.
2. Magee JW, McCalmont TH, Le Boit PE: Overexpression of p53 tumor suppressor protein in porokeratosis. Arch Dermatol 130:187–190, 1994.
3. McCullough TL, Lescher JL Jr: Porokeratosis of Mibelli: Rapid recurrence of a large lesion after carbon dioxide laser treatment. Pediatr Dermatol 11:267–270, 1994.
4. Rodriguez EA, Jakubowicz S, Chinchilla DA, et al: Porokeratosis of Mibelli and HIV-infection. Int J Dermatol 35:402–404, 1996.
5. Tangoren IA, Weinberg JM, Ioffreda M, et al: Penile porokeratosis of Mibelli. J Am Acad Dermatol 36:479–481, 1997.

PATIENT 48

A 59-year-old man with enlarging nodules on his finger and forearm

A 59-year-old man underwent a cadaveric renal transplant 7 months before sustaining a splinter in the right middle finger. Two weeks later, he noted a painless papule, which slowly enlarged. Four months later, he noted several subcutaneous nodules in the right dorsal forearm. He denied fever, chills, and weight loss. Medications included FK 506 (tacrolimus), azathioprine, and prednisone.

Physical Examination: Vital signs: normal. Skin: 1.7 × 1.5 cm, verrucous, crusted nodule with surrounding hyperpigmentation on right middle finger (see figure); several 0.5- to 1.5-cm, subcutaneous nodules on dorsum of right forearm. Lymph nodes: no lymphadenopathy. Abdomen: no hepatosplenomegaly.

Laboratory Findings: KOH examination: negative. Skin biopsy from finger papule, with half of tissue sent for cultures: pending.

Question: What is the differential diagnosis of this clinical presentation?

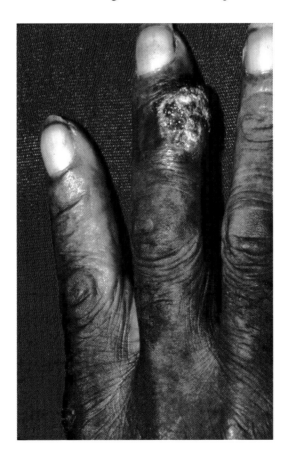

Diagnosis: Phaeohyphomycosis, subcutaneous type

Discussion: Phaeohyphomycosis (PHM) is an infection caused by a dematiaceous (brown or black) fungus that features yeast-like cells, hyphae, pseudohyphae, or a mixture of the three. The term was coined by Ajello and associates in 1974. PHM is classified into four types: (1) superficial PHM includes tinea nigra and black piedra, involves non-viable epithelium, and shows no tissue response; (2) cutaneous and corneal PHM involves keratinized tissues and often shows extensive tissue damage; (3) subcutaneous PHM often is due to traumatic implantation with deep inflammation, which may evolve into microabscesses or cysts (phaeohyphomycotic cysts); (4) systemic PHM disseminates from the lungs and is rare.

Dematiaceous fungi grow in soil, rotten wood (such as old saunas), and decaying vegetation. In addition to PHM, dematiaceous fungi also cause mycetomas (draining sinuses and granulomas) and chromoblastomycosis (verrucous nodules containing muriform or cross-walled cells, which also are known as sclerotic bodies, Medlar bodies, or copper pennies). Dematiaceous fungi are slow-growing and may not be found on culture even when they are seen in tissue.

Subcutaneous PHM begins as a painless papule or nodule at the site of inoculation of the fungus. It slowly enlarges and may undergo central focal necrosis, producing microabscesses with eventual coalescence into a unilocular, fluctuant abscess. If this becomes walled off in the tissues, it is termed a phaeohyphomycotic cyst. Subcutaneous PHM characteristically does not cause lymphadenopathy.

The most common organism producing subcutaneous PHM is *Exophiala jeanselmei*. Patients often are immunosuppressed—either transplant patients on immunosuppressive drugs or patients with AIDS.

Rarely, *E. jeanselmei* causes chromoblastomycosis. Other organisms producing subcutaneous PHM include *Bipolaris spicifera, Exserohilum rostratum, Phielofora rechartsiae, Phielofora verrucosa*, and *Wangiela dermatitidis*.

Because the dematiaceous fungi are brown or black, they may be seen in routine histopathologic sections. They also may be seen on KOH examination. Special stains such as Gomori methenamine-silver nitrate or Fontana-Masson make identification easier. The skin biopsy in the present patient revealed a granulomatous dermatitis with a mixed inflammatory infiltrate, including numerous neutrophils. Microabscesses surrounded the granulomas, and giant cells were present. Pigmented hyphae were seen within the microabscesses and the giant cells.

The *differential diagnosis* of a sporotrichoid presentation such as this includes sporotrichosis, *Mycobacterium marinum*, sporotrichoid pyoderma (e.g., Staphylococcal infection), carcinoma with metastases, other deep fungal infections, nocardiosis, cat scratch fever, primary syphilis, and primary inoculation *M. tuberculosis*.

Treatment of subcutaneous PHM includes surgical drainage or excision if a cyst is present. Intravenous amphotericin B often is required. Combined surgical and antifungal therapy usually is optimal. Other reported therapies include oral ketoconazole, intralesional miconazole, and systemic 5-fluorocytosine. Itraconazole has been used recently with success and may be the best therapeutic option. It is fungistatic and inhibits ergosterol synthesis.

In the present patient, the tissue cultures grew *E. jeanselmei* after 4 weeks. He was treated with IV amphotericin B and 5-fluorocytosine, followed by oral itraconazole for 11 months, with gradual resolution of the lesions.

Clinical Pearls

1. Subcutaneous phaeohyphomycosis is caused by dematiaceous (brown or black) fungi, which may be seen on KOH examination and routine histopathologic sections without special stains.

2. Dematiaceous fungi are saprophytes found in soil, rotten wood, and decaying vegetation.

3. Subcutaneous PHM can produce a sporotrichoid pattern, but does not characteristically produce lymphadenopathy.

REFERENCES

1. Kawachi Y, Tateishi T, Shojima K, et al: Subcutaneous pheomycotic cyst of the finger caused by *Exophiala jeanselmei*: Association with a wooden splinter. Cutis 56:41–43, 1995.
2. Kinkead S, Jancic V, Stasko T, et al: Chromoblastomycosis in a patient with a cardiac transplant. Cutis 58:367–370, 1996.
3. McCown HF, Sahn EE: Subcutaneous phaeohyphomycosis and nocardiosis in a kidney transplant patient. J Am Acad Dermatol 36:863–866, 1997.

PATIENT 49

A 32-year-old woman with multiple, enlarging skin plaques

A 32-year-old woman suffered a flu-like illness with fever, myalgias, and cough 6 weeks after visiting her sister in Ohio. Two months later, she noted several erythematous papules on her back; these had been slowly enlarging. She otherwise was well and was taking no medications.

Physical Examination: Vital signs: normal. Skin: four oval-shaped, verrucous plaques with raised edges; small pustules on the heaped-up edges (see figures). Lymph nodes: no lymphadenopathy. Abdomen: no hepatosplenomegaly. Oral examination: normal.

Laboratory Findings: CBC and serum chemistries: normal. KOH examination of pustule: thick-walled yeast with broad-based budding. Chest radiograph: normal. Skin biopsy and tissue cultures from raised border of plaque: pending.

Questions: What is the most likely diagnosis? How would you manage this patient?

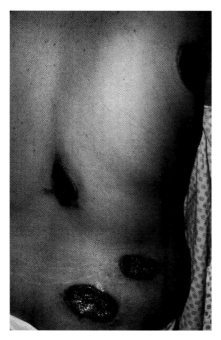
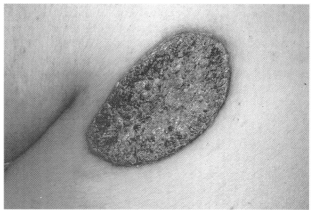

Diagnosis: Blastomycosis (North American)

Discussion: Blastomycosis is a fungal infection caused by *Blastomyces dermatitides*, which is a dimorphic fungus. Other dimorphic fungi include *Coccidioides immitis, Histoplasm capsulatum*, and *Paracoccidioides brasiliensis* (South American blastomycosis). North American blastomycosis is a primary pulmonary mycosis that begins with inhalation of the conidia. Most cases are asymptomatic. Occasionally, there is a flu-like illness with spontaneous recovery; less commonly, more severe disease results. The organism is found in moist, acidic soil, and outbreaks typically are sporadic, although clusters have occurred. It is frequent in dogs. The organism is endemic to the Ohio and Mississippi River valleys in the United States (same endemic areas as for histoplasmosis), and states with endemic areas include Ohio, Wisconsin, Minnesota, Illinois, Kentucky, North Carolina, Arkansas, and Texas. Endemic areas are present in India and Africa, as well.

There are three clinical forms of *Blastomyces dermatitides*. **Primary cutaneous** inoculation is rare and occurs as a laboratory or autopsy accident. No treatment is necessary, as healing is spontaneous. The second type is **pulmonary blastomycosis**, which often is asymptomatic, or resolves spontaneously. Chronic disease may develop, with cavity formation mimicking lung cancer or tuberculosis. The third form is **systemic blastomycosis**, in which spread occurs from the primary pulmonary infection, most commonly disseminating to skin, bone, prostate, or central nervous system. Systemic blastomycosis involves the skin in approximately 70% of patients and features either solitary or multiple verrucous plaques with heaped-up edges containing micropustules. A less common presentation is the ulcerative form. Both types begin as small pustules or papules that slowly enlarge. A subtype of systemic blastomycosis is benign cutaneous blastomycosis, in which there are one or two lesions, generally on the face, and no systemic symptoms.

The *differential diagnosis* of verrucous plaques, such as those seen in this patient, include other types of deep mycoses, particularly chromoblastomycosis and cryptococcosis. Also in the differential are: tuberculosis verrucosa cutis, verrucous carcinoma, halogenoderma, Majocchi's granuloma, hypertrophic discoid lupus erythematosus, pemphigus vegetans, lymphoma, and pyostomatitis vegetans. Blastomycosis-like pyoderma (pyoderma vegetans) is rare and occurs in settings of immunocompromise such as alcoholism, leukemia, chronic prednisone use, radiation therapy, and AIDS. It represents an unusual and exaggerated vegetating reaction to a primary or secondary bacterial infection. Criteria include: (1) large, verrucous plaque with pustules on an elevated border, (2) pseudoepitheliomatous hyperplasia, (3) tissue biopsy growing at least one pathogenic bacteria, (4) negative culture for deep fungi, atypical mycobacteria, and mycobacterium tuberculosis, (5) negative fungal serology test, and (6) normal bromide and iodide levels in the blood.

Pulmonary blastomycosis may not require therapy because it often is self-limited. Primary inoculation cutaneous blastomycosis likewise usually resolves spontaneously. Amphotericin B has been the mainstay of therapy and is still recommended for life-threatening or prolonged illness and certain extrapulmonary manifestations, such as central nervous system involvement. Otherwise, itraconazole is now the treatment of choice, but treatment must continue for at least 6 months. Fluconazole and ketaconazole also have been used successfully. Recurrences are frequent; therefore, follow-up should continue for years.

In the present patient, histologic examination of the skin biopsy revealed a suppurative and granulomatous dermatitis with pseudocarcinomatous hyperplasia of the epidermis. There were intraepidermal abscesses and a mixed infiltrate with neutrophils and multinucleated giant cells in the dermis. On the routine hematoxylin and eosin stain, clear spaces representing spores were seen. On a periodic acid-Schiff stain, single and budding spores were noted within giant cells. These spores were thick-walled, and the attachment of the bud to the spore was broad-based. The tissue culture showed no growth for 3 months, at which time *Blastomyces dermatitides* was identified. Itraconazole was prescribed for her systemic blastomycosis, with gradual resolution of the lesions over 3 months. Hyperpigmentation and cribriform scar formation remained after healing.

Clinical Pearls

1. Benign cutaneous blastomycosis is a type of systemic blastomycosis that is acquired via inhalation of the conidia into the lungs and dissemination from the pulmonary infection.

2. *Blastomyces dermatitides* spores may be seen on KOH exam and routine histopathologic examination. However, they are more evident with periodic-acid Schiff or Gomori's silver stain.

3. When treatment of mild blastomycosis is necessary, itraconazole is the treatment of choice. In severe or life-threatening disease, amphotericin B should be used.

REFERENCES

1. Body BA: Cutaneous manifestations of systemic mycoses. Dermatol Clin 14:125–135, 1996.
2. Bradsher RW: Histoplasmosis and blastomycosis. Clin Infect Dis 22 Suppl 2:102–111, 1996.
3. Shah B, Smith SP, Siegle RJ: North American blastomycosis: The importance of a differential diagnosis. Cutis 58:402–404, 1996.
4. Weil M, Mercurio MG, Brodell RT, et al: Cutaneous lesions provide a clue to mysterious pulmonary process: Pulmonary and cutaneous North American blastomycosis infection. Arch Dermatol 132:822, 824–825, 1996.
5. Minamoto GY, Rosenberg AS: Fungal infections in patients with acquired immunodeficiency syndrome. Med Clin North Am 81:381–409, 1997.

PATIENT 50

A 6-year-old girl with easy bruising and hyperextensible skin

A 6-year-old girl had bruised easily since birth. Pregnancy had been full-term and uneventful. When she began school, her parents were accused of child abuse and were threatened with loss of custody. The child had hyperextensible skin and poor wound healing with abnormal scar formation. There was no family history of similar skin findings. The child was otherwise in good health.

Physical Examination: Vital signs: normal. Skin: soft and velvety, with hyperextensibility of all areas including cheeks and ears (see figures); multiple ecchymoses on buttocks, thighs, and legs; multiple atrophic, wide scars on knees and elbows. Joints: hypermobility of finger joints. Cardiac: no murmurs. Remainder of physical examination: normal.

Laboratory Findings: CBC, platelet count, PT, PTT: normal.

Questions: What is your diagnosis? How would you manage this child?

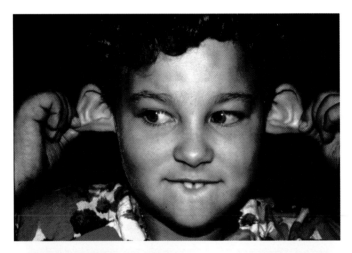

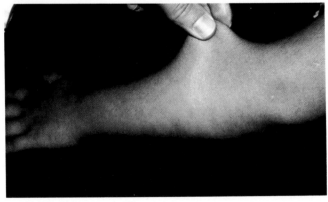

Diagnosis: Ehlers-Danlos syndrome

Discussion: Ehlers-Danlos syndrome (EDS) is a heterogeneous collection of collagen disorders characterized by skin hyperextensibility (with normal recoil), skin fragility, easy bruising, and joint hypermobility. At least 11 subgroups have been characterized, with inheritance patterns including autosomal dominant, autosomal recessive, and X-linked.

Another clinical finding in EDS is abnormal wound healing, such as the formation of "papyraceous" scars (thin, atrophic, cigarette paper–like scars) and bulging, patulous scars called molluscoid pseudotumors (caused by calcification and fibrosis of subcutaneous hematomas). Increased bruising and bleeding is thought to be due to defective blood vessels and skin structures. The extensive bruising frequently leads to suspicion of child abuse. Fifty percent of patients have mitral valve prolapse, and Gorlin's sign—hyperextension of the tongue so that it can touch the tip of the nose—usually is present. Joint laxity can produce frequent dislocations requiring orthopedic intervention. Prematurity frequently is seen in type I or gravis EDS, but is not seen in type II (mitis). This is a major differentiating point.

The pathogenesis of EDS involves mutations in genes for collagen, enzymes affecting collagen, or proteins affecting extracellular matrix. The molecular defect is unknown in EDS types I, II, III, V, and VIII. Type IV shows a decrease in type III collagen. Type VI has decreased lysyl-hydroxylase activity. Type VII features a defective conversion of procollagen to collagen, and in one recent study of this type, mutations in the COL3A1 gene led to abnormally distributed and very small collagen fibrils. Although the molecular defects are unknown for EDS types I, II and III (which together are responsible for at least 90% of EDS cases), new studies have implicated collagen V. A recent report found that mutations in the COL5A1 gene can produce both the EDS I and the EDS II phenotypes. The authors suggested that these two clinical presentations may be allelic disorders.

The *differential diagnosis* of EDS includes cutis laxa and Marfan's syndrome. However, the hyperelastic skin in cutis laxa does not normally recoil back into position after being stretched. Moreover, while joint hypermobility is a characteristic of Marfan's syndrome, skeletal abnormalities and ectopic lenses also are present.

For most patients with EDS, life expectancy is normal. However in type IV, early death may be caused by a catastrophic cardiovascular, gastrointestinal, or pregnancy-related event. Other complications that may be seen in EDS include pneumothorax, congenital hip dislocation, scoliosis, varicose veins, inguinal hernia, diverticula, retinal detachment, and other severe eye problems (type VI).

Treatment of type IV EDS involves prompt recognition and management of potential catastrophic events. Echocardiography or computed tomography (CT) with contrast should be used to monitor for dilatation of the great vessels, and invasive vascular procedures should be strictly avoided. Nonoperative management of these vascular complications is suggested, if possible. Otherwise, simple ligation is better than attempted reconstruction. In the management of the GI complications of perforation and/or massive hemorrhage, total abdominal colectomy with ileostomy is better than primary repair or resection with diversion to prevent reperforation or anastomotic leak. During pregnancy, EDS type IV patients are at risk for premature rupture of membranes and uterine rupture. One patient treated with terbutaline for preterm labor experienced coronary artery dissection and died. Therefore, this type of medication should be avoided in the treatment of preterm labor in EDS. In all types of EDS, sun avoidance is important because the thin skin is extremely susceptible to actinic damage.

All of a patient's first-degree relatives should be examined. Treatment of joint disease with orthopedic and rheumatologic consultation often is necessary. Prevention of trauma and wounds is key in the child, and soccer shin guards have been particularly helpful in avoiding wounds to these areas. Wound may heal better with pressure bandages and judicious placement of adhesive tape. Suturing may need to be done more often, and with strict infection avoidance. Ascorbic acid improves wound healing in type VI EDS, and some physicians advocate its use in all types. Prenatal diagnosis is possible in types IV and VI. Periodontal disease is seen in type VIII; therefore, early referral to a pediatric dentist is recommended.

In the present patient, education on the disease and trauma prevention as well as daily use of soccer shin guards resulted in a marked decrease in the bruising and trauma to the lower extremities. Education of school officials resulted in dismissal of the child abuse charges. She was prescribed ascorbic acid daily. A pediatric gastroenterologist found no evidence of gastrointestinal disease and is following the child yearly.

Clinical Pearls

1. Ehlers-Danlos syndrome types I and II are responsible for 80% of cases. Prematurity occurs only in type I, and this may be a helpful way to distinguish the two types.

2. Patients with EDS type IV are at risk for dilatation and rupture of the great vessels, and careful monitoring with echocardiography or CT scans should be performed instead of invasive vascular procedures.

3. Simple ways to lessen trauma and improve wound healing in all patients with EDS include the use of soccer shin guards and an ascorbic acid oral supplement.

REFERENCES

1. Burrows NP, Nicholls AC, Yates JR, et al: The gene encoding collagen alpha 1(V)(COL5A1) is linked to mixed Ehlers-Danlos syndrome type I/II. J Invest Dermatol 106:1273–1276, 1996.
2. Freeman RK, Swegle J, Sise MJ: The surgical complications of Ehlers-Danlos syndrome. Am Surg 62:869–873, 1996.
3. Solomon JA, Abrams L, Lichtenstein GR: GI manifestations of Ehlers-Danlos syndrome. Am J Gastroenterol 91:2282–2288, 1996.
4. De Paepe A, Nuytinck L, Hausser I, et al: Mutations in the COL5A1 gene are causal in the Ehlers-Danlos syndromes I and II. Am J Hum Genet 60:547–554, 1997.
5. Smith LT, Schwarze U, Goldstein J, et al: Mutations in the COL3A1 gene result in the Ehlers-Danlos syndrome type IV and alterations in the size and distribution of the major collagen fibrils of the dermis. J Invest Dermatol 108:241–247, 1997.

PATIENT 51

A 6-year-old boy with nail dystrophy and white plaques on his tongue

A 6-year-old boy was noted to have nail changes consisting of yellowish discoloration at the age of 6 months. Over the next 6 years, the nails gradually thickened and darkened, with changes most pronounced distally. At the age of 4 years, white plaques developed on the lateral tongue; these did not respond to topical antifungal therapy. His mother and two siblings had similar nail changes.

Physical Examination: General: healthy; normal developmental milestones. Mouth: white plaques along lateral tongue (see figure, *top*). Nails: brown discoloration and distal thickening with subungual debris (see figure, *bottom*). Skin: hyperkeratotic plaques on pressure points of soles. Remainder of physical examination: normal.

Laboratory Findings: Potassium hydroxide (KOH) examination of tongue plaques: negative for hyphal elements. Fungal culture of nails: no growth.

Questions: What is the diagnosis? How would you manage the patient?

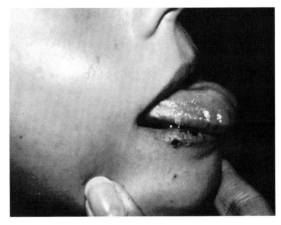

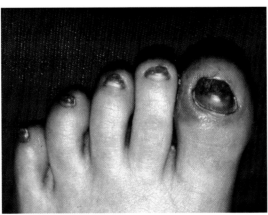

Diagnosis: Pachyonychia congenita

Discussion: Pachyonychia congenita (PC) is a rare disorder of keratinization characterized by thickened nails, oral leukokeratosis, palmoplantar keratoderma, and follicular keratoses. It has been classified into four types: type I is as listed above; type II includes type I plus palmoplantar bullae, natal teeth, and steatocystoma multiplex; type III includes type II plus angular cheilosis and eye changes; type IV includes type III plus laryngeal and hair abnormalities and mental retardation. PC usually is autosomal dominant, with the gene mapped to the keratin cluster on 17q. Specific mutations in the genes for keratins 6, 16, and 17 have been identified.

Nail changes may be present at birth, usually as yellow-brown distal discoloration, or may develop within the first year. All 20 nails gradually thicken due to production of keratotic material under the distal nail. This forces the nail plate to grow upward and outward with an increased transverse curvature, occasionally resulting in a painful tubular or pincer nail. Paronychial infections with candida and staphylococcus as well as shedding of the nail plate may occur.

Oral leukokeratosis may be present at birth or may appear in childhood. Since it resembles candidiasis and often is superinfected with candida, frequent KOH examinations are warranted. Unlike the oral white plaques seen in dyskeratosis congenita, those associated with PC are not premalignant.

Plantar hyperkeratosis may be associated with bullae and may produce pain on walking. Hyperhidrosis and bromhidrosis may accompany plantar hyperkeratosis, adding to the patient's discomfort.

The *differential diagnosis* of PC includes dyskeratosis congenita, onychomycosis, epidermolysis bullosa of certain types, other palmoplantar keratodermas, and occasionally, psoriasis.

Histopathologic examination of the nail unit has shown that the nail plate itself is normal. The nail bed, however, is at least three times thicker than normal, with hard, keratinous debris present. It is this keratinous mass that forces the nail plate upward and outward.

Complications of PC primarily are the nail discomfort and loss of function. Pain and infections in the hyperkeratotic feet are frequent complaints. Eye changes can include opacities and even blindness, although rarely. Squamous cell carcinoma can occur at sites of chronic bulla formation or ulceration.

The management of PC involves periodic grinding or paring of the nails. Surgical excision of the entire nail matrix and bed with matrix ablation can produce a cosmetically and functionally satisfactory result. Treatment of the palmoplantar keratoderma involves lubricants, emollients, and keratolytics. Protective footwear also may be helpful. There are scattered case reports of the successful use of oral retinoids.

In the present patient, no other findings of PC were noted, and his disorder was classified as PC type I. The nails were trimmed, and the surface was ground down with a podiatrist's grinding tool. Other family members also were diagnosed with PC and entered into treatment programs. The patient will be closely followed for the development of oral and eye changes and bullae.

Clinical Pearls

1. Pachyonychia congenita typically is confused with another genodermatosis, dyskeratosis congenita. However, the oral white plaques in PC are not premalignant.

2. The anatomic abnormality in PC is located in the nail bed and can result in painful, tubular nails.

3. Periodic superficial grinding of the nail plates can produce a satisfactory cosmetic and functional outcome.

REFERENCES

1. Corden LD, McLean WH: Human keratin diseases: Hereditary fragility of specific epithelial tissues. Exp Dermatol 5:297–307, 1996.
2. Korge PB, Krieg T: The molecular basis for inherited bullous diseases. J Mol Med 74:59–70, 1996.
3. Mouaci-Midoun N, Cambiaghi S, Abimelec P: Pachyonychia congenita tarda. J Am Acad Dermatol 35:334–335, 1996.
4. Smith FJ, Corden LD, Rugg EL, et al; Missense mutations in keratin 17 cause either pachyonychia congenita type 2 or a phenotype resembling steatocystoma multiplex. J Invest Dermatol 108:220–223, 1997.
5. Sahn EE: Pachyonychia congenita. Clin Dermatol 1(unit 1–33):1–8, 1998.

PATIENT 52

A 10-year-old boy with neck hyperpigmentation and nail dystrophy

A 10-year-old boy was brought in by his parents because of increasing hyperpigmentation which began on his neck and spread to his shoulders and trunk. Scrubbing the area had no effect. On questioning, it was revealed that his nails had been fragile since early childhood. There was no family history of skin or nail abnormalities. He was having trouble keeping up with his schoolwork in the fourth grade.

Physical Examination: Skin: gray-brown, reticulated hyperpigmentation on lateral neck; similar patches on lateral trunk, anterior chest, and upper arms, with hypopigmented macules and scattered telangiectasias (see figure, *top*). Nails: thin and fragile, with longitudinal ridging (see figure, *bottom*). Mouth: white plaques on buccal mucosa bilaterally; periodontal disease and carious teeth.

Laboratory Findings: CBC: normal.

Questions: What is your diagnosis? What are the potential complications?

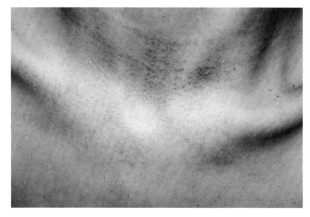

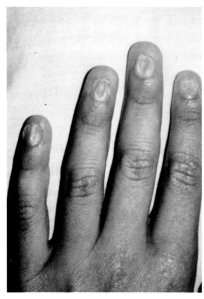

Diagnosis: Dyskeratosis congenita

Discussion: Dyskeratosis congenita (DC) is a rare, X-linked, recessive genodermatosis, characterized by the triad of reticulated hyperpigmentation with hypopigmentation, nail dystrophy, and mucous membrane leukoplakia. The gene locus has been mapped to chromosome Xq28. DC also may be inherited as an autosomal dominant or an autosomal recessive disease, so that girls occasionally are affected.

Clinically, the skin hyperpigmentation almost always begins prior to puberty and is characterized by gray-brown, lacy patches beginning on the upper trunk, neck, shoulders, and thighs. Teachers or parents may at first notice a "dirty neck." Within this hyperpigmentation are hypopigmented macules, telangiectasias, and some atrophy (poikiloderma). Atrophy also occurs over the skin of the hands and feet, producing a characteristic smooth, shiny appearance to the palms and soles, often with a loss of dermatoglyphics. These skin changes may resemble poikiloderma atrophicans vasculare, erythema ab igne, or chronic graft-versus-host disease (GVHD). Additional skin findings include palmoplantar hyperkeratosis, hyperhidrosis, and bullae, which are similar to findings seen in pachyonychia congenita (PC).

The nail changes of DC begin between 6 and 8 years of age and consist of atrophy, onychorrhexis, pterygia, fissuring, pitting, and fragility. Leukoplakia is most commonly seen on the oral mucous membranes, but also can be found on the glans penis, anus, urethra, vagina, and conjunctiva. Unlike the leukoplakia in PC, the leukoplakia in DC carries with it an increased risk of squamous cell carcinoma. Dental abnormalities are frequent and include alveolar bone loss and periodontal disease. Numerous dental caries are common, and patients may be edentulous when first seen. Eye findings include blepharitis, conjunctivitis, ectropion, and lacrimal duct obstruction. The latter produces epiphora or chronic watery eye. Mild mental retardation occurs in about 50% of patients.

Progressive pancytopenia may begin at any age, but most commonly is noted between 12 and 16 years. Thrombocytopenia usually is seen first, followed by anemia and then granulocytopenia. Progressive pancytopenia can occur prior to the skin manifestations and can be rapidly fatal.

The *differential diagnosis* includes PC, poikiloderma atrophicans vasculare, epidermolysis bullosa, anetoderma, palmoplantar keratoderma, chronic GVHD, erythema ab igne, Rothmund-Thomson syndrome, lichen planus, lichen sclerosis et atrophicus, and Fanconi's anemia.

Pathogenesis is unclear, but includes increased chromosome breakages and increased sister chromatid exchanges. There may be a DNA repair defect after exposure to ultraviolet light. The pancytopenia appears related to a bone marrow stem cell defect.

Management begins with anticipation of the skin, eye, dental, oral, and gastrointestinal problems. If pancytopenia occurs, transfusions are the first line of therapy. Bone marrow transplants have been undertaken with variable results. Oral retinoids may lead to regression of the premalignant mucosal leukoplakia. Because there is an increased risk of squamous cell carcinoma, patients should avoid excessive sun exposure and smoking.

DC produces a shortened life span. Most patients die in their 20s or 30s due to pancytopenia-induced opportunistic infection or gastrointestinal bleeding. Malignancy arising in leukoplakia is another cause of premature death in these patients.

In the present patient, skin, nail, and dental abnormalities characteristic of DC confirmed the diagnosis. Mild mental retardation was documented, and he was placed in a more appropriate learning situation. He was referred to a pediatric dentist for management of the periodontal disease and caries. He will be followed carefully and will undergo periodic hematologic examinations.

Clinical Pearls

1. Dyskeratosis congenita frequently is confused with pachyonychia congenita.

2. DC-associated leukoplakia carries an increased risk of squamous cell carcinoma and may be seen on any mucosal surface.

3. Atrophy of the hand and foot skin in DC produces a characteristic smooth, shiny appearance which may include loss of dermatoglyphics.

4. Childhood hyperpigmentation often is misconstrued as a "dirty neck."

5. Epiphora (lacrimal duct obstruction leading to chronic watery eye) is a unique finding.

REFERENCES

1. Knight SW, Vulliamy T, Forni GL, et al: Fine mapping of the dyskeratosis congenita locus in Xq28. J Med Genet 33:993–995, 1996.
2. Yel L, Tezcan I, Sanal O, et al: Dyskeratosis congenita: Unusual onset with isolated neutropenia at an early age. Acta Paediatr Jpn 38:288–290, 1996.
3. Alter BP, Gardner FH, Hall RE: Treatment of dyskeratosis congenita with granulocyte colony-stimulating factor and erythropoietin. Br J Haematol 97:309–311, 1997.
4. Yabe M, Yabe H, Hattori K, et al: Fatal interstitial pulmonary disease in a patient with dyskeratosis congenita after allogeneic bone marrow transplantation. Bone Marrow Transplant 19:389–392, 1997.
5. Sahn EE: Dyskeratosis congenita. Clin Dermatol 1(unit1–34):1–8, 1998.

PATIENT 53

A 10-year-old boy with vesicles and crusts on his trunk, face, and extremities

A 10-year-old boy experienced pruritic vesicles on his chest, which rapidly spread to involve his face, scalp, and extremities. New lesions continued to appear while older ones became crusted. Prior to the eruption, he had a mild fever and malaise for 2 days. He was otherwise in good health.

Physical Examination: Temperature 37.1°C; pulse 88; respirations 26. Skin: scattered 3- to 5-mm vesicles with erythematous bases on face, trunk, extremities, palms, and soles; some lesions crusted. Mouth: two 3-mm ulcerations surrounded by erythematous rims on hard palate.

Laboratory Findings: Tzanck preparation of vesicle: multinucleated giant cells and many steel-gray nuclei.

Questions: What is the most likely diagnosis? What are your management options?

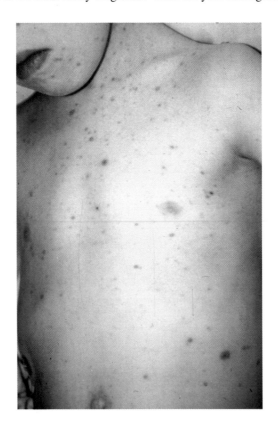

Diagnosis: Varicella

Discussion: Varicella (chicken pox) is a highly contagious disease caused by primary infection with the varicella-zoster virus. Following varicella infection, the virus becomes dormant in dorsal root (sensory) ganglia, with reactivation producing herpes zoster. Varicella exposure leads to infection in approximately 96% of cases. The incubation period is 11–20 days, and the patient is contagious from 2 days before until 8 days after the onset of the eruption.

The clinical appearance of the exanthem is classically described as "a dew drop on a rose petal," referring to the clear vesicle on a red macular base. The exanthem begins on the scalp or trunk and spreads centrifugally. Lesions rapidly crust as new crops appear, so that all stages are present at once.

The disease is more severe in adults and teenagers, infants, and the immunosuppressed patient. Complications include scarring, which is frequent, staphylococcal or streptococcal infection, bullous or hemorrhagic lesions, continuous varicella as seen in HIV infection, otitis media, pneumonia, encephalitis, and Reye syndrome. Reye syndrome has become rare since aspirin is no longer used in varicella treatment. Progressive varicella is a significant cause of morbidity and mortality in children with acute lymphoblastic leukemia. In these children, severe abdominal or back pain may be the presenting complaint, followed later by the exanthem. Children with this history need rapid diagnosis and treatment, often before any skin signs have appeared.

Treatment of varicella in normal children is symptomatic, with relief of pruritus and prevention of secondary infection. Oral acyclovir use in healthy children is controversial. Some recommend its use in sibling contacts, as their disease may be more severe. If oral acyclovir is prescribed, it must be given within 24 hours of the start of the exanthem to be effective. Intravenous acyclovir is used for varicella in neonates, immunocompromised patients, and patients with varicella pneumonia. Varicella zoster immunoglobulin provides passive immunization in certain clinical settings, such as neonatal exposure or exposure of immunocompromised patients. The live, attenuated varicella vaccine is used safely both in normal children and children with leukemia.

In the present patient, Tzanck preparation demonstrated herpes virus infection, confirming the diagnosis of chicken pox. He cleared within 3 weeks on oral antihistamines and topical lotions, but was left with several 3-mm, depressed scars on the trunk and face.

Clinical Pearls

1. Varicella is *not* an innocuous disease, and many complications can occur—some of which may be fatal. Although rare, these complications may be seen in healthy children as well as in immunocompromised individuals.

2. Untreated progressive varicella, with a mortality rate of 20%, is a significant cause of morbidity and mortality in acute lymphoblastic leukemia. Severe abdominal or back pain may be the only presenting sign.

3. The use of oral acyclovir in healthy children with varicella is controversial. For attenuation of varicella, the drug must be given within 24 hours of the onset of the exanthem.

REFERENCES

1. Rowland P, Wald ER, Mirro JR Jr, et al: Progressive varicella presenting with pain and minimal skin involvement in children with acute lymphoblastic leukemia. J Clin Oncol 13:1697–1703, 1995.
2. Ogilvie MM: Antiviral prophylaxis and treatment in chickenpox: A review prepared for the UK Advisory Group on Chickenpox, on behalf of the British Society for the Study of Infection. J Infect 36 Suppl 1:31–38, 1998.
3. Tarlow MJ, Walters S: Chickenpox in childhood: A review prepared for the UK Advisory Group on Chickenpox, on behalf of the British Society for the Study of Infection. J Infect 36 Suppl 1:39–47, 1998.

PATIENT 54

A 57-year-old man with a black nodule on his back

A 57-year-old, white veteran was noted to have a black nodule on his back during a chest examination for chronic obstructive pulmonary disease. He had sustained heavy ultraviolet exposure during his career as a sailor. He had smoked two packs of cigarettes per day for 40 years. Other than his chronic cough, he had no other complaints.

Physical Examination: Vital signs: normal. Eye: no retinal lesions. Skin: 2-cm, black, smooth nodule with extension from superior surface on left upper back (see figure); lesion not ulcerated. Abdomen: no hepatosplenomegaly. Lymph nodes: no lymphadenopathy.

Laboratory Findings: Chest radiograph: changes consistent with chronic obstructive pulmonary disease. Excisional skin biopsy of nodule: pending.

Question: What is the most likely diagnosis?

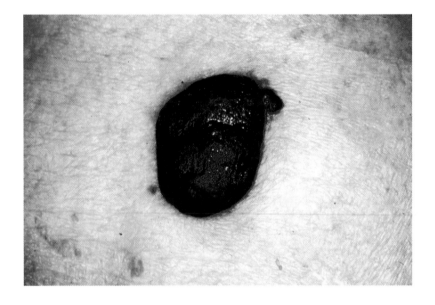

Diagnosis: Malignant melanoma

Discussion: The incidence of malignant melanoma has increased rapidly in recent years, so that the lifetime risk is 1:80 (1.25%) in a Caucasian person born in the United States today. Risk factors for the development of melanoma include: (1) the presence of dysplastic (clinically atypical) nevi, which feature three or more of these five characteristics—diameter ≥ 5 mm, an indistinct border, asymmetry, irregular pigment, and erythema; (2) the presence of the dysplastic nevus syndrome, which is defined as the presence of both melanoma and one or more clinically atypical nevi; (3) the presence of the familial dysplastic nevus syndrome (familial atypical multiple mole–melanoma syndrome [FAMM]), meaning that the patient plus one or more close relatives have melanoma and other relatives have atypical nevi; (4) the presence of giant congenital nevi, (5) excessive ultraviolet exposure, (6) skin type I with red hair, freckling, and inability to tan, and (7) multiple benign nevi. In FAMM, the risk of melanoma approaches 100%.

Key features in the clinical diagnosis of melanoma can be recalled using the mnemonic "ABCD." *A* refers to asymmetry; *B* to border irregularities, particularly notching; *C* refers to variegation of color, particularly the presence of red, white, and blue; and *D* refers to a diameter greater than 0.6 cm. Epiluminescence (cutaneous surface) microscopy is an important aid to the clinical diagnosis of melanoma, but it is operator-dependent and requires much experience. Several recent articles describe findings such as "pseudopods"—which may be the same as "radial streaming"—and "black dots" that are helpful in making the diagnosis of melanoma.

Malignant melanoma often is classified into four types. **Superficial spreading melanoma** is the most common type, representing about 70% of all melanomas. It develops from in situ melanoma and has a long radial growth phase before entering the vertical growth phase. **Lentigo maligna melanoma** is found on sun-exposed skin of the elderly and develops from a lentigo maligna (Hutchinson freckle or in situ melanoma). **Acrolentiginous melanoma**, found on the palms and soles, represents 8% of all melanomas in Caucasians, but represents a higher proportion in African-Americans, Orientals, and Hispanics because their incidence of melanoma is lower. **Nodular melanoma** shows rapid and early vertical growth and may have a worse prognosis than superficial spreading melanoma.

The *differential diagnosis* of malignant melanoma includes an unusual or atypical nevus, an irritated seborrheic keratosis or wart, hemorrhage in the skin, a thrombosed hemangioma, and other less common types of skin neoplasms.

A patient with one primary melanoma has a 5% chance of developing a second primary, much higher than would be expected by chance alone. Other factors that may increase this risk include genetic predisposition, long-term exposure to an environmental carcinogen, such as ultraviolet light, and growth of micrometastases from the primary lesion. Recent studies have linked mutations in the tumor-suppressor gene CDKN2A with familial melanoma. More recently, it has been reported that some patients with multiple primary melanomas but no family history also have germ-line mutations of the CDKN2A gene. Therefore, family members of a patient with multiple primary melanomas may be at increased risk of melanoma even if no one else in the family has melanoma. They may benefit from close surveillance.

Prognosis in malignant melanoma depends on many factors. The most important are the Breslow thickness and the mitotic rate. Melanoma in situ has a 10-year survival rate greater than 99% with a limited excision. Malignant melanoma less than 0.76 mm in thickness has a 97.9% 5-year survival rate. Other prognostic factors include age, sex, level of invasion, histologic type, location, and presence of ulceration or regression.

Therapy of primary melanoma includes complete excision with at least 1-cm margins for lesions thinner than 1 mm and 3-cm margins for lesions greater than 2 mm in thickness. The purpose of complete excision is to prevent local recurrence. Sentinel lymph node biopsy currently is being evaluated. A radioactive tracer is injected at the site of the primary melanoma before wide excision is undertaken. The tracer travels via the lymphatics to the first draining (sentinel) node. This node is then removed and evaluated for micrometastases. This procedure may be helpful in determining which patients would benefit from elective lymph node dissection. Currently, there is insufficient data to support elective lymph node dissection for the improvement of survival. Sentinel lymph node evaluation helps provide accurate staging of the disease and is reassuring to those patients whose sentinel nodes are found to be free of disease. Other modalities that appear to be helpful include the use of high-dose interferon alpha-2b therapy, which improves relapse-free survival rate, and the use of melanoma vaccines.

In the present patient, the excisional biopsy showed a nodular melanoma with a Breslow thickness of 2.4 mm. He underwent wide excision with skin grafting, but refused sentinel lymph node biopsy. All melanoma patients require long-term follow-up, since they are at increased risk of developing a second primary melanoma, and late metastases may occur even after excision of thin melanomas.

Clinical Pearls

1. The lifetime risk of a melanoma for a white person in the U.S. is currently 1 in 80, or 1.25%. About 5% of patients with one melanoma develop an additional primary melanoma.

2. Mutations in the tumor-suppressor gene CDKN2A are linked with familial melanoma and with nonfamilial multiple primary melanomas.

3. Sentinel lymph node biopsy followed by elective lymph node dissection may improve survival in melanoma patients.

REFERENCES

1. Menzies SW, Crotty KA, McCarthy WH: The morphologic criteria of the pseudopod in surface microscopy. Arch Dermatol 131:436–440, 1995.
2. Piepkorn M, Barnhill RL: A factual, not arbitrary, basis for choice of resection margins in melanoma. Arch Dermatol 132:811–814, 1996.
3. Brady MS, Coit DG: Sentinel lymph node evaluation in melanoma. Arch Dermatol 133:1014–1020, 1997.
4. Piepkorn M, Weinstock MA, Barnhill RL: Theoretical and empirical arguments in relation to elective lymph node dissection for melanoma. Arch Dermatol 133:995–1002, 1997.
5. Monzon J, Ling L, Brill H, et al: CDKN2A mutations in multiple primary melanomas. N Engl J Med 338:879–887, 1998.

PATIENT 55

A 7-year-old boy with a pruritic, erythematous, scaly eruption

A 7-year-old boy sustained a pruritic, erythematous, generalized eruption at 3 months of age. His mother smoked during pregnancy and did not breast-feed. His parents had been to numerous health practitioners, but no diagnosis had been made, and there was no sustained improvement in his symptoms. He performed well in school, but was distracted by the constant pruritus. Other than seasonal respiratory allergies, he was in good health. Both parents likewise suffered from allergic rhinitis.

Physical Examination: Vital signs: normal. Skin: poorly defined erythematous plaques, with scale and some crusting, over extremities and trunk—particularly anticubital and popliteal fossae; erythema and scale on face; double folds under eyelids; eyebrows sparse and broken off; fine scale throughout scalp (see figures). Lymph nodes: shotty axillary and inguinal lymphadenopathy. Nails: shiny and buffed secondary to scratching.

Laboratory Findings: CBC and IgE: normal.

Questions: What is the differential diagnosis? How would you counsel the parents?

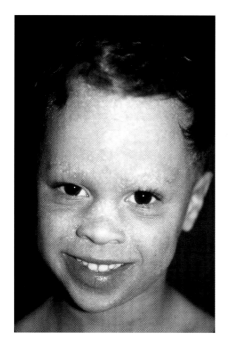
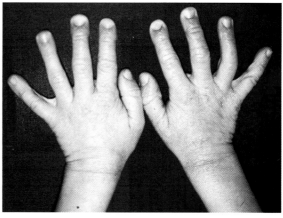

Diagnosis: Atopic dermatitis

Discussion: Atopic dermatitis is a chronic inflammatory disease of the skin related to hereditary and environmental factors but with an unknown etiology and pathogenesis. Atopic diseases refer to atopic dermatitis, asthma, and allergic rhinitis. Patients with atopic dermatitis have an increased incidence of atopic diseases in their family history. The onset is most often at around 3 months of age, when the "itch-scratch" mechanism develops, thus supporting the theory that atopic dermatitis is "an itch that rashes" (Jaquet). However, erythema and dry scaling may be seen as early as 2 weeks in some infants.

The diagnosis of atopic dermatitis is made clinically on the basis of major and minor criteria. Hanifin and Lobitz have put forth the following **major diagnostic criteria:** pruritus; chronicity with tendency to relapse; personal or family history of atopic disease; and typical morphology and distribution. Typical morphology in the acute phase includes erythema, scale, vesicles, and crusts; the chronic stage includes lichenification (thickening with increased skin markings), scale, and pigmentary alterations. Typical distribution in infancy involves cheeks, scalp, and extensor extremities, with sparing of the diaper area (protected from scratching and usually moist). Distribution in childhood involves flexural areas. Adolescent and adult distribution can be more diffuse or can be localized to hand eczema.

Minor diagnostic criteria have been the subject of much discussion and controversy. One recent study of 24 established minor criteria found only the following nine to be significant: xerosis; early onset; increased skin infections; Dennie-Morgan infraorbital folds; facial erythema; itch when sweating; wool intolerance; white dermatographism; and delayed blanch phenomenon. These authors found an additional significant minor criterion, diffuse scalp scaling. They also noted that two signs frequently mentioned, infra-auricular fissuring and the Hertoghe sign (loss of lateral eyebrows), were *not* significant as minor diagnostic criteria in atopic dermatitis. Other minor criteria frequently mentioned are ichthyosis vulgaris, hyperlinear palms, keratosis pilaris, pityriasis alba, lichen spinulosis, keratoconjunctivitis, cataracts, keratoconus, central facial pallor, infraorbital darkening ("atopic shiners"), cheilitis, perifollicular accentuation, and elevated IgE levels.

Breast feeding may be protective against the development of atopic dermatitis. Two recent studies have reported that exclusive breast feeding for 1 or more months and prolonged breast feeding for 6 months protects against the development of atopic dermatitis as well as respiratory and food allergy. These studies involved over 200 children followed for up to 17 years. Another study of 678 preschool children showed that smoking during pregnancy and/or lactation greatly increased the incidence of atopic dermatitis in the child.

The *differential diagnosis* of atopic dermatitis includes contact dermatitis, seborrheic dermatitis, scabies, psoriasis, and ichthyosis. Much less often, the following diseases may mimic atopic dermatitis: acrodermatitis enteropathica, agammaglobulinemia, ataxia telangiectasia, Wiscott-Aldrich syndrome, gluten-sensitivity enteropathy, Netherton syndrome, pityriasis rubra pilaris, drug eruption, nutritional deficiency, histiocytosis X, Leiner disease, phenylketonuria, prolidase deficiency, pemphigus erythematosus, and lymphoreticular malignancy. In addition, contact dermatitis can occur in association with atopic dermatitis. A recent report showed that children with atopic dermatitis are at least as likely as unaffected children to experience allergic or irritant contact dermatitis. The presence of atopic dermatitis is not a contraindication to patch testing, if indicated.

Therapy for atopic dermatitis includes education of the parents and patient, topical corticosteroids and oral antihistamines for the pruritus, emollients for xerosis, tar preparations, and antibiotics for secondary infection. Phototherapy with UVB and topical or oral photochemotherapy (PUVA) are important therapeutic options. For severe atopic dermatitis, cyclosporine and interferon-alpha and gamma have proven helpful in some cases. Less successful therapies that have been tried recently include disodium chromoglycolate, evening primrose oil, thymopoietin, and Chinese herbs.

Atopic dermatitis is a chronic inflammatory disease despite clinical remissions and requires long-term management. This is underscored by a recent study of soluble HLA-1 heterodimers in children with atopic dermatitis. Soluble HLA-1 (sHLA-1) is elevated in viral infection, organ transplant, and autoimmune disease—conditions with activated T-cells. It also is elevated in children with severe atopic dermatitis and does not fall even with clinical improvement following successful therapy.

The prognosis in atopic dermatitis is guarded. While most children improve with age, a significant number develop allergic rhinitis or asthma. Many have chronic hand eczema as adults. Those with severe atopic dermatitis as children should receive occupational counseling so that they avoid occupations in which workers are subject to frequent irritant or allergic contact dermatitis (e.g., hair dressers, florists, electricians, plumbers).

The parents of the present patient were counseled extensively regarding the diagnosis, long-term outlook, and treatment options. The patient cleared substantially using topical corticosteroids, emollients, daily baths, and oral antihistamines over 2 months. Three months later he experienced a severe flare when his topical therapy was interrupted while visiting his grandparents.

Clinical Pearls

1. The diagnosis of atopic dermatitis is made clinically and depends upon major and minor diagnostic criteria. A new helpful minor criterion is diffuse scalp scaling. Findings which are not helpful include infra-auricular fissuring and the Hertoghe sign.

2. Breast-feeding and avoidance of smoking during pregnancy and lactation may be protective against the development of atopic dermatitis in children.

3. Allergic and irritant contact dermatitis occur as frequently in patients with atopic dermatitis as they do in patients without atopic dermatitis.

REFERENCES

1. Saarinen UM, Kajosaari M: Breast feeding as prophylaxis against atopic disease: Prospective follow-up study until 17 years old. Lancet 346:1065–1069, 1995.
2. Klas PA, Corey G, Storrs FJ, et al: Allergic and irritant patch test reactions and atopic disease. Contact Dermatitis 34:121–124, 1996.
3. Nagaraja, Kanwar AJ, Dhar S, et al: Frequency and significance of minor clinical features in various age-related subgroups of atopic dermatitis in children. Pediatr Dermatol 13:10–13, 1996.
4. Moore C, Ehlayel M, Inostroza J, et al: Elevated levels of soluble HLA class I (sHLA-I) in children with severe atopic dermatitis. Ann Allergy Asthma Immunol 79:113–118, 1997.
5. Schäfer T, Dirschedl P, Kunz B, et al: Maternal smoking during pregnancy and lactation increases the risk for atopic eczema in the offspring. J Am Acad Dermatol 36:550–556, 1997.

PATIENT 56

A 2-year-old boy with sudden onset of annular skin lesions

A 2-year-old child was brought in by his father with the sudden appearance 2 weeks before of multiple annular lesions on the trunk, back, and shoulders. The child was in good health otherwise, but did not yet talk. The child's mother had been killed in an auto accident 1 year previously, and the father was raising the patient and his 13-year-old brother alone.

Physical Examination: General: fearful, withdrawn. Vital signs: normal. Skin: multiple hyper-pigmented, slightly scaly, annular plaques over trunk and back; some overlapping (see figures). Abdomen: soft and nontender. Genitalia: no lesions or abnormalities. Funduscopic examination: no retinal hemorrhages. Ears: no tympanic hemorrhage.

Laboratory Findings: Radiographic skeletal survey: no fractures.

Question: What is your diagnosis and immediate course of action?

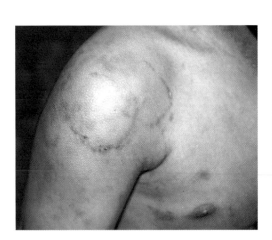
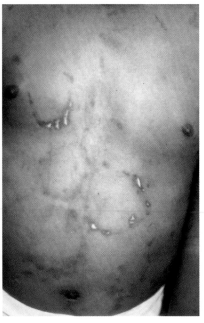

Diagnosis: Child abuse

Discussion: Child abuse has been increasingly recognized since Kempe, Silverman, and Steele introduced the term "battered child syndrome" in 1962. In order for the physician to appropriately intervene for the child's protection, the signs of child abuse must be familiar.

There are many physical signs of child abuse. **Unexplained ecchymosis** (bruising), the most common sign, frequently is multiple and found in areas not usually bruised in children, such as the genitalia and buttocks. If multiple, the ecchymoses may be in different stages of healing. Linear bruising follows trauma with a straight object, such as a rod or stick. Chronic subungual hematomas can be markers of trauma to the fingers and toes. Loop marks are due to hitting with small cords, such as electric cords, and represent the single most characteristic finding of child abuse. Belt buckles leave a characteristic imprint, as do pinches.

Bite marks have been used in forensic cases to identify the perpetrator. Human bites produce a crushing injury, in contrast to animal bites, which produce puncture wounds. An adult dental arch width equals or exceeds 4 cm, so it can be easily differentiated from a child's bite.

Thermal burns can produce several characteristic marks. Cigarette burns leave wounds and scars of a specific size, as do other branding injuries. Dunking an extremity in hot water produces a "glove" or "stocking" injury. Forcing a child to sit in scalding water in a bath tub can produce characteristic "doughnut sparing" in the buttock area.

Traumatic alopecia due to yanking of the hair most commonly is seen in the occipital area and may be accompanied by scalp hemorrhage. **Binding injuries** produce lesions at the wrists and ankles. **Blunt trauma** can produce severe or fatal injuries if delivered to the abdomen. Slaps produce broken capillaries between where the fingers hit, which then result in a pattern of bruises outlining the perpetrators' hand. **Shaking** can produce severe brain injury, with retinal hemorrhages and subdural hematoma.

Other physical findings that support the diagnosis of child abuse include multiple fractures at different stages of healing on radiographic examination and failure to thrive. These children often are neglected and abused in nonphysical ways, too; typically, routine health care appointments are missed, and immunizations are not obtained.

Management of suspected child abuse includes removal of the child from the abusing environment and immediate reporting to the child protective services in the area. Appropriate work-up may include CBC, VDRL, cultures to exclude sexually transmitted disease and HIV, and radiographs. Photographs must be taken and careful documentation performed. Younger children who are nonverbal are the most often abused.

The *differential diagnosis* of child abuse includes the following: Ehlers Danlos syndrome, lichen sclerosis et atrophicus and osteogenesis imperfecta (bone mineral density studies and skin biopsy for collagen analysis may be helpful in differentiating the two), streptococcal toxic shock syndrome, painful and disabling granuloma annulare (recent case report of Munchausen by proxy in a 6-year-old), Gardner-Diamond syndrome, Mongolian spots, phytophotodermatitis, erythema multiforme, and platelet or clotting abnormalities. Certain Asian cultures have medical practices that may be confused with child abuse. These practices include cupping, coining (heated coins applied to the skin produce round areas of purpura), cao gio (coin rubbing), and moxibustion (the burning of a tuft of soft, combustible material on the skin surface).

Once abused, a child is likely to be abused again; therefore, he or she *must not be returned to the same environment without active intervention.* Abused children are likely to become abusing parents, and intervention offers the possibility of avoiding this vicious cycle.

The present patient was seen by the child protective services agency within 2 hours and removed from the home environment to the home of relatives. Investigation over the next several days revealed that the 13-year-old brother was left alone with the patient daily while the father worked, and he had applied heated rings to the patient's skin. The lesions faded with time, but left hyperpigmented scars.

Clinical Pearls

1. The single most characteristic finding in child abuse is a loop mark secondary to hitting with a cord.

2. Human adult bite marks are characterized by crushing injury and at least a 4-cm dental arch width.

3. Asian culture medical practices such as moxibustion, cao gio, coining, and cupping are not markers of child abuse.

REFERENCES

1. Gavin LA, Lanz MJ, Leung DY, et al: Chronic subungual hematomas: A presumed immunologic puzzle resolved with child abuse. Arch Pediatr Adolesc Med 151:103–105, 1997.
2. Look KM, Look RM: Skin scraping, cupping, and moxibustion that may mimic physical abuse. J Forensic Sci 42:103–105, 1997.
3. Weston WL, Morelli JG: "Painful and disabling granuloma annulare": A case of Munchausen by proxy. Pediatr Dermatol 14:363–364, 1997.
4. Ablin DS: Osteogenesis imperfecta: A review. Can Assoc Radiol J 49:110–123, 1998.
5. Nields H, Kessler SC, Boisot S, et al: Streptococcal toxic shock syndrome presenting as a suspected child abuse. Am J Forensic Med Pathol 19:93–97, 1998.

PATIENT 57

**An 11-month-old boy with closed comedones and erythematous papules
on his face**

An 11-month-old infant was noted to have closed comedones on the nose at birth. These spread to involve the cheeks and chin and were accompanied by the appearance of erythematous, white papules and an occasional pustule. Both parents had had severe acne vulgaris as teenagers. The child was in excellent health and was not taking medications. The parents were not applying topical agents to his face.

Physical Examination: Vital signs: normal. Skin: numerous closed comedones scattered over nose and cheeks; small erythematous papules on both cheeks with some pustules (see figure); no pubic or axillary hair; normal distribution of scalp hair. Abdomen: no masses. Testes: normal.

Question: How would you manage this problem?

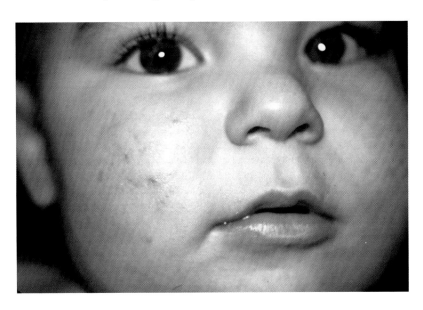

Diagnosis: Infantile acne vulgaris

Discussion: Infantile acne begins 3–6 months after birth and consists of comedones, papules, pustules, nodules, and cysts. It may follow neonatal acne or begin de novo and usually persists to ages 2–5. However, it can continue into childhood and adolescence. It is much less common than neonatal acne, which occurs in up to 20% of newborns. Neonatal acne usually consists of comedones alone and resolves spontaneously by 6 months of age.

Neonatal acne is thought to be caused by sebaceous gland stimulation from maternal and neonatal androgens derived from hyperactive adrenal glands. Testicular androgens may play a part in male neonates, explaining the increased prevalence in males. In normal males, testosterone levels rise during the first 3 months of life and then fall to normal preadolescent levels by 6 or 7 months. In female infants, however, testosterone levels fall immediately after birth until about 2 weeks of age.

The *differential diagnosis* of infantile acne includes congenital adrenal hyperplasia (most commonly due to 21-hydroxylase deficiency); acne venenata infantum (caused by the application of comedogenic preparations, usually moisturizers); steroid acne (topical or systemic); chloracne (exposure to dioxins, producing symmetric malar comedones with occasional comedones of the trunk and extremities); fetal hydantoin syndrome (maternal ingestion of hydantoin also causes hypoplastic terminal phalanges, craniofacial dysmorphism, and mental retardation); maternal ingestion of lithium; androluteoma syndrome of pregnancy (virilizing luteoma of pregnancy); neonatal sebaceous gland hyperplasia (small, yellow-white, follicular papules on the nose and cheeks without comedones); oral vitamin D_2 used to prevent rickets; and virilizing adrenal, testicular, or ovarian tumors.

Androgen excess may produce acne in early childhood and is associated with three conditions: (1) Early adrenarche. Adrenarche occurs when the adrenal gland develops the ability to respond to ACTH with secretion of 17-ketosteroids. At this point, normally between the ages of 6 and 8, the adrenal androgens DHEA and DHEA-S increase. (2) A genetic defect in steroidogenic enzymes (most commonly 21-hydroxylase with congenital adrenal hyperplasia). (3) An androgen-producing tumor. In one study of 15 children aged 5–10 years, early-onset acne was associated with an increase in DHEA-S in seven. Only two of these seven had a 21-hydroxylase deficiency, and these two had either clitoromegaly or advanced bone age on hand and wrist radiographs. Increased androgens were found only in those with early pubic hair development (pubarche).

The management of infantile acne includes a hormonal evaluation if the acne is unusually severe or resistant to therapy, or there are signs of androgen excess (i.e., pubarche, clitoromegaly, or advanced bone age). Free and total testosterone, DHEA, DHEA-S, luteinizing hormone, follicle-stimulating hormone, and prolactin are measured. In most cases, hormonal evaluation is not indicated, and treatment can be undertaken with topical azelaic acid, low-strength benzoyl peroxide, topical antibiotics, or low-strength tretinoin cream or gel. More severe cases require oral antibiotics (not tetracycline, which may stain teeth), and some clinicians advocate intralesional corticosteroid injections of cysts to prevent scarring. In severe cystic acne or acne conglobata infantum, systemic retinoids may be required. The prognosis of infantile acne is guarded, as there is an increased risk of severe adolescent acne.

In the present patient, low-strength benzoyl peroxide, tretinoin cream, and topical antibiotics were all required to produce clearing. He will be followed closely for signs of childhood or adolescent acne.

Clinical Pearls

1. Neonatal acne is common, occurring in up to 20% of newborns, while infantile acne is much less common. Infantile acne can demonstrate severe lesions including nodules, cysts, and scarring, and may portend severe adolescent acne.

2. A hormonal evaluation is indicated in infantile acne if it is unusually severe or resistant to therapy, or there are signs of androgen excess.

3. Pubarche in infantile acne may be a reliable sign of androgen excess.

REFERENCES

1. Rosenfield RL, Lucky AW: Acne, hirsutism and alopecia in adolescent girls: Clinical expressions of androgen excess. Adol Endocr Metabol Clin North Am 22:507–527, 1993.
2. De Raeve L, De Schepper J, Smitz J: Prepubertal acne: A cutaneous marker of androgen excess? J Am Acad Dermatol 32:181–184, 1995.
3. Tabata N, Terui T, Watanabe M, et al: Infantile acne associated with a high plasma testosterone level in a 21-month-old boy. J Am Acad Dermatol 33:676–678, 1995.
4. Jansen T, Burgdorf W, Plewig G: Pathogenesis and treatment of acne in childhood. Pediatr Dermatol 14:17–21, 1997.

PATIENT 58

An 11-year-old, mentally retarded girl with a nodule on the shoulder

An 11-year-old girl with an asymptomatic nodule on the shoulder was referred from a psychiatric hospital, where she had been admitted for "emotional problems and mental retardation." There was no record of seizures. Additional history, including family history, was unavailable from her foster parents.

Physical Examination: Blood pressure 95/65. Neurologic: mild mental retardation; bland affect, but cooperative. Skin: 2-cm, firm nodule on anterior shoulder, with surrounding hyperpigmentation (see figure, *left*); large café au lait macule on flank and five additional café au lait macules 1.5–2 cm in diameter (see figure, *right*); numerous small, brown freckles in axillae. Breasts: nipples widely spaced. Funduscopic: normal. Skeletal: mild scoliosis.

Laboratory Findings: CBC with differential: normal. Skin biopsy of right shoulder nodule: pending. MRI of brain and slit-lamp examination: pending.

Questions: What is your diagnosis? How would you manage this child?

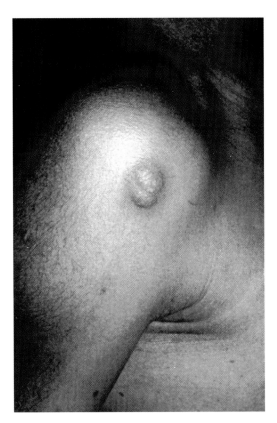 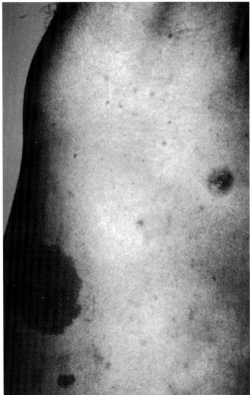

Diagnosis: Neurofibromatosis type 1

Discussion: Neurofibromatosis type 1 (NF 1) is one of the most common genodermatoses, with an incidence of approximately 1:3000 individuals. It is characterized by skin, nervous system, bone, and soft tissue abnormalities. The diagnostic criteria have been established by the National Institutes of Health.

The classic clinical findings in NF 1 are neurofibromas, café au lait macules, and Lisch nodules. **Neurofibromas** usually arise at puberty and may be of three types: cutaneous or dermal neurofibromas are soft and rubbery and, if small, may be invaginated into the underlying dermal defect ("button-hole sign"); subcutaneous neurofibromas are hard, with the consistency of a pencil-eraser; plexiform neurofibromas resemble a nerve plexus or "bag of worms." Plexiform neurofibromas typically affect the trigeminal or upper cervical nerves and present as elongated, beaded masses running along the course of a nerve. There may be overlying hyperpigmentation or hypertrichosis, which can resemble a congenital melanocytic nevus. A hair whorl over the spine may be a marker of paraspinal plexiform neurofibroma (Riccardi sign).

Café au lait macules may be present at birth or appear in infancy. New ones may appear as late as adolescence. Five or six café au lait macules of 0.5-cm diameter in young children and 1.5-cm diameter in adults frequently are indicative of neurofibromatosis. Axillary (Crowe sign) or other fold freckles develop during childhood, and 80% of adult patients with NF 1 show freckling in the folds.

Lisch nodules are melanocytic hamartomas of the iris. They present in 5% of 3-year-olds and 100% of 21-year-olds with NF 1. Slit-lamp examination may be necessary to visualize Lisch nodules, although some may be visualized on ophthalmoscopy.

Endocrine disorders occur in 1–3% of all patients with NF 1. Pheochromocytoma is the most common, occurring in 1% of adult patients. In children, central precocious puberty occurs in 3% (versus 0.6% in the general pediatric population). Optic chiasm gliomas sometimes are found in these patients. Growth hormone deficiency has a prevalence of 2.5% in children with NF 1.

Tumors found in NF 1 include neural fibrosarcomas, brain tumors (astrocytoma, meningioma), sarcomas, liposarcomas, and rhabdomyosarcomas. The incidence of malignant tumors in NF 1 varies from 2–16%, probably a low estimate because many cases of asymptomatic NF 1 are undiagnosed. Carcinoid and pheochromocytomas are reported. Unilateral acoustic neuromas (bilateral occur in neurofibromatosis 2) can produce deafness. Optic nerve gliomas were found to occur in 19% of 176 children with NF 1. These are diagnosed on MRI, and 80% are present by the age of 10. In children with NF 1 and multiple juvenile xanthogranulomas, the incidence of juvenile chronic myelogenous leukemia is 32 times greater than in those children with NF 1 and no juvenile xanthogranuloma.

The gene responsible for neurofibromatosis 1 is located on the long arm of chromosome 17 (17_q). The neurofibromatosis-2 gene is located on the long arm of chromosome 22 (22_q). The protein product of the NF-1 gene is neurofibromin, which acts as a tumor suppressor through negative feedback control on the *ras*GAP (guanosine diphosphotase-activating) protein system. Mutations in neurofibromin allow the *ras*GAP protein to remain active or overactive, producing Schwann cell hyperplasia. *Ras* mutations are known to stimulate tumor angiogenesis. Therefore, angiogenesis inhibitors may prove to be beneficial in the treatment of neurofibromas as well as malignant tumors. A recent study of spontaneous neurofibromas and those from patients with NF 1 found that neurofibromas are highly vascular despite their grossly white appearance. These authors found a high level of vascular endothelial growth factor in the perivascular cells of the neurofibromas. The authors concluded that the marked vascularity of neurofibromas may be mediated by the high levels of this angiogenic factor, which could be related to *ras* mutations.

The inheritance of the NF-1 gene is autosomal dominant, with approximately 50% new mutations. There is a recent report of germ-line mosaicism in a clinically normal father who transmitted NF 1 to his offspring. Ten per cent of the father's sperm carried the same NF-1 deletion as the affected children, but it was not present in his peripheral cells. Therefore, future children of this father could be affected.

The *differential diagnosis* of a child with one large café au lait macule includes McCune-Albright syndrome (polyostotic fibrous dysplasia), in which the irregular macule borders are noted to resemble the coast of Maine. These café au lait macules usually respect the midline. Hyperpigmentation or hypertrichosis overlying a plexiform neurofibroma can resemble a congenital melanocytic nevus. Café au lait macules can be seen in multiple syndromes, including Bloome, Bannayan-Riley-Ruvalcaba, Watson, LEOPARD, Russell-Silver, Noonan, ataxia-telangiectasia, Maffucci, and Fanconi.

In the present patient, histologic examination of the shoulder nodule specimen revealed a neurofibroma with thin, wavy collagen fibers containing many embedded oval- to spindle-shaped nuclei.

Special nerve stains demonstrated a small number of nerve fibers, consistent with a neurofibroma. An MRI of her cranial vault and orbits showed bilateral optic nerve gliomas. A slit-lamp examination revealed six Lisch nodules on the irises. A hearing test was normal. IQ testing revealed moderate mental retardation. She will be carefully followed with blood pressure and head circumference measurements, periodic ophthalmologic examinations, and MRIs as indicated. She will be observed for the development of malignancies, skeletal abnormalities, and psychological disabilities.

Clinical Pearls

1. Neurofibromatosis 1 is one of the most common genodermatoses; nevertheless, the diagnosis frequently is delayed.

2. Angiogenesis inhibitors may prove to be beneficial in NF 1 in the treatment of neurofibromas as well as malignant tumors.

3. The presence of multiple juvenile xanthogranulomas in a child with NF 1 greatly increases the risk of the child developing juvenile chronic myelogenous leukemia.

REFERENCES

1. Zvulunov A, Barak Y, Metzler A: Juvenile xanthogranuloma, neurofibromatosis, and juvenile myelogenous leukemia: World statistical analysis. Arch Dermatol 131:904–908, 1995.
2. Cnossen MH, Stam EN, Cooiman L, et al: Endocrinologic disorders and optic pathway gliomas in children with neurofibromatosis type 1. Pediatr 100:667–670, 1997.
3. Pivnick EK, Lobe TE, Fitch SJ, et al: Hair whorl as an indicator of a mediastinal plexiform neurofibroma. Pediatr Dermatol 14:196–198, 1997.
4. Arbiser JL, Flynn E, Barnhill RL: Analysis of vascularity of human neurofibromas. J Am Acad Dermatol 39:950–954, 1998.
5. Menor F, Marti-Bonmati L, Arana E, et al: Neurofibromatosis type 1 in children: MR imaging and follow-up studies of central nervous system findings. Eur J Radiol 26:121–131, 1998.

PATIENT 59

A 19-year-old boy with a slowly growing hyperkeratotic nodule
on his toe

A 19-year-old boy noticed a rough papule on the plantar surface of his second toe 6 months previously. The papule slowly enlarged and began causing discomfort when he walked.

Physical Examination: Skin: tender, hyperkeratotic nodule with collarette of raised skin at base on plantar surface of second toe (see figure).

Laboratory Findings: Biopsy of papule: pending.

Question: What are the diagnosis and differential diagnosis of this lesion?

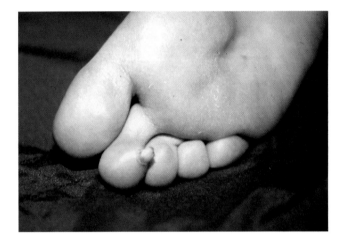

Diagnosis: Acquired digital fibrokeratoma

Discussion: Acquired digital fibrokeratoma is a benign hyperkeratotic papule or nodule most commonly seen on the fingers or toes of adults. It may be elongated, resembling a cutaneous horn, or dome-shaped. There is a collarette of slightly raised skin at the base. In addition to the digits, an acquired fibrokeratoma has been reported on the plantar surface of the heel. The lesions are solitary.

Histopathologic examination of an acquired digital fibrokeratoma reveals epidermal hyperkeratosis and acanthosis, which may be accompanied by thick and branching rete ridges. The core of the lesion consists of vertically oriented collagen bundles, which often are highly vascularized.

The *differential diagnosis* of enlarging lesions on the digits includes recurrent digital fibroma of childhood, also known as recurrent infantile digital fibroma or digital fibrous tumor of childhood. This is a benign, painless, skin-colored nodule that often is located near a nail but spares the thumb and great toe. Nodules typically are multiple. Biopsy shows characteristic perinuclear, intracytoplasmic, eosinophilic inclusion bodies. These bodies originate from desmin, vimentin, and actin, confirming that the cells are myofibroblasts. These tumors spontaneously involute. Recurrences, reported in up to 75% of cases, are now thought to be due to attempted excision.

Rudimentary supernumerary digit presents as a smooth or verrucous papule located on the medial surface of the base of the fifth digit and is present at birth. These are traumatic neuromas resulting from either in utero amputation or postnatal removal. Histopathologic examination of these papules reveals scattered peripheral nerve bundles surrounded by a capsule composed of collagen and perineural cells.

Malignancy must be included in the differential diagnosis if the clinical appearance is not classic.

In the present patient, biopsy results demonstrated epidermal hyperkeratosis and acanthosis, with branching rete ridges. Thus, the diagnosis of acquired digital fibrokeratoma was confirmed. Treatment was accomplished with local anesthesia, a shave excision, and hemostasis obtained with aluminum chloride. There was no recurrence.

Clinical Pearls

1. The first occurrence of acquired digital fibrokeratoma usually is in adulthood, while the first occurrence of recurrent infantile digital fibroma (digital fibrous tumor of childhood, recurrent digital fibroma of childhood) is in infancy or childhood.

2. Acquired digital fibrokeratoma clinically resembles rudimentary supernumerary digit, but the latter is present from birth and occurs at the base of the fifth finger(s).

3. Acquired digital fibrokeratoma shows a core of vertical collagen bundles on histopathologic examination, while rudimentary supernumerary digit features numerous nerve bundles.

REFERENCES
1. Berger RS, Spielvogel RL: Dermal papule on a distal digit: Acquired digital fibrokeratoma. Arch Dermatol 124:1559–1560, 1562–1563, 1988.
2. Spitalny AD, Lavery LA: Acquired fibrokeratoma of the heel. J Foot Surg 31:509–511, 1992.

PATIENT 60

A 70-year-old man with an expanding annular plaque on his forehead

A 70-year-old man noticed a forehead papule 6 months previously, which developed into an annular, enlarging plaque. He had been a farmer most of his life and had received intense sun exposure. He was in good health otherwise, with no pulmonary complaints.

Physical Examination: Vital signs: normal. Skin: 3-cm, annular, skin-colored plaque on forehead; plaque has raised, shiny border and normal-appearing skin in center (see figure). Chest: clear. Lymph nodes: no lymphadenopathy. Abdomen: no hepatosplenomegaly.

Laboratory Findings: Chest radiograph: normal. Angiotensin-converting enzyme level: normal. Excisional biopsy: pending.

Question: What is the differential diagnosis in this case?

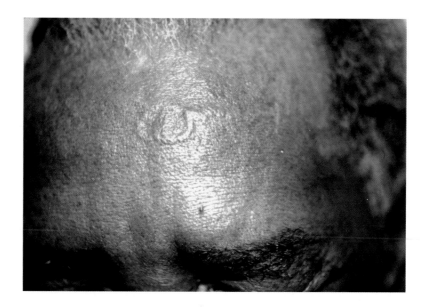

Diagnosis: Annular elastolytic granuloma

Discussion: Annular elastolytic giant-cell granuloma, also known as actinic granuloma or Miescher's granuloma, is a localized, chronic, inflammatory reaction consisting of slowly enlarging annular plaques on sun-exposed areas. It is rare, more common in fair-skinned individuals, and occasionally seen on areas not exposed to the sun.

The pathogenesis is controversial. Some believe that annular elastolytic granuloma is a variant of granuloma annulare. Others believe that it is a response to damaged elastic tissue (solar elastosis), because this focal granulomatous reaction results in resorption of elastic fibers by histiocytic giant cells. Other conditions in which abnormal elastic tissue is associated with a granulomatous reaction include pseudoxanthoma elasticum and elastosis perforans serpiginosa.

Clinically, skin-colored or erythematous papules or annular plaques are the primary lesions. They may have a pearly border, and the center may be normal or atrophic and hypopigmented. The plaques are asymptomatic and usually resolve spontaneously over months to years without scarring.

The diagnosis is confirmed on histopathologic examination of a radial biopsy that shows a typical "triple zone." Skin outside the annulus shows elastolytic tissue consistent with actinic elastosis (basophilic degeneration). The raised border reveals consumption of elastic fibers and fragments (elastophagocytosis) by foreign body giant cells. The granulomatous infiltrate may damage eccrine structures, leading to squamous syringometoplasia. There is no necrosis, palisading of histiocytes, lipid, or mucin. The central zone may show hypopigmentation and atrophy.

The *differential diagnosis* includes the following diseases that can present with annular plaques: granuloma annulare, sarcoidosis, necrobiosis lipoidica, tuberculoid leprosy, granuloma multiforme, secondary syphilis, elastosis perforans serpiginosa, discoid lupus erythematosus, and morphea. The histopathologic differential diagnosis includes granuloma annulare, necrobiosis lipoidica, and mid-dermal elastolysis. Biopsy in a recently reported case showed features of mid-dermal elastolysis in the center of the annular plaque and features of annular elastolytic giant-cell granuloma in the border, leading the authors to postulate that the two diseases may represent differing stages of one disease.

Treatment of annular elastolytic granuloma includes the use of sunscreens and sun avoidance. Some authors have reported success with intralesional corticosteroids, oral cyclosporin A, topical cryotherapy with liquid nitrogen, and dapsone. Since spontaneous resolution is the rule, the lesion may be watched. There is a report of concurrent annular elastolytic giant-cell granuloma and adult T-cell leukemia in a 74-year-old man. The disorder also has been reported to coexist with hepatitis C virus antibody positivity.

In the present patient, the biopsy demonstrated characteristic "triple zone" findings. Age-appropriate screening tests showed no underlying diseases. He is being treated with sun avoidance and sunscreens.

Clinical Pearls

1. Annular elastic granuloma is rare, but should be included in the differential diagnosis of sarcoidosis and granuloma annulare on sun-exposed skin.

2. The diagnosis is made by a radial skin biopsy across the raised border which shows typical findings in three areas: outside the border, within the border, and in the center of the annular plaque.

3. Annular elastolytic giant-cell granuloma is benign and usually resolves spontaneously. There are reports of concurrent adult T-cell leukemia in one patient and hepatitis C virus positivity in another patient.

REFERENCES

1. Helton JL, Metcalf JS: Squamous syringometaplasia in association with annular elastolytic granuloma. Am J Dermatopathol 17:407–409, 1995.
2. Revenga F, Rovira I, Pimentel J, et al: Annular elastolytic giant cell granuloma: Actinic granuloma? Clin Exp Dermatol 21:51–53, 1996.
3. Hohenleutner S, Wlotzke U, Landthaler M, et al: [Elastolysis of the mid-dermis and annular elastolytic giant cell granuloma: different stages in the clinical spectrum of dermal elastolysis? Case report and review of the literature. Hautarzt 48:45–50, 1997.
4. Igawa K, Maruyama R, Katayama I, et al: Anti-oxidative therapy with oral dapsone improved HCV antibody positive annular elastolytic giant cell granuloma. J Dermatol 24:238–241, 1997.
5. Sahn E: Annular elastolytic giant-cell granuloma, actinic granuloma, granulomatosis disciformis chronica et progressiva (Miescher's granulomatosis). Clin Dermatol 1(unit 4):9, 1998.

PATIENT 61

A 31-year-old woman with an itchy, red spot on the buttock

A 31-year-old woman with hidradenitis suppurativa was placed on trimethoprim-sulphamethoxazole (TMP-SMX) for a draining cyst. Within 6 hours, she noticed a pruritic, erythematous patch on her right buttock. She recalled that 1 year previously, when she had been treated with the same drug, a similar lesion had appeared in the same area.

Physical Examination: Vital signs: normal. Skin: 3-cm, slightly edematous plaque with sharp demarcation located on right buttock (see figure); several tender, erythematous papules and a draining 1-cm cyst located in inguinal creases.

Question: What is the most likely diagnosis? How would you manage this patient?

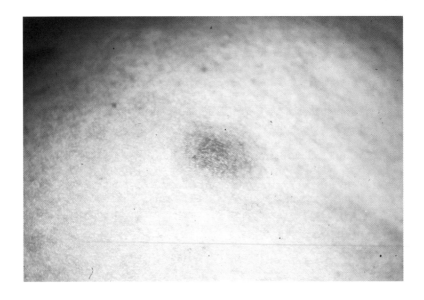

Diagnosis: Fixed drug eruption

Discussion: Fixed drug eruption most commonly presents as a solitary, round or oval, pruritic patch that is dusky red to violaceous and recurs at the same site after ingesting the offending drug. First described by Bourns in 1989, Brocq later used the term "fixed drug eruption." The lesions may be multiple or bullous and typically resolve in 10–14 days, with marked and prolonged postinflammatory hyperpigmentation. Typical sites affected are the lips, genitalia, and sacrum.

Histopathology reveals similarities to erythema multiforme; therefore, fixed drug eruption is thought to be a localized form of erythema multiforme. Characteristics include vacuolar changes in the basal cell layer of the epidermis, with pigmentary incontinence leading to melanin-laden macrophages in the dermis; Civatte bodies (dysplastic eosinophilic keratinocytes in the epidermis); and eosinophils in the dermal infiltrate. Some investigators think that the drug acts as a hapten, binding to the basal keratinocyte or the melanocyte and producing a cell-mediated response. Others believe that antibody-dependent cellular cytotoxicity plays a part in the keratinocyte destruction. It has been suggested that the particular location of the reaction might be a site of previous cutaneous injury or inflammation.

The drugs most commonly implicated in fixed drug eruption include sulfonamides, oral contraceptives, aspirin, phenolphthalein, tetracycline, barbiturates, phenylbutazone, and carbamazepine. Less common causes include fluoroquinolones and amoxicillin. A recent report of fixed drug eruption to tartrazine yellow dye underscores the importance of considering artificial flavors, colors, and preservatives as possible etiologic agents. A man with known allergy to TMP-SMX developed a fixed drug eruption after sexual intercourse with his wife, who was taking the drug. The authors suggested that exposure to the drug in the vaginal fluid produced the recurrent reaction.

Fixed drug eruption may be nonpigmenting, in which case the most common presentation is tender, symmetrical, erythematous plaques that resolve without pigmentation. Nonpigmenting fixed drug eruption in solitary form resembles the typical epidermal type of fixed drug eruption. There have been several recent reports of pseudoephedrine producing a nonpigmenting fixed drug eruption. The authors speculate that this occurrence is secondary to drug hypersensitivity that is dermal rather than epidermal. Pseudoephedrine can produce typical pigmenting fixed drug eruption, as well.

Management includes avoidance of the offending drug. Confirmation of the diagnosis can be made by re-exposure, in which case oral provocation produces rapid reappearance of the lesion or lesions within 30 minutes to 8 hours. If oral rechallenge is refused, topical open provocation may reproduce the lesion. Subsequent episodes of fixed drug eruption may be more severe and produce darker hyperpigmentation.

In the present patient, the offending medication was discontinued, and the lesion gradually cleared over several weeks. It left a hyperpigmented patch that persisted for several months. The patient's hidradenitis suppurativa was controlled with oral cephalothin, and she was advised to avoid TMP-SMX.

Clinical Pearls

1. Fixed drug eruption may represent a localized form of erythema multiforme, because it demonstrates similar clinical and histopathologic features.

2. Fixed drug eruption may be nonpigmenting, in which case the typical postinflammatory hyperpigmentation is not seen. Pseudoephedrine recently has been implicated as a cause of nonpigmenting fixed drug eruption.

3. Tartrazine yellow dye has been reported to be causative; in determining the etiology of fixed drug eruption, artificial flavors, colors, and preservatives should be considered.

REFERENCES

1. Gruber F, Stasic A, Lenkovic M, et al: Postcoital fixed drug eruption in man sensitive to trimethoprim-sulphamethoxazole. Clin Exp Dermatol 22:144–145, 1997.
2. Orchard DC, Varigos GA: Fixed drug eruption to tartrazine. Australas J Dermatol 38:212–214, 1997.
3. Hindioğlu U, Sahin S: Nonpigmenting solitary fixed drug eruption caused by pseudoephedrine hydrochloride. J Am Acad Dermatol 38:499–500, 1998.
4. Vidal C, Prieto A, Perez-Carral C, et al: Nonpigmenting fixed drug eruption due to pseudoephedrine. Ann Allergy Asthma Immunol 80:309–310, 1998.

PATIENT 62

A 28-year-old man with a 10-year history of hair loss

A 28-year-old man complained of increasing hair loss beginning 10 years previously. He noted intermittent itching, but otherwise was asymptomatic. He had not observed any skin lesions and considered himself to be in good health. He took no medications. There was no family history of alopecia.

Physical Examination: Scalp: patchy, scarring alopecia; follicular plugs and papules in some areas; smooth scalp with loss of follicular openings in other areas (see figure); mild, violaceous erythema with scaling. Nails: no pterygium. Skin: no violaceous, flat-topped papules. Mouth: lacy, white, reticulated plaques on buccal mucosa. Genitalia: no lesions.

Laboratory Findings: Scalp biopsy from edge of scarred patch: pending.

Question: What is the most likely diagnosis?

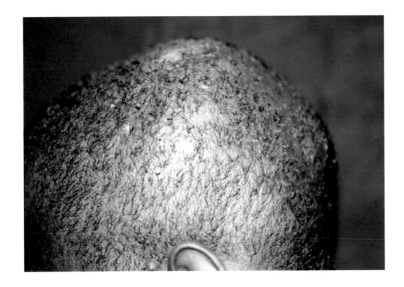

Diagnosis: Lichen planopilaris

Discussion: Lichen planopilaris is a variant of lichen planus, which has been called follicular lichen planus or Graham-Little syndrome. It is a triad consisting of scarring alopecia of the scalp (with or without atrophy), follicular papules, and mucocutaneous lesions of lichen planus. The scalp involvement consists of patchy, violaceous, and acuminate (cone-shaped) follicular papules, some with erythema and scaling. Lichen planopilaris is more common in adult females than males, but also has been reported in children.

Lichen planopilaris often is associated with lichen planus, requiring a search for the typical nail changes (i.e., onychorrhexis, onychoschizia, pterygium, and anonychia), mucous membrane abnormalities (white, reticulated, lacy papules on the buccal mucosa), and skin lesions (flat-topped, violaceous papules on flexural sites, such as wrists, as well as legs and genitalia). The latter are pruritic and show the Koebner phenomenon. Occasionally, lichen planopilaris may be seen elsewhere than the scalp, particularly in the axilla, and it can occur (although rarely) with ulcerative lichen planus of the feet.

The *differential diagnosis* includes other causes of scarring alopecia, such as chronic discoid lupus erythematosus (deep patchy infiltrate, vacuolar degeneration, and extensive hyperkeratosis), morphea (collagen thickening and homogenization), folliculitis decalvans (intrafollicular pustules, neutrophilic infiltrate, deep folliculitis, and granulomatous changes), and pseudopellade of Brocq (always limited to scalp; may be idiopathic or secondary to several other diseases including folliculitis decalvans, discoid lupus erythematosus, and lichen planus). Other causes of scarring alopecia that occasionally resemble lichen planopilaris include kerion (tinea capitis), sarcoid, dissecting cellulitis, idiopathic fibrosing alopecia, pemphigus vulgaris

or foliaceous, bullous pemphigoid (Brunsting-Perry type of cicatricial pemphigoid, which affects scalp, head, neck, and oral mucosa), hot comb/oil alopecia, carcinoma metastases, necrobiosis lipoidica diabeticorum, and acne keloidalis. Noninflammatory scalp scarring can result from trauma, herpes zoster, or aplasia cutis congenita.

It is noteworthy that in the late stage of lichen planopilaris, the histopathologic examination is indistinguishable from that of pseudopellade of Brocq. In pseudopellade of Brocq, the inflammatory infiltrate is present only transiently and often is missed. In lichen planopilaris, it persists much longer and extends into the lower third of the hair follicle as well as into the dermis.

A recent histopathologic study of frontal fibrosing alopecia in postmenopausal women found the biopsies to be identical to those of lichen planopilaris. In the former entity, there is progressive loss of the frontal hairline as well as of the eyebrows. The authors conclude that it is a variant of lichen planopilaris. Other recent reports describe lichen planopilaris of the face and lichen planopilaris associated with dermatitis herpetiformis.

Treatment of lichen planopilaris frequently is unsatisfactory. Occasionally during the inflammatory stage, topical, intralesional, or oral corticosteroids may produce improvement. Systemic retinoids have met with some success.

In the present patient, histologic examination of the scalp biopsy revealed a band-like mononuclear infiltrate concentrated around hair follicles, particularly the dermal hair papillae, below the epidermis. Some areas showed obliteration of the hair, with absence of sebaceous glands, flattened epidermis, and dermal fibrosis. In one location, dilated hair follicles were plugged with keratin. Intralesional corticosteroids produced minimal improvement over several months.

Clinical Pearls

1. Lichen planopilaris frequently is associated with lichen planus; thus, a thorough examination of nails, mucous membranes, and skin is necessary.

2. Frontal fibrosing alopecia in postmenopausal women with progressive loss of the frontal hairline and scarring alopecia of the eyebrows is probably a variant of lichen planopilaris.

3. When lichen planopilaris is considered, a scalp biopsy should be done to exclude treatable causes of scarring alopecia.

REFERENCES

1. Issac M, McNeely MC: Dermatitis herpetiformis associated with lichen planopilaris. J Am Acad Dermatol 33:1050–1051, 1995.
2. Headington JT: Cicatricial alopecia. Dermatol Clin 14:773–782, 1996.
3. Kossard S, Lee MS, Wilkinson B: Postmenopausal frontal fibrosing alopecia: A frontal variant of lichen planopilaris. J Am Acad Dermatol 36:59–66, 1997.
4. Gerritsen MJ, de Jong EM, van de Kerkhof PC: Linear lichen planopilaris of the face. J Am Acad Dermatol 38:633–635, 1998.

PATIENT 63

A 6-year-old boy with flat papules on the face and scalp

A 6-year-old boy sustained flat papules on his forehead 1 year previously. The papules increased in number to include areas of his scalp and the extensor surfaces of his arms. There was no consanguinity or similar lesions noted in any family members. The child was in good health otherwise and had done well in his first-grade class.

Physical Examination: Skin: widely disseminated, 2- to 3-mm, flat-topped papules—skin-colored and hypopigmented—distributed over forehead and scalp (see figure); some confluent into small plaques; scattered lesions on lower face, shoulders, extensor surfaces of arms, and dorsum of hands. Remainder of examination: normal.

Laboratory Findings: HIV test: negative. CBC with differential: normal. Antinuclear antibody: negative.

Question: What are your recommendations to the parents?

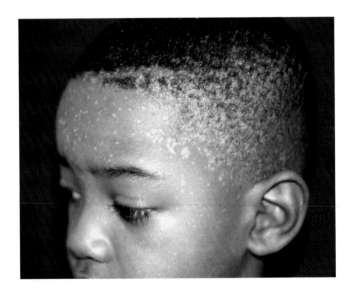

Diagnosis: Epidermodysplasia verruciformis

Discussion: Epidermodysplasia verruciformis (EV) is a rare, probably autosomal recessive genodermatosis in which there is an increased susceptibility of the skin to human papillomavirus (HPV) infections. The HPV types seen are not those common in the general population. HPV5 is observed most frequently, but also seen are 8, 9, 12, 14, 15, 17, and 19–25. Less common but reported types include 2, 3, 10, 26–30, and 38. The clinical appearance features widespread verrucae planae with white, pink, or skin-colored, flat-topped papules located on the face, trunk, extremities, and dorsum of the hands and feet. Occasionally, lesions may be red-brown, scaly macules and patches resembling tinea versicolor. Onset after sunburn has been reported, and Koebnerization may produce linear lesions. The oral cavity, palms, and soles usually are spared. Onset typically is during childhood. Malignant transformation occurs in 30–50% of patients with EV, most often squamous cell carcinoma and Bowen's disease on sun-exposed skin. These lesions usually are nonmetastasizing.

Histopathologic examination reveals swollen, irregular keratinocytes with abundant, basophilic cytoplasm containing many keratohyalin granules in the upper layer of the epidermis. Nuclei are pale and enlarged, with marginal distribution of chromatin. Intranuclear vacuoles (clear spaces) are pathognomonic. Occasional dyskeratotic cells are seen in the lower epidermis.

The *differential diagnosis* includes acquired EV-like presentations due to HIV infection, systemic lupus erythematosus, and immunosuppression secondary to chemotherapy or drugs used in transplantation. Other diseases that occasionally resemble EV include acrokeratosis verruciformis of Hopf (localized, with palmar hyperkeratosis), Darier-White disease (greasy scale, typical distribution), and epidermal nevus (distribution in Blaschko's lines).

Recent research has focused attention on EV as a model of cutaneous oncogenesis. EV-specific HPVs have been identified in immunosuppressed individuals—for example, in skin tumors of transplant recipients—as well as in cutaneous tumors in the general population. Some investigators believe that these EV-specific HPV types play a role in skin cancer pathogenesis. Another recent study implicates psoriasis as a reservoir for HPV5, which up until this time had been detected only rarely in patients without EV. This study looked at antibodies to HPV5 virus–like particles in 335 patients. Significantly higher levels were found in psoriasis patients than in controls, which included renal transplant and atopic dermatitis patients. P53 gene mutations have been looked for in a patient with EV, since p53 (tumor suppressor gene) mutations are one of the most common genetic lesions of human cancers; however, this mutation was not found.

Management of these patients includes sun avoidance and photoprotection, as well as careful surveillance for cutaneous malignancy. Malignancies should prompt surgical treatment. 5-fluoracil has been useful, as have systemic retinoids, although the latter does not clear the lesions but merely improves them. Parents should be counseled that the risk to future siblings is up to 25%.

In the present patient, photoprotection with sunscreens, hats, and sun avoidance was instituted. He was treated with 5-fluoracil, and his lesions flattened and decreased. He is being followed closely.

Clinical Pearls

1. Epidermodysplasia verruciformis is a rare, autosomal recessive, genetic susceptibility of the skin to specific types of human papillomavirus infections.

2. An EV-like presentation can be seen with HIV infection, systemic lupus erythematosus, and immunosuppression secondary to chemotherapy or transplantation.

3. Photoprotection and surveillance for cutaneous malignancy are imperative.

REFERENCES

1. Kanekura T, Kanzaki T, Kanekura S, et al: p53 gene mutations in skin cancers with underlying disorders. J Dermatol Sci 9:209–214, 1995.
2. Harris AJ, Purdie K, Leigh IM, et al: A novel human papillomavirus identified in epidermodysplasia verruciformis. Br J Dermatol 136:587–591, 1997.
3. Hopfl R, Bens G, Wieland U, et al: Human papillomavirus DNA in nonmelanoma skin cancers of a renal transplant recipient: Detection of a new sequence related to epidermodysplasia verruciformis–associated types. J Invest Dermatol 108:53–56, 1997.
4. Majewski S, Jablonska S: Human papillomavirus-associated tumors of the skin and mucosa. J Am Acad Dermatol 36:659–685, 1997.
5. Favre M, Orth G, Majewski S, Baloul S, et al: Psoriasis: A possible reservoir for human papillomavirus type 5, the virus associated with skin carcinomas of epidermodysplasia verruciformis. J Invest Dermatol 110:311–317, 1998.

PATIENT 64

A 27-year-old man with red spots on the chest

A 27-year-old man noted pruritic, erythematous macules on his chest 2 years ago. They increased in number and spread to his face and proximal arms. He was in excellent health and was not receiving medications. He denied excessive alcohol intake.

Physical Examination: Temperature 36.8°C; pulse 68; blood pressure 118/76. Skin: numerous blanchable, erythematous macules containing wiry telangiectasias scattered over chest, face, and proximal arms (see figures); light brown hyperpigmentation; some telangiectasias with mat-like appearance; no wheal elicited by vigorous stroking of lesions. Mouth: no telangiectasias. Eyes: no scleral telangiectasias. Abdomen: no hepatosplenomegaly.

Laboratory Findings: CBC with differential: normal. Liver function tests: normal. Bone scan: no lesions. Skin biopsy: pending.

Question: What is your diagnosis?

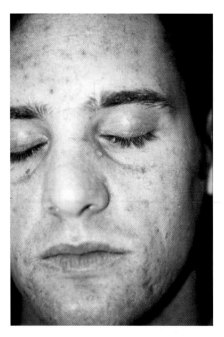

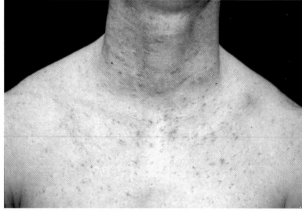

Diagnosis: Telangiectasia macularis eruptiva perstans

Discussion: Telangiectasia macularis eruptiva perstans (TMEP) is a rare form of cutaneous mastocytosis that typically develops in adults. Numerous, hyperpigmented, telangiectatic macules arise on the trunk, particularly the chest, but also on the extremities and, less often, the face. There is a background erythema, which may obscure the underlying hyperpigmentation. Characteristically, these lesions do not show Darier's sign, unlike other forms of cutaneous mastocytosis. They may urticate, however, with firm stroking or pressure. Dermatographism also may be seen. Pruritus may be present or the lesions may be asymptomatic. Bone lesions and peptic ulcer disease can be seen in association with this form of mastocytosis.

The *differential diagnosis* of multiple telangiectasias includes generalized essential telangiectasia (essential progressive telangiectasia), which usually starts on the legs and moves upward and is more common in women. One case was successfully treated with tetracycline. Localized forms include angioma serpiginosum and unilateral nevoid telangiectasia. Liver disease, such as alcoholic cirrhosis, can produce increased venous pressure as well as decreased metabolism of estrogen and lead to extensive telangiectasias. In addition to liver disease, estrogen therapy, pregnancy, and menarche can be associated with the appearance of telangiectasias. In one recent report, TMEP appeared in a pregnant woman who then suffered an anaphylactoid reaction and went into preterm labor. The authors suggested that elevated histamine levels may have induced the preterm labor.

Hereditary hemorrhagic telangiectasia (Rondu-Osler-Weber) presents with epistaxis during childhood; skin and mucous membrane telangiectasias occur later. Radiodermatitis is characterized by multiple telangiectasias. Telangiectasias are seen in poikiloderma atrophicans vasculare (PAV). PAV can be idiopathic or can be associated with connective tissue disease (e.g., systemic lupus erythematosus, dermatomyositis, or scleroderma); cutaneous T-cell lymphoma or Hodgkin's lymphoma; or a genodermatosis (e.g., Rothmund-Thomson syndrome, dyskeratosis congenita, Bloom syndrome, Cockayne syndrome, pseudoxanthoma elasticum, xeroderma pigmentosum). Ataxia telangiectasia features progressive cerebellar ataxia beginning early, usually at 1–2 years of age, as well as oculocutaneous and pinnae telangiectasia. Corticosteroid therapy frequently induces telangiectasias.

The histopathologic findings in TMEP can be subtle. Vascular ectasias are seen, with mast cells located only in the upper third of the dermis and around capillaries. There may be only a slight increase in numbers of mast cells, and specific stains such as Giemsa, toluidine blue, or the Leder method should be requested.

Treatment of TMEP that is pruritic can be attempted with antihistamines, topical steroids, or psoralens plus UVA (PUVA). Successful treatment of the telangiectasia has been accomplished using the 585-nm flashlamp-pulsed tuneable dye laser. In one recent report, all telangiectasias resolved following laser treatment, but there was recurrence 14 months later; it was stressed that H1 and H2 receptor blockade must be undertaken preoperatively and postoperatively to avoid laser-induced mast cell mediator release.

In the present patient, study of the Giemsa-stained specimen revealed vascular ectasias and characteristic location of mast cells. There was no evidence of systemic disease, and 24-hour urine collection for the histamine metabolite N-methyl-imidazole-acetic acid (N-MIAA) revealed no elevation. Since his major concern was the cosmetic appearance, particularly on the face, treatment was undertaken using the pulsed tuneable dye laser. An excellent cosmetic result was obtained. However, he was warned that recurrence was likely.

Clinical Pearls

1. When TMEP occurs in pregnancy, the increased histamine levels may induce preterm labor.

2. Successful treatment of the telangiectasias has been accomplished with the 585-nm flashlamp-pulsed tuneable dye laser. Unfortunately, good results are temporary.

3. If laser therapy is undertaken, H1 and H2 receptor blockade must be accomplished in order to prevent massive mast cell degranulation.

REFERENCES

1. Donahue JG, Lupton JB, Golichowski AM: Cutaneous mastocytosis complicating pregnancy. Obstet Gynecol 85:813–815, 1995.
2. Ellis DL: Treatment of telangiectasia macularis eruptiva perstans with the 585-nm flashlamp-pumped dye laser. Dermatol Surg 22:33–37, 1996.

PATIENT 65

A 7-year-old boy with recurrent blisters on the elbow

A 7-year-old boy sustained a cluster of vesicles and blisters 1 year previously. It was treated with oral antibiotics and resolved in 1 week. He experienced recurrence of the blisters in the same location on three more occasions; each occurrence was treated with topical antibiotics or antifungals, achieving prompt resolution. A new episode developed 4 days ago, and he was referred by his pediatrician to the Dermatology Service. He was asymptomatic, in good health, and on no medications.

Physical Examination: Vital signs: normal. Ophthalmologic: normal. Intraoral: no lesions. Skin: cluster of 3- to 5-mm vesicles and vesicopustules on red base confined to one elbow (see figure).

Laboratory Findings: CBC with differential: normal. Bacterial and fungal cultures: no growth. Tzanck preparation and viral cultures: pending.

Questions: What is the most likely diagnosis? What complications are possible?

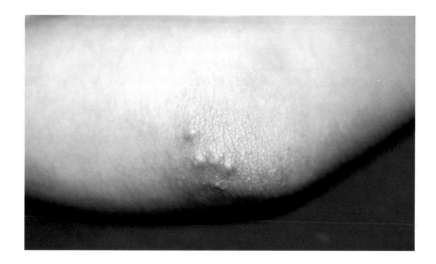

Diagnosis: Recurrent herpes simplex virus infection

Discussion: The Herpesvirus family includes varicella-zoster, cytomegalovirus, herpes simplex viruses (types I and II), Epstein-Barr virus, and human herpesvirus VI and VII. All have a nucleic acid core surrounded by a capsid and covered with glycoprotein. Herpes simplex virus (HSV) eventually infects most human beings. It enters through skin, mucous membrane, lungs, or eyes and travels along peripheral nerves to the regional sensory nerve ganglion, where it remains for the life of the individual. Stimuli such as UV light, immunosuppression, fever, and trauma reactivate the virus.

HSV infection presents clinically as grouped vesicles on a red, edematous base. There may be an abnormal sensation in the area prior to the outbreak. The vesicles are intact for a short while, often only 1 day, and may become pustular. Erosions, crusting, and re-epithelialization follow within about 1 week.

Recurrent HSV infection can be seen at any site where the primary infection was located. Most primary infections are subclinical or mild, but occasionally are severe. In young children, the severe reaction usually is seen in the mouth as primary herpetic gingivostomatis, but it can occur on the skin. The lesions of primary infection are more inflammatory, last longer, and have a greater association with systemic symptoms than do the lesions of recurrent disease.

The diagnosis is made clinically. A Tzanck preparation is performed on a new blister by removing the blister roof and scraping the base of the lesion and the underside of the roof. Giemsa or Wright stain reveals the multinucleated giant cells (keratinocytes) that are diagnostic of herpes virus infection and are not seen in other blister-producing viral diseases. Nuclei may be swollen and smudged. Viral cultures confirm the diagnosis and differentiate the types. Polymerase chain reaction amplification of viral DNA is extremely sensitive, but is not routinely available.

Histopathologic examination reveals intraepidermal vesicles produced by balloon or reticular degeneration of keratinocytes; marked acantholysis; and keratinocyte multinucleated giant cells. The nuclei are large, swollen, and slate-gray and may contain eosinophilic inclusion bodies. There is a dermal inflammatory infiltrate, and leukocytoclastic vasculitis is present in about half of the cases.

The *differential diagnosis* of recurrent blisters in the same location includes bullous mastocytoma, impetigo, contact dermatitis, and bullous fixed drug eruption.

Various complications of HSV infection have been reported. Kaposi varicelliform eruption, in which widespread HSV infection develops in patients with underlying skin diseases such as atopic dermatitis, Darier's disease, or ichthyosis, can occur. The eye can be the location of primary or recurrent HSV infection, characterized by pain, blurred vision, conjunctivitis, chorioretinitis, corneal dendrytic ulcers, and blindness. HSV pneumonia usually is associated with oropharyngeal HSV, but may rarely occur by hematogenous spread. HSV encephalitis is rare, but is the most frequent and devastating viral infection of the brain in the United States. The mortality rate is high, and survivors often have significant disabilities. Recurrent HSV-associated erythema multiforme typically is not severe and can be precipitated by sun exposure. It can be prevented by prophylactic acyclovir therapy, but one recent study showed that individual episodes may not respond.

Management of recurrent HSV may require oral suppressive antiviral agents, such as acyclovir, or may only require symptomatic treatment when episodes occur. Prophylactic acyclovir also has been useful in the prevention of recurrent disease following neonatal HSV.

In the present patient, the herpes culture revealed HSV type I. He was treated with compresses and antibacterial ointment, with prompt resolution. It was stressed that precipitating factors include sunlight and trauma and these should be strictly avoided. On follow-up examination 1 year later, he had no further recurrences.

Clinical Pearls

1. The multinucleated giant cells seen on Tzanck smear are diagnostic of herpes virus infection and are not seen in other blister-producing viral diseases.

2. HSV infects almost everyone, and recurrences are common.

3. Prophylactic, continuous acyclovir has proved useful in the prevention of recurrent HSV disease following neonatal herpes simplex.

REFERENCES
1. Weston WL, Morelli JG: Herpes simplex virus-associated erythema multiforme in prepubertal children. Arch Pediatr Adolesc Med 151:1014–1016, 1997.
2. Jacobs RF: Neonatal herpes simplex virus infections. Semin Perinatol 22:64–71, 1998.
3. Kesson AM: Use of acyclovir in herpes simplex virus infections. J Paediatr Child Health 34:9–13, 1998.

PATIENT 66

A 63-year-old man with a chronic, pruritic, scaly eruption

A 63-year-old man experienced a skin eruption during his late teen years. The eruption was widespread, pruritic, and malodorous. He had undergone many different unsuccessful therapies until he was prescribed an oral medication 2 years previously that resulted in substantial clearing. However, he discontinued the medication 1 year later due to financial reasons. He was in good health otherwise.

Physical Examination: Vital signs: normal. Skin: widespread, symmetric, red-brown, and rough papules and plaques widely distributed over face and ears, neck, trunk, and extremities (see figure). Nails: subungual hyperkeratotic material, distal notches, and both red and white longitudinal bands. Oral mucosa: cobblestone papules.

Laboratory Findings: CBC with differential, serum chemistries, and urinalysis: normal.

Questions: What is the most likely diagnosis? How would you treat this patient?

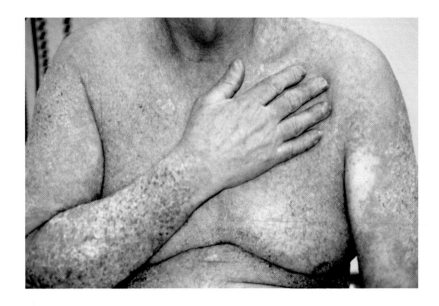

Diagnosis: Darier's disease (Darier-White, keratosis follicularis)

Discussion: Darier's disease is an autosomal dominant skin disease characterized by slowly progressive, symmetrical, red-brown papules that are greasy, hyperkeratotic, and crusted and have a waxy scale. Removal of the crust reveals central umbilication. These papules may coalesce into crusted plaques. They most commonly are located in a seborrheic distribution on the face, neck, chest, back, extremities, and scalp, particularly the scalp margins. Distribution is both follicular and nonfollicular.

The palms and soles are involved, with punctate pits and papules, in 85% of patients. The oral mucosa shows typical white, cobblestone papules. The dorsa of the hands and feet may show skin-colored or brown, flat-topped, warty papules without scale, which resemble acrokeratosis verruciformis of Hopf. The nails are thin and friable, producing a nail that is wider than it is long. Because of the fragility, distal, V-shaped notches are present. Nails also show red and white longitudinal subungual bands, subungual hyperkeratoses, and subungual splinter hemorrhages. Nail changes are present in more than 90% of patients.

Less common clinical findings include hemorrhagic macules and blisters, a flexural instead of a seborrheic distribution, and zosteriform or unilateral distributions. When Darier's disease is localized or unilateral, the average age of onset is older, about 27 years, and the most common site is the trunk. This variant may be a manifestation of genetic mosaicism, although there has not yet been a report of a patient with unilateral or localized Darier's producing offspring with Darier's disease.

Typical onset of Darier's disease is between the ages of 8 and 15 years, but it may begin any time from late childhood through early adulthood. Heat, sweating, sunlight, and exercise aggravate the disease. There often is photodistribution of the lesions. Patients frequently complain of pruritus and malodor. The latter is related to maceration in intertriginous areas and bacterial superinfection. The gene responsible for Darier's disease has been mapped to the long arm of chromosome 12 (12q23-24.1). In 50% of patients, there is no family history, suggesting a new mutation.

The pathogenesis is thought to be related to a defect in the synthesis, organization, or maturation of the tonofilament-desmosome complex. Dissolution of the desmosomal plaque proteins (desmoplakin I and II, plakoglobin, and desmoglein) results in deficient tonofilament-desmosome attachment, producing tonofilament clumping and vesicle formation. This loss of adhesion between the epidermal cells along with abnormal keratinization produces the typical histopathologic findings. The dyskeratosis is manifested as corps ronds and grains, seen in the upper layers of the epidermis and stratum corneum. Suprabasilar acantholysis is manifested as suprabasal clefts or lacunae with villi (dermal papillae lined with a single layer of basal cells protruding up into the lacunae). There also is papillomatosis, acanthosis, and hyperkeratosis.

Frequent complications include impetiginization, which occasionally has resulted in acute streptococcal glomerulonephritis and subsequent chronic renal failure. Kaposi's varicelliform eruption is not rare, and patients should strictly avoid contact with individuals infected with herpes simplex or varicella-zoster virus. There are several reports of Darier's disease associated with psychiatric disturbances, including psychosis, suicidal ideation, and intellectual deficiencies. It is unclear whether there is a valid association between the two.

The diagnosis of Darier's disease usually is straightforward when the disease is fully developed. At the onset, however, it may be confused with several other diseases. The *differential diagnosis* includes atopic dermatitis, seborrheic dermatitis, acrokeratosis verruciformis of Hopf, flat warts, epidermodysplasia verruciformis, benign familial pemphigus (Hailey-Hailey disease), acneiform eruptions, keratosis pilaris, epidermal nevi, ichthyosiform disorders, pityriasis lichenoides chronica, and histiocytosis.

Treatment begins with daily sunscreen and sun avoidance. Antibacterial soaps may reduce the incidence of impetiginization. Any infection should be treated promptly with oral antibiotics. Since the most common cause of infection is staphylococcus, appropriate antibiotics need to be chosen to cover the staphylococcus. Topical isotretinoin and tretinoin helped in some cases. Recently, a topical retinoid, tazarotene gel, was reported to be successful in a patient resistant to oral retinoids. In females with premenstrual flares, oral contraceptives may be helpful. Topical 5-fluorouracil achieved complete clearing in two patients resistant to systemic retinoids.

In the present patient, investigation revealed that he had been taking oral retinoids. Systemic retinoids were restarted. He was placed on sunscreen and a daily antibacterial soap. Three months later, his skin had cleared substantially.

Clinical Pearls

1. Darier's disease is autosomal dominant, but with a 50% new mutation rate.

2. The unilateral or zosteriform variants of Darier's disease may be an example of genetic mosaicism: there may be a risk of widespread disease transmission to offspring.

3. Superinfection of skin lesions in Darier's disease is a major problem. Streptococcal impetigo may result in acute glomerulonephritis and chronic renal failure. Staphylococcus is the most common cause of infection.

4. Many patients with Darier's disease require systemic retinoid therapy for control.

REFERENCES

1. Knulst AC, De La Faille HB, Van Vloten WA: Topical 5-fluorouracil in the treatment of Darier's disease. Br J Dermatol 133:463–466, 1995.
2. Hellwig B, Hesslinger R, Walden J: Darier's disease and psychosis. Psychiatry Res 64:205–207, 1996.
3. O'Malley MP, Bassat AS, Honer WG, et al: Linkage analysis between schizophrenia and Darier's disease region on 12q. Psychiatr Genet 6:187–190, 1996.
4. O'Malley MP, Haake A, Goldsmith L, et al: Localized Darier disease: Implications for genetic studies. Arch Dermatol 133:1134–1138, 1997.
5. Burkhart CG, Burkhart CN: Tazarotene gel for Darier's disease. J Am Acad Dermatol 38:1001–1002, 1998.

PATIENT 67

A 7-year-old boy with pruritic pustules on the hand

A 7-year-old boy had been playing in the dirt in a playground 2 days previously when he developed sharp pain in multiple areas of the hand. No arthropods were observed. His parents noted several pruritic, red papules on the hand several hours later. In addition, a large bullous lesion was noted on one finger. The parents sought medical attention because the lesions appeared to be worsening. He was in good health otherwise and was without systemic symptoms.

Physical Examination: Vital signs: normal; no angioedema. Skin: pustules on red base on right thumb and proximal third and fifth fingers; large, irregular bulla with small fissure on proximal fourth finger (see figure). Chest: no wheezing. Remainder of examination: normal.

Laboratory Findings: Cultures of bulla and pustule: no growth.

Question: What is your diagnosis?

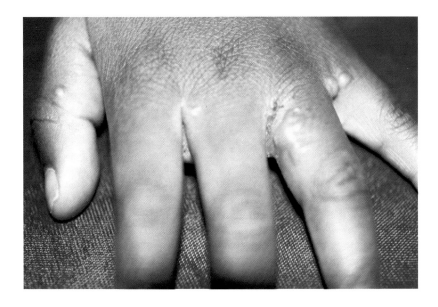

Diagnosis: Fire ant stings

Discussion: Fire ants belong to the order Hymenoptera, which includes bees, wasps, and ants. The fire ant species is Solenopsis, which is one of several ant species in the superfamily Formicoidee. There are four native species of fire ants in the United States and two imported species; the latter are *Solenopsis invicta* (red) and *Solenopsis richteri* (black). *S. invicta* is the species most commonly producing stings in humans. Imported fire ants were brought to the United States on ships and introduced into Alabama in the 1930s.

The classic clinical picture of fire ant stings is related to the stinging process. First the ant bites the victim, grasping the skin with its mandible. It then pivots its abdominal stinger (ovipositor apparatus) in a circle, stinging as it turns. This results in a circle of pustules with two hemorrhagic puncta in the center. Immediate pain is felt, but rapidly subsides. A wheal and a vesicle subsequently form within 4 hours. Within 24 hours, the classic pruritic pustule with central umbilication on a red base develops. Healing occurs over several days unless complications, which can include secondary infection, scarring, and pigmentary changes, ensue. Pustules are the most common reaction. Edema, erythema, pain, and pruritus usually resolve within hours. The reaction usually is nonallergic.

Extensive local reactions occur in about 10% of stings, with severe prolonged edema and redness lasting from 24 hours to a week. Systemic reactions to fire ant stings occur in 4 out of 100,000 exposures and range from urticaria, pruritus, malaise, and angioedema to anaphylaxis and even, rarely, death. Most deaths are related to multiple stings, and several case reports of alcoholics suffering multiple stings have been noted in the literature. Late systemic reactions include serum sickness, thrombocytopenic purpura, acute tubular necrosis, and liver failure.

The magnitude of the problem of fire ant sting reactions often is underestimated. In areas epidemic for imported fire ants, mainly the southeastern U.S., fire ant stings are the most frequent cause of Hymenoptera hypersensitivity. There appears to be a high attack rate. One recent study found that 50% of 107 medical students temporarily trained in an endemic area (San Antonio, Texas) for 3 weeks suffered stings. There has been progressive spread and increased colony density of imported fire ants in the southeastern U.S. and there is not yet a successful means of control. Fire ants live in large colonies, with mounds measuring up to 3 feet in diameter, usually in field, yard, and playground soil.

There have been several reports of fire ant colonies living in inhabited houses; one bed-bound patient was attacked at home.

Fire ant venom consists mainly of piperidine alkaloids and is bacteriocidal, hemolytic, cytotoxic, and insecticidal. Research on fire ant venom has identified the allergens of *S. invicta* venom, which are termed SOL 1 through 4. The venoms of all fire ant species are highly cross-reactive, so that it is only necessary to do testing with the imported fire ant venom if considering hyposensitization immunotherapy for allergic reactions to any of the fire ant species.

The venom skin test is the most sensitive and specific for diagnosing fire ant allergy. The majority of patients with a history of an allergic reaction to fire ant stings and a positive skin test have venom-specific IgE titers on the radioallergosorbent test (RAST). The RAST is not as specific as the skin test, however. Even with a positive skin test and a history of a systemic reaction, only 60% of patients will react to future stings. Most allergists use skin testing to diagnose fire ant allergy, and most (97% in one survey) treat with immunotherapy. Even with hyposensitization, in those patients with severe systemic reactions and a positive venom skin test, the estimated incidence of a future reaction is 7–16%.

The management of fire ant stings includes immediate treatment for anaphylaxis, if present. Patients who have had a severe systemic reaction should carry an epinephrine injection kit at all times. Otherwise, local care—ice, elevation, cleansing to avoid secondary infection, and high-potency topical corticosteroids to control the itching—is all that is necessary. In severe local reactions, a short course of oral corticosteroids is required. Destruction of fire ant mounds and avoidance in the future should be stressed to the family. Hyposensitization, when undertaken, represents a lifelong commitment of time and money and does not prevent all future reactions. Controversy exists over the use of fire ant venom versus whole body fire ant extract for the diagnosis and treatment of fire ant allergy.

In the present patient, the classic clinical picture of a pruritic pustule plus a history of playground activity suggested fire ant stings. Since he showed no signs of a systemic reaction, he was treated with strong topical corticosteroid cream and oral antihistamines for 3 days, with resolution of all symptoms. On returning to the local playground, the father noted three large fire ant mounds, which subsequently were destroyed.

Clinical Pearls

1. In areas endemic for the imported fire ant, mainly the southeastern United States, the most frequent cause of Hymenoptera hypersensitivity is the imported fire ant.

2. The classic clinical picture of fire ant stings is related to the novel method the insect uses to sting its victim.

3. The venom skin test is the most sensitive and specific for confirming fire ant venom allergy in a patient with a history of a hypersensitivity reaction. The RAST may identify venom-specific IgE titers, but is not as specific as the skin test.

4. Hyposensitization may be undertaken in patients with a severe systemic reaction to fire ant venom and a positive venom skin test, but the cost and time commitment is high and reaction prevention is not 100%.

REFERENCES

1. DeShazo RD, Williams DF: Multiple fire ant stings indoors. South Med J 88:712–715, 1995.
2. Tracy JM, Demain JG, Quinn JM, et al: The natural history of exposure to the imported fire ant (*Solenopsis invicta*). J Allergy Clin Immunol 95:824–828, 1995.
3. Stafford CT: Hypersensitivity to fire ant venom. Ann Allergy Asthma Immunol 77:87–95, 1996.
4. Freeman TM: Hymenoptera hypersensitivity in an imported fire ant endemic area. Ann Allergy Asthma Immunol 78:369–372, 1997.
5. Hoffman DR: Reactions to less common species of fire ants. J Allergy Clin Immunol 100:679–683, 1997.

PATIENT 68

A 5-year-old girl with erythematous patches on the tongue

A 5-year-old girl was noted to have red patches on her tongue for 6 months. The patches changed shape daily, and she intermittently complained of tongue discomfort. She was in good health otherwise, with no scalp, skin, nail, or joint complaints.

Physical Examination: Vital signs: normal. Tongue: three smooth, erythematous patches on dorsum of tongue; no fissuring; white, hyperkeratotic borders; no lacy reticulated plaques on buccal mucosa. Scalp: no erythema or scale. Hair: no loss or thinning. Eyes: no conjunctivitis. Joints: normal. Nails: no onycholysis, subungal debris, or "oil spots."

Laboratory Findings: No tests performed.

Question: What is the most likely diagnosis?

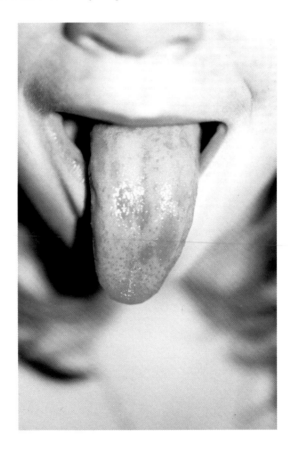

Diagnosis: Geographic tongue

Discussion: Geographic tongue also is known as annulus migrans, benign migratory glossitis, and exfoliato areata migrans. It is a benign, idiopathic, inherited, and inflammatory condition of the anterior two-thirds of the dorsum of the tongue. The condition is characterized by erythematous, single or multiple, circinate or irregularly-shaped patches that may have elevated, grey-white, advancing borders. There may be similar skin lesions elsewhere in the mouth, in which case the term "stomatitis areata migrans" is used. The patches usually are asymptomatic, but glossodynia (burning) may be present. Occasionally, spicy or hot foods produce pain. The patches may be fixed or migratory.

Geographic tongue is more common in children, usually older children, but it has been reported in infants as young as 3 months of age. The overall incidence in the population is said to be 2%, and the mode of inheritance is thought to be polygenic. Half the individuals with geographic tongue also have fissured tongue (lingua plicata). Geographic tongue has been reported in association with psoriasis, atopic dermatitis, seborrheic dermatitis, and respiratory disorders.

A biopsy of the advancing raised border demonstrates hyperkeratosis, parakeratosis, and regular acanthosis. The center of the patch shows epithelial suprapapillary thinning, transepithelial migration of neutrophils, and spongiform pustules of Kogoj in the upper epithelium. The lamina propria reveals a superficial perivascular infiltrate, which contains lymphocytes, histiocytes, and neutrophils. The clinical picture is produced by transient atrophy of the epithelium and filiform papillae. These rapidly regenerate so that the edges of the patches migrate at the rate of several millimeters per hour.

The *differential diagnosis* of geographic tongue includes pustular psoriasis and Reiter's disease. The histologic picture of these entities, with spongiform pustules of Kogoj, acanthosis, parakeratosis, and a mixed inflammatory infiltrate, resemble that of geographic tongue. Some authors believe that geographic tongue is an abortive form of pustular psoriasis. Also in the differential diagnosis is contact stomatitis, leukoplakia, lichen planus, secondary syphilis (mucous patches), fissured tongue (which shows deep furrows and is a common anatomic variant), candidiasis, and smooth tongue (nutritional deficiencies, for example of iron, riboflavin, vitamin B-12, or folic acid, can produce large areas of atrophy of filiform papillae).

Management of geographic tongue primarily includes reassurance, since the lesion is benign. Biopsy usually is not necessary. However, patients should be informed that the condition may last for months to years. Aggravating or irritating substances should be avoided. For symptomatic relief, topical corticosteroids or topical retinoid gel may be helpful. Antifungal therapy occasionally is useful, and "magic mouthwash" (various combinations of antibiotics, antifungals, antihistamines, and corticosteroids) or oral rinses with cold apple juice may provide relief.

In the present patient, reassurance and avoidance of hot or spicy food were all that was necessary.

Clinical Pearls

1. Geographic tongue, also known as annulus migrans, is an inherited condition frequently seen in association with fissured tongue.

2. Lesions elsewhere in the mouth that are clinically similar to those of geographic tongue are termed stomatitis areata migrans.

3. Geographic tongue may be an abortive form of pustular psoriasis, since the histologic pictures are similar.

REFERENCES

1. Gonzaga HF, Torres EA, Alchorne MM, et al: Both psoriasis and benign migratory glossitis are associated with HLA-Cw6. Br J Dermatol 135:368–370, 1996.
2. Zhu JF, Kaminski MJ, Pulitzer DR, et al: Psoriasis: Pathophysiology and oral manifestations. Oral Dis 2:135–144, 1996.
3. Drezner DA, Schaffer SR: Geographic tongue. Otolaryngol Head Neck Surg 117:291, 1997.

PATIENT 69

A 59-year-old man with malodorous feet

A 59-year-old man had had hyperhidrosis of the palms and soles since adolescence. He worked as an FBI agent and wore occlusive boots 12–24 hours at a time. The palmar sweating especially bothered him while he was handling his gun. He also had been bothered by malodorous feet since moving to a subtropical climate 5 years ago.

Physical Findings: Skin: excessive moisture of the palms and soles, palmar skin otherwise normal; tiny crateriform pits over volar surface of toes, weight-bearing plantar surface of foot, and heel (see figure). Remainder of physical examination: normal.

Laboratory Findings: Gram stain of thin shaving of sole's stratum corneum: pending.

Questions: What is your diagnosis? How would you treat this man?

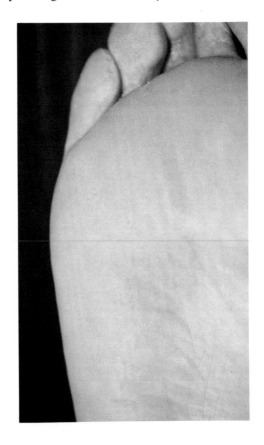

Diagnosis: Pitted keratolysis

Discussion: Pitted keratolysis (keratolysis plantara sulcarum) originally was described by Castelanni in 1910. Zais, et al. provided the name "pitted keratolysis" in 1965 for this superficial skin infection characterized by shallow, discrete crateriform defects or pits in the stratum corneum. The punched-out areas measure 1–7 mm in diameter, and they may appear brown or "dirty." The pits may coalesce to form erosions that are painful in severe cases. Fissures or crevices may develop as well.

The sites most commonly affected by pitted keratolysis are the weight-bearing areas of the feet, typically the heels, ball of the foot, and volar pads of the toes. The lesions may be seen between the toes where friction is present. The instep is spared. Rarely, pitted keratolysis involves the hands.

Factors that contribute to the development of pitted keratolysis include **hyperhidrosis**; humidity, such as in a tropical or subtropical climate; occlusive footwear, such as boots; prolonged emersion; and a living environment in which the custom is to go barefoot in wet and muddy conditions. In a recent study of 53 adults with pitted keratolysis, the most common symptom was hyperhidrosis; also common were complaints of malodor and sliminess of the skin. Many patients are asymptomatic, however.

The diagnosis can be made clinically, or the organism can be revealed by a Gram stain of a thin shaving of stratum corneum. The organism is a gram-positive, filamentous, branching Corynebacterium species, such as *C. minutissimum*. Dermatophilus and Streptomyces species also have been implicated as causative. When skin biopsies have been done, the pits are noted to involve the stratum corneum. Tissue gram stains reveal the organism in the walls and floors of the pits.

The *differential diagnosis* of pitted keratolysis includes tinea pedis, plantar warts, and eczematous conditions such as contact dermatitis and atopic dermatitis. Conditions that produce palmar pits, including basal cell nevus syndrome, Darier-White disease, palmoplantar keratosis secondary to arsenic, esophageal cancer or other cancers, and certain palmoplantar keratodermas, may cause some confusion, but rarely.

Treatment of pitted keratolysis includes control of hyperhidrosis and antibacterial therapy. Aluminum chloride 20% solution, Whitfield's ointment (benzoic and salicylic acids), and 40% formaldehyde all have been used successfully. Topical antibiotics such as erythromycin or mupirocin also have achieved good results. Rarely, oral antibiotics are used.

In the present patient, Gram stain demonstrated *C. minutissimum*. He was treated with aluminum chloride 20% solution to both the palms and soles and erythromycin solution to the soles. On follow-up visit 1 month later, the pitted keratolysis had cleared completely. The patient was very pleased with the resolution of the hyperhidrosis of the palms and soles.

Clinical Pearls

1. The most common complaints of patients with pitted keratolysis are hyperhidrosis, malodor, and slimy skin.

2. Pitted keratolysis can be diagnosed clinically or by finding the bacterium in a Gram-stained sliver of stratum corneum.

3. Pitted keratolysis is easily treated with measures to control hyperhidrosis and topical antibiotics.

REFERENCES
1. Vazquez-Lopez F, Perez-Oliva N: Mupirocin ointment for symptomatic pitted keratolysis. Infection 24:55, 1996.
2. Takama H, Tamada Y, Yano K, et al: Pitted keratolysis: Clinical manifestations in 53 cases. Br J Dermatol 137:282–285, 1997.

PATIENT 70

A 6-month-old girl with an ulcerated red plaque

The parents of a 6-month-old girl noticed a white spot on her right buttock at 2 weeks of age. Telangiectasias were noted within this area. The lesion rapidly enlarged and developed a painful ulcer 2 weeks ago. The child had been treated with compresses and oral antibiotics with partial resolution. The parents wanted a definitive diagnosis and treatment.

Physical Examination: Vital signs: normal. Skin: brightly erythematous plaque on buttock containing pale areas and a central tender, crusted ulcer (see figure); no other lesions. Abdomen: no hepatosplenomegaly.

Laboratory Findings: No tests performed.

Questions: How would you counsel the parents? What treatment would you offer for rapid relief of the child's symptoms?

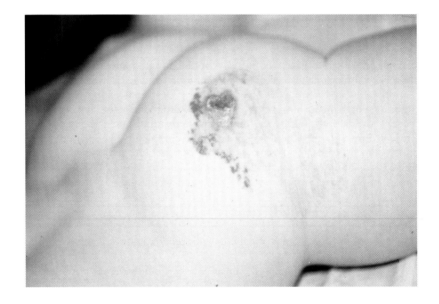

Diagnosis: Superficial hemangioma with ulceration

Discussion: Hemangiomas are benign vascular tumors of childhood (vascular birthmarks) characterized by proliferating vascular endothelium. They are different from a second type of vascular birthmark, the vascular malformation, which includes the port wine stain. Vascular malformations do not show endothelial proliferation, and they represent a structural abnormality of vasculature. Hemangiomas are classified into superficial, mixed, or deep types. The superficial type previously was termed "strawberry" or "capillary" hemangioma, but since all hemangiomas are composed of capillaries, these terms are redundant. Deep hemangiomas previously were called "cavernous." Mixed hemangiomas contain both deep and superficial elements and are probably the most common type of hemangioma. Superficial hemangiomas are the next most common, and deep hemangiomas are the least common variety.

The natural history of hemangiomas is well studied and involves a changing clinical appearance. Approximately 30% of hemangiomas are present at birth, but most are first noticed at 3–5 weeks of age. They may begin as a white or pale macule containing wiry telangiectasias, or as a red macule resembling a port wine stain. Rapid growth occurs for the next 6–8 months, resulting in a raised, brightly erythematous or purple, lobulated tumor. Maximum growth is reached by 10–12 months and is followed by slow involution. As regression begins, the bright color fades and grey-white areas appear within the tumor. Complete regression occurs in 50% of patients by the age of 5 years, 70% by the age of 7, 90% by the age of 9, and up to 97% by the age of 12. Residual changes following regression include atrophic or redundant skin, scarring, telangiectasias, and hypopigmentation.

The incidence of hemangiomas is high, with 2.6% of all newborns having at least one hemangioma by the age of 1 year. Incidence in Caucasian infants is 10–12%, and girls are affected three times more frequently than boys. There is a positive family history of hemangiomas in at least 10% of affected individuals. Sites most commonly affected are the head and neck, and the next most common site is the trunk.

Complications include ulceration, which occurs in about 10%, and infection, bleeding, and scarring, which occur less often. Hemangiomas may be markers of internal disease. Large facial hemangiomas have been reported in association with ipsilateral cerebellar hypoplasia and the Dandy-Walker malformation. Midline spinal hemangiomas can be markers of spinal dysraphism or the tethered cord syndrome. Interference with a vital function by the hemangioma requires intervention. Large or internal hemangiomas may produce airway obstruction, feeding difficulties, or visual occlusion. Diffuse neonatal hemangiomatosis involves numerous skin hemangiomas in association with internal organ hemangiomas, most often liver, lungs, gastrointestinal tract, and central nervous system. The Kasabach-Merritt syndrome is due to platelet sequestration and clotting within a rapidly enlarging hemangioma accompanied by thrombocytopenia, hemolytic anemia, and disseminated intravascular coagulation.

Therapy of hemangiomas, because of their natural history, may be expectant and conservative in most cases. The natural history should be discussed in detail with the parents. When systemic therapy is required, intralesional or oral corticosteroids often provide excellent results, especially in superficial and mixed hemangiomas requiring treatment. Deep hemangiomas do not respond as well. Oral corticosteroids are the first choice for many of the complications of hemangiomas, as well. When high-dose oral corticosteroids are ineffective, interferon alpha-2a has produced good results. One recent study reported success using interferon alpha-2b. Side effects of interferon include fever, neutropenia, skin necrosis, and elevated liver function tests.

Use of the pulsed tuneable-dye laser in the treatment of hemangiomas is controversial. Studies have shown good results on superficial hemangiomas treated early, particularly when they are still macular. However, many of these lesions are expected to spontaneously involute. The laser has produced excellent results in increasing the healing and decreasing the pain of ulcerated superficial hemangiomas and good results in improving the appearance of cosmetically undesirable hemangiomas of the face, nose, and hands.

In the present patient, topical compresses and zinc oxide paste in conjunction with oral antibiotics did not produce resolution of the pain and ulcer. Therefore, the pulsed tuneable-dye laser was applied. After two treatment sessions, all symptoms completely resolved and clinical appearance improved.

Clinical Pearls

1. Vascular birthmarks are classified into two types: hemangiomas, which consist of proliferating vascular endothelium, and vascular malformations, which show no endothelial proliferation.

2. Hemangiomas are classified as superficial, deep, or mixed. The terms "capillary," "strawberry," and "cavernous" are of historical interest. All hemangiomas consist of capillaries, and most hemangiomas develop larger vascular channels as they age.

3. The natural history of hemangiomas should be considered when contemplating use of the newer treatment technologies.

REFERENCES

1. Scheepers JH, Quaba AA: Does the pulsed tunable dye laser have a role in the management of infantile hemangiomas? Observations based on 3 years' experience. Plast Reconstr Surg 95:305–312, 1995.
2. Gangopadhyay AN, Sinha CK, Gopal SC, et al: Role of steroid in childhood haemangioma: A 10-year review. Int Surg 82:49–51, 1997.
3. Matsui T, Ono T, Kito M, et al: Extensive facial strawberry mark associated with cerebellar hypoplasia and vascular abnormalities. J Dermatol 24:113–116, 1997.
4. Tamayo L, Ortiz DM, Orozco-Covarrubias L, et al: Therapeutic efficacy of interferon alpha-2b in infants with life-threatening giant hemangiomas. Arch Dermatol 133:1567–1571, 1997.
5. Jackson R: The natural history of strawberry naevi. J Cutan Med Surg 2:187–189, 1998.

PATIENT 71

A 2-year-old boy with a pruritic eruption under the right arm

A 2-year-old boy experienced a mildly pruritic eruption under his right arm, which spread to involve his medial arm, flank, and chest within several days. His pediatrician prescribed topical steroids; however, the eruption progressively spread onto his left periaxillary area. He had a mild cough and rhinorrhea 1 week previously, but was currently without respiratory symptoms.

Physical Examination: Temperature 36.8°C. Skin: erythematous papules and plaques with scale and poorly defined border over right flank and medial upper arm (see figure); scattered erythematous papules and fine scale on left flank.

Laboratory Findings: KOH examination: negative for hyphal elements. CBC: mild lymphocytosis.

Questions: What is your diagnosis? How would you counsel the parents?

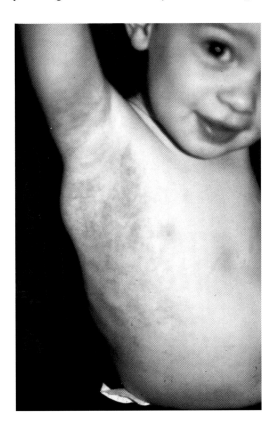

Diagnosis: Unilateral laterothoracic exanthem

Discussion: Unilateral laterothoracic exanthem, also known as asymmetric periflexural exanthem of childhood, is a recently described exanthem of young children that has an unusual distribution. The primary lesions are erythematous macules and papules (morbilliform eruption), which may coalesce into circinate, annular, or reticulate patterns. The eruption becomes eczematous or scarlatiniform and ends with a fine, branny (wheat bran–like) desquamation. The eruption begins on one side of the trunk close to the axilla or, less often, the inguinal crease and then spreads centrifugally to become bilateral, retaining a unilateral predominance. There are no excoriations or lichenification.

Most cases are seen in children under the age of 3 years, and the mean age of onset is 2 years. However, there have been recent case reports of unilateral laterothoracic exanthem occurring in adults. There is a female predominance of 2:1. The eruption resolves spontaneously in a mean of 5 weeks (range 4–6 weeks), but may last up to 4 months. Brief recurrences may be seen months after resolution.

Although termed a rare and recently described childhood exanthem, unilateral laterothoracic exanthem may have been reported in the 1960s as lichen miliaris. Some authors give credit to Bodemer and DePrest for the first descriptions of asymmetric, periflexural exanthem of childhood.

Although skin biopsies are unnecessary because of the typical clinical presentation, histologic study reveals a unique, eccrine, lymphocytic infiltrate.

The cause of unilateral laterothoracic exanthem is suspected to be viral. It may represent a specific skin reaction to one or more infectious agents. There often are signs of a preceding infection, including fever, upper respiratory tract symptoms, pharyngitis, otitis, vomiting, and diarrhea.

The *differential diagnosis* of unilateral laterothoracic exanthem includes tinea corporis and contact dermatitis. Also consider atopic dermatitis, drug eruption, scabies, scarlet fever, miliaria, and atypical pityriasis rosea.

Treatment is unnecessary, since the disease is self-limited with spontaneous resolution. If pruritus is present, oral antihistamines and topical emollients usually suffice. Topical steroids usually are not helpful. There is a single report of unilateral laterothoracic exanthem in a 6-year-old girl with acute lymphoblastic leukemia, but no other evidence to date that unilateral laterothoracic exanthem is associated with more serious conditions.

In the present patient, topical antihistamines and a soothing emollient relieved the itching. The eruption spread to the groin area bilaterally and subsequently faded. It resolved with mild desquamation by 10 weeks.

Clinical Pearls

1. Unilateral laterothoracic exanthem, also known as asymmetric periflexural exanthem of childhood, is easily confused with contact dermatitis and tinea corporis at the onset.
2. Unilateral laterothoracic exanthem may have a prolonged course of up to 4 months.
3. Asymmetric periflexural exanthem of childhood has now been reported to occur in adults.

REFERENCES
1. McCuaig CC, Russ P, Powell J, et al: Unilateral laterothoracic exanthem: A clinicopathologic study of 48 patients. J Am Acad Dermatol 34:979–984, 1996.
2. Gutzmer R, Herbst RA, Kiehl P, et al: Unilateral laterothoracic exanthem (asymmetrical periflexural exanthem of childhood): Report of an adult patient. J Am Acad Dermatol 37:484–485, 1997.
3. Fort DW, Greer KE: Unilateral laterothoracic exanthem in a child with acute lymphoblastic leukemia. Pediatr Dermatol 15:51–52, 1998.
4. Pride HB: Pediatric dermatoses commonly seen, uncommonly recognized. Pediatr Ann 27:129–130, 1998.

PATIENT 72

A 10-year-old girl with an erythematous nodule on the lower lip

A 10-year-old girl sustained an erythematous, soft, friable nodule on her lip 1 year previously. It bled easily whenever she brushed her teeth or ate. It was excised, but rapidly regrew to its present size.

Physical Examination: Skin: 1-cm, darkly erythematous, soft, and slightly pedunculated nodule with collarette at base located on middle of lower lip (see figure); no satellite lesions. Lymph nodes: no lymphadenopathy.

Laboratory Findings: No tests performed.

Question: What is the differential diagnosis?

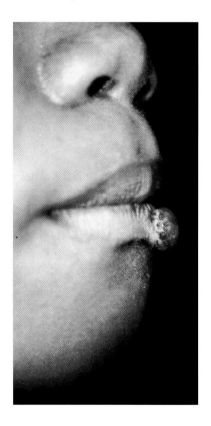

Diagnosis: Pyogenic granuloma

Discussion: Pyogenic granuloma (lobular capillary hemangioma) is a benign vascular growth, usually solitary, varying from 1 mm to 2 cm in size. It occurs most often on the face or fingers, but can be seen anywhere on the skin. Crocker provided the name granuloma pyogenicum in 1903, because he thought these lesions were of bacterial origin. The lesion is friable, so that oozing and bleeding occur frequently, especially following trauma. Erosions, ulcerations, and crusting commonly are present.

Pyogenic granuloma frequently occurs in the oral cavity, most often on the gingiva. Pregnancy is a precipitating factor, and the lesion often is termed **"pregnancy gingivitis"** or **"pregnancy tumor."** Although unusual, severe bleeding necessitating induction of labor has occurred in pregnancy.

Recurrent pyogenic granuloma with multiple satellite lesions (Warner and Wilson-Jones syndrome) occurs rarely. It is benign but may cause concern because of its "pseudo-metastatic" appearance. It occurs after removal or mechanical irritation of a pyogenic granuloma. Curiously, most cases of recurrent pyogenic granuloma with multiple satellitosis have been reported in children with lesions on the trunk and in the region of the scapula.

The *differential diagnosis* of pyogenic granuloma includes amelanotic melanoma, early lesions of Kaposi's sarcoma, angiosarcoma, papular angioplasia, capillary hemangioma, excessive granulation tissue, and early cherry hemangioma.

Treatment may be accomplished with a superficial shave followed by electrodessication of the base under local anesthesia. Other options include cryotherapy and multiple pulses of the pulsed-dye laser. Excision with suture placement is not required and should not be done. If a destructive method is chosen, a biopsy should be performed to exclude amelanotic melanoma. If satellite lesions occur following removal, observation is warranted, as most will spontaneously involute within 6–12 months.

In the present patient, a shave biopsy with electrodesiccation was performed under local anesthesia. Histopathologic examination revealed a pedunculated nodule composed of a proliferation of endothelial cells and capillary lumina. At the base was an inward growth of epidermis producing an epidermal collarette. There was stromal edema without an inflammatory infiltrate. There was no recurrence.

Clinical Pearls

1. Bleeding is common in pyogenic granuloma, but rarely is severe. Severe bleeding has been reported in a pregnant patient with a gingival pyogenic granuloma.

2. Recurrent pyogenic granuloma with multiple satellite lesions occurs most commonly in children in the region of the scapula. Satellite lesions usually resolve spontaneously.

3. The 585-nm pulsed-dye laser is a safe, effective treatment for pyogenic granuloma. However, a biopsy must be done first to exclude amelanotic melanoma.

REFERENCES

1. González S, Vibhagool C, Falo LD, Jr, et al: Treatment of pyogenic granulomas with the 585-nm pulsed-dye laser. J Am Acad Dermatol 35:428–431, 1996.
2. Le meur Y, Bedane C, Clavere P, et al: A proliferative vascular tumor of the skin in a kidney-transplant recipient (recurrent pyogenic granuloma with satellitosis). Nephrol Dial Transplant 12:1271–1273, 1997.
3. Senser M, Derancourt C, Blanc D, et al: Recurrent pyogenic granuloma or Warner and Wilson-Jones syndrome. Arch Pediatr 4:653–655, 1997.
4. Wang PH, Chao HT, Lee WL, et al: Severe bleeding from a pregnancy tumor: A case report. J Reprod Med 42:359–362, 1997.

PATIENT 73

A 59-year-old man with itchy, red bumps

A 59-year-old man opened his wooden-sided hot tub for the first time in several months and soaked for 2 hours. He noted that "the bromine level was too low." Two days later itchy papules rapidly developed over his trunk, buttocks, and extremities. He was otherwise in good health.

Physical Examination: Vital signs: normal. Skin: erythematous, 3- to 6-mm, follicular papules with superimposed pinpoint pustules scattered over trunk, buttocks, arms, and legs (see figure).

Laboratory Findings: CBC: normal. Culture of pustule: *Pseudomonas aeruginosa*. Culture from water of hot tub: *P. aeruginosa*.

Questions: What is your diagnosis? How would you manage this entity?

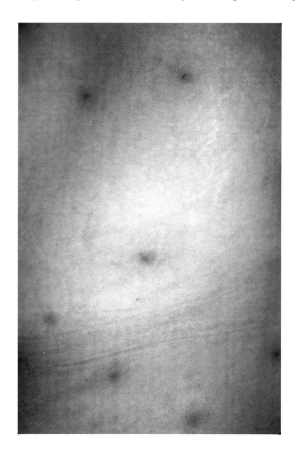

Diagnosis: Hot tub folliculitis

Discussion: Hot tub folliculitis is a superficial infection caused by *Pseudomonas aeruginosa*. Outbreaks of this folliculitis were reported in the 1970s and 1980s due to contaminated health spas and whirlpools. The eruption characteristically begins 6 hours to 5 days after the use of a contaminated hot tub and features pruritic, urticarial papules and deep pustules, usually on red bases. The eruption is distributed over the trunk, buttocks, legs and arms, but the head and neck usually are spared.

While bathing in contaminated water, for example in hot tubs, spas, and swimming pools, is the most common cause of hot tub folliculitis, **Pseudomonas folliculitis** has resulted from other factors, as well. The use of contaminated objects while bathing has produced Pseudomonas folliculitis. In a study of 13 patients, commercial bathing sponges were found to contain the same serogroup of *P. aeruginosa* as was recovered from the affected patients. These authors noted that serogroup O:11 is the most common type of *P. aeruginosa* implicated in hot tub folliculitis. In their group of patients they also found subgroups O:3 and O:6, not previously reported as sources. The different strains of *P. aeruginosa* were identified using O-serogrouping and pyocin typing and subtyping. Another report implicated the use of commercial diving suits as a cause of Pseudomonas folliculitis. Pseudomonas folliculitis after shaving of legs is well known to dermatologists. A recent report stated that a contaminated sponge used to wash the legs after depilation was the source of the *P. aeruginosa*. Pseudomonas folliculitis unrelated to hot tubs, spas, or pools occurs in hospitalized patients.

The *differential diagnosis* of Pseudomonas folliculitis includes: other gram-positive and gram-negative causes of folliculitis; infundibulofolliculitis (spongiosis in the follicle, associated with atopic dermatitis); follicular pityriasis rosea (more common in blacks); follicular eczema; follicular drug eruption (e.g., phenobarbital, dilantin, lithium, iodides, steroids); sarcoid; secondary syphilis; chloracne (e.g., agent orange, dioxin exposure); agminate folliculitis (*Trichophyton verrucosum*); eruptive vellus hair cysts; pityrosporum folliculitis; viral folliculitis; perforating folliculitis; follicular cutaneous T-cell lymphoma; lichen spinulosus; eosinophilic folliculitis; phrynoderma (vitamin A deficiency); and lichen scrofulasorum.

Management of hot tub folliculitis only requires removal of the contaminated source. Most cases heal spontaneously in 7–10 days. Occasionally, there are residual, postinflammatory pigmentary changes. Recurrences have been reported up to 2 months after resolution.

In the present patient, the eruption resolved spontaneously in 5 days with no therapy. He had the bromine level in his hot tub elevated appropriately.

Clinical Pearls

1. Hot tub folliculitis is caused by *Pseudomonas aeruginosa*, most often serogroup O:11, which can be cultured from the patient's pustules and the water or walls of the hot tub.

2. *P. aeruginosa* strains are differentiated on the basis of O-serogrouping and pyocin typing and subtyping.

3. Hot tub folliculitis is self-limited, with spontaneous healing in 7–10 days.

REFERENCES

1. Agger WA, Mardan A: *Pseudomonas aeruginosa* infections of intact skin. Clin Infect Dis 20:302–308, 1995.
2. Maniatis AN, Karkavitsas C, Maniatis NA, et al: *Pseudomonas aeruginosa* folliculitis due to non-O:11 serogroups: Acquisition through use of contaminated synthetic sponges. Clin Infect Dis 21:437–439, 1995.
3. De La Cuadra J, Gil-Mateo P, Llucian R: *Pseudomonas aeruginosa* folliculitis after depilation. Ann Dermatol Venereol 123:268–270, 1996.
4. Hogan PA: Pseudomonas folliculitis. Australas J Dermatol 38:93–94, 1997.
5. Saltzer KR, Schutzer PJ, Weinberg JM, et al: Diving suit dermatitis: A manifestation of Pseudomonas folliculitis. Cutis 59:245–246, 1997.

PATIENT 74

A 2-year-old boy with a pruritic, erythematous, linear lesion

A 2-year-old boy sustained an itchy, red papule on his leg, which then spread in a linear and serpiginous fashion. He had not visited the beach or played outside in the dirt; however, he attended daycare, where there was a large, open sandbox. The child was otherwise asymptomatic and in good health. Topical steroid creams had been tried without success.

Physical Examination: Vital signs: normal. Skin: erythematous, serpiginous track, approximately 2- to 3-mm wide, extending from front of left leg around to back of calf (see figure); frontal lesion raised, bright red, and edematous; lateral lesion flatter and pinker; some areas of serpiginous linear hypopigmentation on posterior calf.

Laboratory Findings: CBC: mild eosinophilia.

Questions: What is the most likely diagnosis? What is the most appropriate treatment?

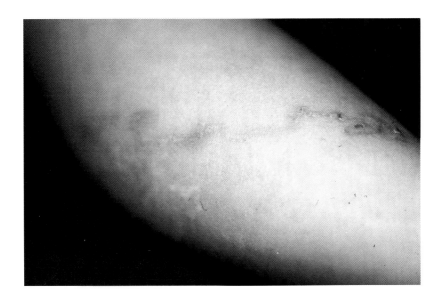

Diagnosis: Cutaneous larva migrans

Discussion: Cutaneous larva migrans ("creeping eruption") is due to the migration through the skin of filiform larvae of several **roundworm species** that usually do not parasitize humans. Clinically, an erythematous, itchy papule develops within a few hours of penetration by the larvae. After a brief incubation period of up to 2 days, the larvae begin moving through the epidermis, producing a 2- to 3-mm wide, thread-like track that is elevated, erythematous, and serpiginous and that corresponds to the burrow. The migration rate is a few mm to 1–2 cm per day. The track may be edematous or vesicular, and urticaria and peripheral eosinophilia may be present. Older lesions become dry and crusted, with gradual resolution. Postinflammatory pigmentary changes may occur.

The causative organism of cutaneous larva migrans is most commonly the dog and cat hookworm, *Ancylostoma braziliense*. Other common causes include *A. caninum, A. caylanicum, Uncinaria stenocephala,* and *Bunostomum phlebotomum*. Another possible organism is *Dirofilaria conjunctiva*, and atypical, rare, or abortive forms may be caused by the human hookworms *Necator americanus* and *A. duodenali*. The hookworm lives in the intestines of the dog or cat, and ova are deposited in their feces. The eggs hatch best in a shady, sandy, and warm environment (tropical or subtropical areas) and grow to 500–700 microns in length. After several molts, third-stage filariform larvae develop, which can penetrate human skin. Occasionally, they may penetrate through clothing and beach towels as well.

The most common infected sites include the feet, buttocks, and hands, which reflect the areas that come into contact with contaminated soil or sand. Lesions can be seen on plumber's or electrician's knees, children's buttocks secondary to sitting in sandboxes, or on beachwalker's soles.

Several days after the larvae penetrate the skin, probably through eccrine ducts or hair follicles, they burrow through the skin. They cannot penetrate the human dermis and therefore are unable to complete their life cycle. The larvae die within weeks to months. In the normal host (dog or cat), after penetration of the dermis, the larvae migrate to the lungs via the vasculature and lymphatic channels and then travel to the trachea, where they are coughed up and swallowed. Once in the gastrointestinal tract, the larvae molt again to become adult worms. The larvae in skin are approximately 0.5 mm long. They are not located in the erythematous, thread-like lesion, but are within 1 to 2 cm of the advancing edge of the track.

Complications from cutaneous larva migrans include secondary bacterial infection due to the intense pruritus and scratching. This secondary infection may obscure the primary lesion. Rarely, the larvae penetrate the dermis and complete their life cycle in the human. This unusual occurrence may result in Loeffler's syndrome or transitory pulmonary infiltrates with peripheral eosinophilia.

The *differential diagnosis* usually is not problematic. Scabies and impetigo occasionally need to be excluded. Larva currens, named from the Latin word for "running," spreads much more rapidly, up to 10 cm per day. It is caused by *Strongyloides stercoralis* and is seen in parts of the world where humans defecate on the ground and do not wear shoes. The organism enters through the feet, arrives in the gastrointestinal tract, and produces lesions beginning in the perianal area. Pruritic, urticarial, perianal bands that rapidly extend over the abdomen, buttocks, and thighs form the classic clinical picture.

Gnathostomiasis, seen in Southeast Asia, also is known as larva migrans profundus or eosinophilic nodular migratory panniculitis. It is caused by a parasite in the gastrointestinal tracts of leopards, tigers, cats, and dogs and requires passage through an aquatic intermediate host. Humans usually acquire it from eating raw fish. A recent report described six Japanese men who developed gnathostomiasis from eating the raw flesh of a poisonous snake. The clinical presentation is subcutaneous, pruritic, urticarial plaques that may be migratory. A biopsy reveals eosinophilic panniculitis.

Migratory myiasis is due to fly larvae in the skin. The usual presentation is a boil-like lesion with a central, draining opening; the lesion often moves spontaneously. The fly larvae are much larger than the larvae that cause cutaneous larva migrans: the outlines of fly larvae can be detected through the skin. Antibodies to the various parasites may be measured using the Ouchterlony method or an enzyme-linked immunosorbent assay to confirm the diagnosis.

Management of cutaneous larva migrans typically is straightforward. Topical thiabendazole 10–15% cream or suspension, or the oral suspension used topically, 4 to 6 times/day for 1 week usually is sufficient. Even without treatment, spontaneous resolution occurs in 1–2 months (80% cleared within 4 weeks in one study and 50% cleared within 12 weeks in another study). Most organisms produce an increased inflammatory reaction when they die; however, the roundworms of cutaneous larva migrans cause no reaction when they die. Instead, the migratory track stops moving, fades, and resolves. In widespread or noncompliant cases, oral medication may be used. Thiabendazole is successful, but new reports of albendazole show that it may be more efficacious and require a shorter course. Invermectin has been extremely successful as a single dose. The older method of liquid nitrogen destruction of the larva is not reliable, since it is difficult to localize the worm accurately. Even in healthy individuals, topical therapy occasionally fails. There is a single report of failure for almost 2 years, which may have been due to the organism residing deep in the hair follicle, where the medication did not penetrate.

In the present patient, histopathologic examination revealed the parasite, thought to have been acquired from the sandbox at the child's daycare center. He was treated with topical thiabendazole cream 15% applied q.i.d. for 1 week. Spread of the lesion stopped within 24 hours, and the track became dry and scaly. The skin disorder resolved with minimal postinflammatory hypopigmentation.

Clinical Pearls

1. The larva causing cutaneous larva migrans is not located in the erythematous, serpiginous burrow, but rather is within a 1- to 2-cm radius of the advancing edge of the track.

2. Unlike many other organisms that produce human disease, death of the larva causing cutaneous larva migrans does not produce an inflammatory reaction in the skin.

3. Although topical treatment usually is sufficient for cutaneous larva migrans, there are reports of treatment failure. In these cases, the medication may not have penetrated deeply into hair follicles.

REFERENCES

1. Chabasse D, Le Clec'h C, de Gentile L, et al: Larva migrans. Sante 5:341–345, 1995.
2. Richey TK, Gentry RH, Fitzpatrick JE, et al: Persistent cutaneous larva migrans due to Ancylostoma species. South Med J 89:609–611, 1996.
3. Rizzitelli G, Scarabelli G, Veraldi S: Albendazole: A new therapeutic regimen in cutaneous larva migrans. Int J Dermatol 36:700–703, 1997.
4. Elgart ML: Creeping eruption. Arch Dermatol 134:619–620, 1998.
5. Kurokawa M, Ogata K, Sagawa MS, et al: Cutaneous and visceral larva migrans due to Gnathostoma doloresi infection via an unusual route. Arch Dermatol 134:638–639, 1998.

PATIENT 75

A 65-year-old woman with hand and foot eruptions

A 65-year-old woman suffered an intermittent, tender, erythematous, and pustular eruption on her palms and soles 4 years previously. The paronychial skin and nails were severely involved. This eruption was treated with keratolytics and superpotent topical steroids, without satisfactory improvement. She had a 20-year history of small, erythematous, scaling papules and plaques over the elbows, knees, and legs. These lesion were controlled with topical steroid applications. Her only medication was a beta-blocker for hypertension.

Physical Examination: Vital signs: normal. Palms and soles: erythematous, scaly plaques containing pustules (see figure). Nails: thickening, onycholysis, subungual debris, and paronychial erythema, edema, and tenderness. Skin: faintly erythematous, scaly papules and plaques over elbows, knees, and anterior legs. Remainder of skin examination, including eyes, mouth, and genitalia: normal.

Laboratory Findings: Routine patch testing: negative. KOH examination: no fungus. Fungal culture: no growth. Skin biopsies of leg papule and foot pustule: pending.

Question: What therapeutic intervention would you recommend?

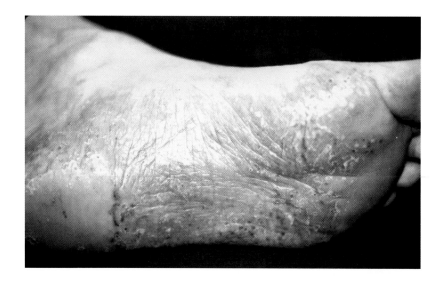

Diagnosis: Acrodermatitis continua of Hallopeau

Discussion: Acrodermatitis continua of Hallopeau is a form of pustular or erosive psoriasis. Pustular psoriasis can be divided into localized and generalized varieties. **Generalized pustular psoriasis** of von Zumbusch usually occurs suddenly in patients with pre-existing psoriasis. It is accompanied by hypocalcemia and can be precipitated by systemic medications, notably corticosteroids, penicillin, nystatin, progesterone, salicylates, and iodide. Generalized pustular psoriasis occurring during the third trimester of pregnancy, known as impetigo herpetiformis, also is accompanied by hypocalcemia and features increased maternal and fetal morbidity and mortality. **Localized pustular psoriasis** can be divided into three types: pustules that develop within existing plaques of typical psoriasis vulgaris; pustular psoriasis of the palms and soles—the most common localized type; and acrodermatitis continua of Hallopeau, the third and rarest type of localized pustular psoriasis, considered to be synonymous with dermatitis repens.

Pustular psoriasis of the palms and soles (pustulosis palmaris et plantaris of Barber) is characterized by sterile pustules of the volar skin and digits, most commonly located in the mid palms, thenar eminences of the hands, and the heels and insteps of the feet. There usually are papulosquamous lesions of psoriasis elsewhere. The acral portions of the fingers and toes typically are *not* involved. As the lesions resolve, the pustules form brown macules. Clinically identical to this entity is pustular bacterid of Andrews, which in the 1930s was thought to represent a reaction to an infectious focus elsewhere in the body.

Acrodermatitis continua of Hallopeau may have accompanying systemic symptoms and lesions elsewhere. The nails and acral areas of the digits are primarily involved. Inflammation may be so great that resulting erythema, erosions, and pustules resemble acute paronychial infection. Suppurative changes may be accompanied by radiographic changes in the distal phalanges. Atrophy of the skin of the digits and permanent loss of the nails may follow.

Histologic examination of both localized and generalized pustular psoriasis reveals unilocular intraepidermal pustules filled with neutrophils. These sterile pustules are called **spongiform pustules of Kogoj**. The term spongiform refers to the sponge-like network formed from degenerated and thinned keratinocytes around the border of the pustule. The keratinocytes undergo complete cytolysis in the center of the cavity, resulting in large macropustules. Also characteristic of pustular psoriasis are **Monroe's microabscesses**. As the spongiform pustule moves up into the stratum corneum, the neutrophils become pyknotic, producing a characteristic pattern. Other histopathologic findings of typical psoriasis are parakeratosis, acanthosis with elongation of rete ridges, and a neutrophilic dermal infiltrate with increased dermal vascularity.

The *differential diagnosis* of scaly, red plaques on the palms and soles with nail involvement includes tinea manuum and pedis, onychomycocis, and paronychial infection. The most common cause of tinea pedis accompanied by vesicles is *Trichophyton mentagrophytes* of the granular variant. An eczematous process, such as an id reaction, dyshidrotic eczema, or contact dermatitis, also should be considered. Reiter's syndrome can produce pustules that later become crusted, hyperkeratotic plaques on the palms and soles (keratoderma blennorrhagicum). Reiter's syndrome most often is seen in young males and is characterized by urethritis, conjunctivitis, and arthritis.

Management of localized pustular psoriasis can be difficult. Keratolytics and superpotent steroids can be tried, but they often are not adequate. Some authors have found calcipotriol or tazarotene to produce good symptomatic relief. Black Cat—equal parts crude coal tar, acetone, and collodion that is painted onto the skin—has produced good results in some cases (personal communication from Richard L. Dobson, M.D.). Systemic therapies often are required, and good results have been obtained with psoralen plus ultraviolet A (PUVA) therapy, including hand and foot bath PUVA. Other systemic therapies include retinoids or the combination of PUVA with retinoids; cyclosporin-A; and methotrexate. A recent report from Japan noted marked improvement using oral itraconazole. Pustulation stopped in seven patients after 2 weeks on oral itraconazole, but all patients experienced relapses when the itraconazole was discontinued. Itraconazole is known to have immunosuppressive properties, such as suppression of chemotaxis, random movement of neutrophils, and mitogen-induced transformation of lymphocytes.

In the present patient, acrodermatitis continua of Hallopeau was pinpointed by the primary involvement of the nails and acral portions of the digits, as well as the characteristic findings on skin biopsy. The development of the patient's hand and foot disease paralleled the use of the beta-blocker. Since beta-blockers can aggravate psoriasis, it was discontinued. She was started on PUVA therapy three times per week, and good results were obtained within several months.

Clinical Pearls

1. Acrodermatitis continua of Hallopeau is a rare type of localized pustular psoriasis characterized by severe involvement of the tips of the toes and fingers, nails, and paronychial skin.

2. Medications implicated in the precipitation or aggravation of pustular psoriasis include iodides, salicylates, tar, anthralins, progesterone, birth control pills, lithium, penicillin, and nystatin.

3. Treatment of localized pustular psoriasis is problematic. Aside from keratolytics and potent topical corticosteroids, topical agents that might be used include Black Cat, calcipotriene, and tazarotene. PUVA and systemic retinoids are the mainstay of systemic therapy. Oral itraconazole may prove beneficial in the future.

REFERENCES

1. Emtestam L, Weden U: Successful treatment for acrodermatitis continua of Hallopeau using topical calcipotriol. Br J Dermatol 135:644–646, 1996.
2. Kuijpers AL, van Dooren-Greebe RJ, van de Kerkhof PC: Acrodermatitis continua of Hallopeau: Response to combined treatment with acitretin and calcipotriol ointment. Dermatology 192:357–359, 1996.
3. Behrens S, von Kobyletzki G, Hoffman K, et al: PUVA-bath photochemotherapy in Hallopeau's acrodermatitis continua suppurativa. Hautarzt 48:824–827, 1997.
4. Mihara M, Hagari Y, Morimura T, et al: Itraconazole as a new treatment for pustulosis palmaris et plantaris. Arch Dermatol 134:639–640, 1998.
5. Mooser G, Pillekamp H, Peter RU: Suppurative acrodermatitis continua of Hallopeau: A differential diagnosis of paronychia. Dtsch Med Wochenschr 123:386–390, 1998.

PATIENT 76

An 8-year-old girl with numerous red and skin-colored papules

An 8-year-old girl was noted to have papules on her face since birth. The papules had been previously diagnosed as milia, miliaria, dermatitis, or infantile acne. Her parents were concerned because small pitted scars had appeared on her face. The child was completely symptomatic and in good health.

Physical Examination: Skin: symmetrical distribution of numerous 1- to 2-mm, follicular papules; erythematous and skin-colored; most pronounced over cheeks, but also on chin, eyebrows, ears, and neck (see figure); tiny, reticulated, pitted scars on both cheeks; follicular papules in eyebrows with thinning of lateral brows. Nails, teeth, and scalp: normal.

Laboratory Findings: No tests performed.

Question: What is your diagnosis?

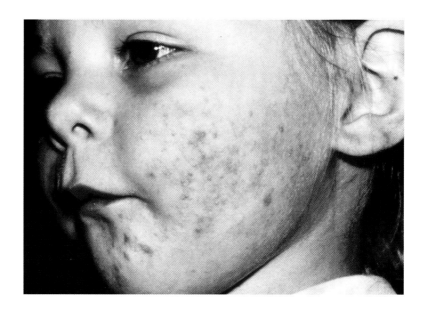

Diagnosis: Keratosis pilaris atrophicans faciei

Discussion: Keratosis pilaris and its many variants, classified together under the term "scarring keratosis pilaris," are inherited disorders of keratinization. Keratosis pilaris is an extremely common disorder characterized by hyperkeratotic follicular papules on the extensor surfaces of the upper arms and thighs. The papules may be associated with atopic dermatitis or ichthyosis vulgaris. Scarring keratosis pilaris variants are a group of inflammatory, follicular, atrophic conditions characterized by inflammation early and reticulated, follicular atrophy later.

The classification and nomenclature of this group of disorders has not been clarified in the literature, and there is disagreement among experts concerning proper terminology. The term keratosis pilaris atrophicans was first used by Rand and Baden in 1983 to describe keratosis pilaris with inflammation followed by atrophy. At that time, they grouped together other terms within this category. Other authors insist that these entities be considered separately. Keratosis pilaris atrophicans faciei (KPAF) and ulerythema ophryogenes are synonymous according to many authorities. Other terms used for KPAF include folliculitis rubra, atrophoderma vermiculata, and erythromelanosis follicularis faciei et coli. KPAF consists of rough follicular papules on an erythematous base in the lateral eyebrows and on the cheeks of children. As the follicular plug is shed, pitted scars with a honeycomb pattern result. There may or may not be loss of eyebrows. KPAF is thought to be autosomal dominant. It occasionally is associated with Noonan syndrome.

Atrophoderma vermiculatum (-a), also called atrophoderma vermicullaris or acne vermoulante (from the Latin "vermis," meaning worm), begins between the ages of 5 and 12 years. There is inflammation and follicular plugging followed by erythematous pits, with numerous ridges of normal skin between the pits producing a worm-like atrophy, also described as cribriform (sieve-like) or honeycomb scarring or atrophy. There may be background telangiectasia as well.

Keratosis follicularis spinulosa decalvans (keratosis pilaris decalvans, follicular ichthyosis) is noninflammatory and features skin-colored hyperkeratotic papules that appear in childhood or infancy on the face, trunk, and extremities (extensive keratosis pilaris). Often infants show numerous milia. Scarring alopecia then develops, usually during adolescence, although some authors report improvement at puberty. Eyebrows and occasionally eyelashes are lost, as well. There is no erythema, however, as is seen in ulerythema ophryogenes.

Keratosis follicularis spinulosa decalvans is associated with corneal defects and photophobia. It is thought to be X-linked recessive, and in one family the gene was mapped to the Xp 22 locus.

All of these disorders of keratinization primarily affect the pilosebaceous follicle. On histopathologic examination, follicles are acanthotic, dilated, and filled with keratinous material. There is a perivascular and follicular infiltrate of lymphocytes and vascular dilatation. In the scarring or atrophic variants, there is sclerosis of dermal collagen, with atrophy of dermal ridges and sebaceous glands. Horn cysts may be present.

The *differential diagnosis* usually can be narrowed readily. Acne vulgaris features open and closed comedones and erythematous papules and cysts, and it most often presents at puberty. Lichen spinulosis is an acquired, self-limited, discrete patch of spiny papules. Pityriasis rubra pilaris initially can show spiny papules over the knees, elbows, and knuckles, which later coalesce to form plaques. Keratosis pilaris frequently is seen with atopic dermatitis and ichthyosis vulgaris, so these must be considered as well. Syndromes that are seen in association with keratosis pilaris include Noonan syndrome, Howel-Evans syndrome (hereditary palmoplantar keratoderma), Bushke-Ollendorff syndrome (disseminated dermatofibrosis with osteopoikilosis), cardiofaciocutaneous syndrome (probably a subset of Noonan syndrome with high forehead, koilonychia, and curly hair), and Rombo syndrome (milia, basal cell carcinoma, hypotrichosis). Recently, other syndromes have been reported to be associated with keratosis pilaris, including Olmsted syndrome (palmoplantar keratoderma, hyperkeratotic plaques around orifices) and two as yet unnamed syndromes, one of which demonstrates keratosis pilaris, keratoderma, hypertrichosis, and leukonychia and the other of which features keratosis pilaris, ectodermal dysplasia, corkscrew hairs, and mental retardation.

Most of the variants listed above are chronic, but tend to spontaneously improve. Topical emollients and corticosteroids sometimes can provide symptomatic relief. Other treatment options include keratolytics such as urea, alpha-glycolic acids, lactic acid, and topical retinoids. Dermabrasion occasionally is used for reticulated atrophy, which does not resolve during adolescence. Calcipotriol ointment was found to be unhelpful in one study of nine patients; it is a bioactive form of vitamin D3 that modulates epidermal proliferation and differentiation. Another study found that calcipotriol enhanced epidermal differentiation in some diseases of keratinization, such as Darier's disease and erythrodermic lamellar ichthyosis, but did not enhance epidermal differentiation in keratosis pilaris.

In the present patient, the use of sunscreens and sun avoidance was stressed to decrease the background erythema. Lactic acid lotion was tried for several months, but was unsatisfactory due to stinging. Topical tretinoin was then used, with satisfactory improvement. Complete clearing was not achieved.

Clinical Pearls

1. The atrophic or scarring variants of keratosis pilaris are genodermatoses characterized as disorders of keratinization.

2. Keratosis pilaris atrophicans faciei (ulerythema ophryogenes) is a chronic disorder seen on the faces of children that tends to improve spontaneously; thus, scarring often resolves by adulthood.

3. Keratosis pilaris atrophicans faciei in children seems to respond well to topical retinoids.

REFERENCES

1. Basaran E, Yilmaz E, Alpsoy E, et al: Keratoderma, hypotrichosis and leukonychia totalis: A new syndrome? Br J Dermatol 133:636–638, 1995.
2. Kragballe K, Steijlen PM, Ibsen HH, et al: Efficacy, tolerability, and safety of calcipotriol ointment in disorders of keratinization: Results of a randomized, double-blind, vehicle-controlled, right/left comparative study. Arch Dermatol 131:556–560, 1995.
3. Perry HO, Su WP: Olmsted syndrome. Semin Dermatol 14:145–151, 1995.
4. Lucker GP, Steijen PM, Suykerbuyk EJ, et al: Flow-cytometric investigation of epidermal cell characteristics in monogenic disorders of keratinization and their modulation by topical calcipotriol treatment. Acta Derm Venereol 76:97–101, 1996.
5. Argenziano G, Monsurro MR, Pazineza R, et al: A case of probable autosomal recessive ectodermal dysplasia with corkscrew hairs and mental retardation in a family with tuberous sclerosis. J Am Acad Dermatol 38:344–348, 1998.

PATIENT 77

A 4-year-old girl with white papules on the face

A 4-year-old girl was noted to have an increasing number of white papules on her face for the past 3 months. The lesions were asymptomatic. She was in excellent health and attended daycare with 30 other children. No family member had similar lesions.

Physical Examination: Skin: numerous 1- to 2-mm, white papules without surrounding inflammation scattered over face, particularly right periocular area, left cheek, and perioral area; central umbilification of some larger lesions. Lymph nodes: no cervical lymphadenopathy. Conjunctiva: clear. Oral examination: no lesions.

Questions: What is your diagnosis? What are the treatment options?

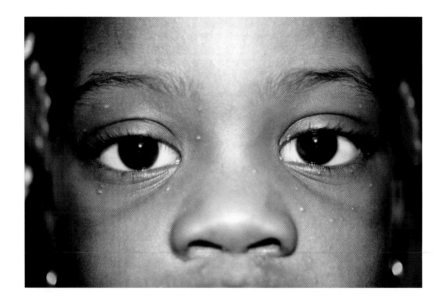

Diagnosis: Molluscum contagiosum

Discussion: Molluscum contagiosum is a common viral disease in children, and though it is contagious, it is benign. It typically is seen in those under 5 years of age and has been reported in a 1-week-old neonate. It also is seen in sexually active adults and in immunocompromised individuals. Molluscum contagiosum virus is a double-stranded DNA of the **poxvirus family**. It is brick-shaped and is the largest virus known to cause disease in humans. The only other poxvirus species specific for humans is variola virus, which is thought to have been eradicated.

Clinically, molluscum contagiosum presents as single or multiple, pearly or waxy, dome-shaped, umbilicated papules. They most commonly involve the face and trunk; less often, the extremities and genital area. They range in size from 1 mm to 15 mm (the largest ones are termed "giant molluscum"), and they may be pink, white, or skin-colored. They usually are asymptomatic, but occasionally are pruritic or tender. In 10% of patients, an eczematous eruption, termed "molluscum eczema," surrounds the papule. Additional atypical appearances include a translucent vesicular appearance, a milia-like picture, pedunculated or tag-like lesions, folliculitis, and furuncle-like lesions. The lesions are self-limited in healthy individuals, with resolution typically occurring in 6–12 months, although occasionally they may last for a longer period of time.

The molluscum contagiosum virus is spread by skin-to-skin contact as well as by fomites, including water and autoinoculation. Mechanical trauma facilitates transmission. Breaks in the epidermis as well as shaving facilitate the spread. The incubation period is approximately 2–8 weeks.

Two serious complications are seen in molluscum contagiosum infection. Conjunctival molluscum contagiosum can produce a severe toxic conjunctivitis that may permanently damage the eye. Widespread, disfiguring, and recalcitrant molluscum contagiosum may develop in immunodeficiency states, including atopic dermatitis, topical and systemic steroid use, and congenital immunodeficiency and lymphoproliferative disorders. Severe cases have been reported in HIV-infected patients. The prevalence of molluscum contagiosum in HIV-infected patients is 5–18%. Extensive molluscum contagiosum, in which giant or hyperkeratotic molluscum may be present, is a marker for advanced HIV infection. One recent report noted severe molluscum folliculitis of the beard area in a man with HIV infection. This clinical presentation probably reflected the spread of the lesions produced by the trauma of shaving.

Histopathologic examination reveals epidermal hyperplasia, with the epidermis growing down into the dermis. The epidermal cells are filled with intracytoplasmic inclusion bodies (called Henderson-Patterson or molluscum bodies). These bodies are diagnostic and may be demonstrated by Gram, Giemsa, or Wright stain. Large (up to 35 μm), ovoid structures,which tend to be eosinophilic in the lower epidermis but become basophilic in the mid and upper epidermis and the stratum corneum, are seen. The basal cell layer does not contain molluscum bodies. The bodies increase in size as they move from the lower to the upper epidermal layers. The stratum corneum in the center of the lesion eventually disintegrates, releasing the molluscum bodies and forming the characteristic craters seen clinically. Molluscum contagiosum can be detected on polymerase chain reaction from either fresh or formalin-fixed tissue, and by this method the three common molluscum contagiosum virus types can be determined: 1, 1v, and 2.

The molluscum contagiosum virus genome has been sequenced and found to encode approximately 163 proteins. One of these is a type I topoisomerase enzyme. Other poxviruses sequenced to date also encode type I topoisomerase enzymes. In vaccinia virus, for example, topoisomerase is required for viral replication. If this also is true for molluscum contagiosum virus, then topoisomerase inhibitors might provide medical therapy for molluscum contagiosum. At least six topoisomerase inhibitors have been identified to date.

Multiple treatments have been reported to be successful in molluscum contagiosum, but waiting for spontaneous resolution sometimes is the best management. Success has been obtained with benzoyl peroxide, tretinoin, cantharidin, podophyllin, topical 5-fluorouracil, cimetadine, isotretinoin, photochemotherapy, intralesional interferon, and even electron beam therapy. In one recent study of 13 children, complete clearing was achieved in 75% of patients with cimetadine, the H_2 receptor blocker with immunomodulatory effects. The dose used was 40 mg/kg/d given for 2 months. Locally destructive methods that have been applied successfully include expression of the molluscum body, curettage, cryosurgery, light electrodesiccation, and trichloracetic acid peel. Destructive methods often are inappropriate in fearful children, on the face or eyelids, or in extensive or recurrent disease. The 585-nm tunable pulsed-dye laser was used in the treatment of an AIDS patient with widespread, recalcitrant molluscum contagiosum. Another author reported success in treating healthy children with the pulsed-dye laser. Cidofovir, a nucleotide analog of deoxycytidine monophosphate with known broad-spectrum anti-DNA virus activity, was used intravenously or topically to treat three AIDS patients with extensive molluscum contagiosum. Other antiviral agents were used simultaneously. This new medication may prove to be a specific anti-molluscum contagiosum viral agent, after further clinical trials.

In the present patient, tretinoin cream was applied to many of the lesions. Resolution was achieved after 3 months.

Clinical Pearls

1. Severe, widespread, disfiguring, or recalcitrant molluscum contagiosum may be seen in HIV infection, congenital immunodeficiency states, lymphoproliferative disorders, and atopic dermatitis, as well as following the use of systemic and even topical steroid use.

2. The molluscum contagiosum viral genome has been found to encode a type I topoisomerase enzyme,which may be necessary for viral replication. Therefore, topoisomerase inhibitors might provide specific medical therapy for extensive molluscum contagiosum.

3. Cidofovir, a nucleotide analog of deoxycytidine monophosphate, may provide specific activity against molluscum contagiosum virus.

4. Cimetadine, which is useful in verruca vulgaris, also may be helpful in the therapy of molluscum contagiosum.

REFERENCES

1. Dohil M, Prendiville JS: Treatment of molluscum contagiosum with oral cimetadine: Clinical appearance in 13 patients. Pediatr Dermatol 13:310–312, 1996.
2. Meadows KP, Tyring SK, Pavia AT, et al: Resolution of recalcitrant molluscum contagiosum virus lesions in HIV-infected patients treated with cidofovir. Arch Dermatol 133:987–990, 1039–1041, 1997.
3. Myskowski PL: Molluscum contagiosum: New insights, new directions. Arch Dermatol 133:1039–1041, 983–986, 987–990, 1997.
4. Hughes PS: Treatment of molluscum contagiosum with the 585-nm pulsed-dye laser. Dermatol Surg 24:229–230, 1998.
5. Hwang Y, Wang B, Bushman FD: Molluscum contagiosum virus topoisomerase: Purification, activities, and response to inhibitors. J Virol 72:3401–3406, 1998.
6. Nehal KS, Sarnoff DS, Gotkin RH, et al: Pulsed-dye laser treatment of molluscum contagiosum in a patient with AIDS. Dermatol Surg 24:533–535, 1998.

PATIENT 78

A 9-month-old girl with an expanding ulcer on the mons pubis

A 9-month-old infant suffered an erythematous papule with a blister on her mons pubis. Despite oral antibiotic therapy, the lesion enlarged and ulcerated, and a second lesion developed on her right buttock.

Physical Examination: Temperature 38.5°C; height and weight less than 5th percentile. Skin: 2.5 × 3.0 cm ulcer on mons pubis (see figure) and 1.5-cm ulcer on right perianal area; both ulcers surrounded by purple, raised, undermined border; center of larger ulcer covered with dried, black eschar. Lymph nodes: submandibular and inguinal lymphadenopathy. Abdomen: liver palpable 8 cm below right costal margin.

Laboratory Findings: Cultures from ulcer base: scant growth of mixed fecal bacteria. HIV antibody titers: positive on enzyme-linked immunosorbent assay and Western blot analysis. T-cell subsets: T4/T8 ratio 0.5.

Questions: What is your differential diagnosis? How would you establish a diagnosis?

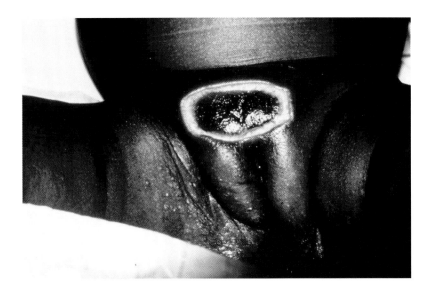

Diagnosis: Pyoderma gangrenosum in a child with HIV infection

Discussion: Pyoderma gangrenosum (PG) is a rare skin disease of unknown cause characterized by a painful, purulent, necrotizing, and expanding ulcer surrounded by a raised and undermined purple or dusky border. Ulcers may be multiple, often persist and recur, and heal with a characteristic cribriform scar. The name is a misnomer since the disease is not a pyoderma, although colonizing bacteria frequently are present. The most common location is the lower leg and foot.

Pathergy is a characteristic feature of PG, in which trauma produces expansion of the lesion. The bullous variant is probably related to Sweet's syndrome, as seen in patients with myeloproliferative disease.

Histopathologic examination is nonspecific. There is necrosis and usually a neutrophilic vascular reaction. Neutrophil dust and vasculitis may be present. There is a deep, mixed or mononuclear infiltrate.

Although deep incisional biopsy may induce pathergy, it is helpful in differentiating PG from other diseases with a similar clinical appearance. It is important to exclude infections, which can be done with tissue cultures for bacterial, fungal, mycobacterial (including atypicals), and viral organisms. A Tzanck preparation can be useful in excluding herpes simplex (HSV) or varicella-zoster virus. Other diseases to be considered include connective tissue diseases, such as systemic lupus erythematosus and rheumatoid arthritis; vasculitis or vasculitic syndromes, such as Behçets, Wegener's, and granulomatosis polyarteritis nodosum; factitial ulcers; halogenodermas; and malignancy, such as squamous cell carcinoma.

PG is idiopathic in up to 50% of patients. Inflammatory bowel disease, either ulcerative colitis or Crohn's disease, is associated in up to 15% of patients. Other possible associations include rheumatoid or other polyarthritis; chronic, active (or persistent) hepatitis; myeloproliferative diseases, such as leukemia; and immunodeficient states, such as hypogammaglobulinemia, IgA deficiency, leukocyte adhesion deficiencies, chronic granulomatous disease, hyper-IgE syndrome, and HIV infection.

Treatment of PG often is problematic. Any underlying disease should be treated. Local care, including wet compresses, topical antibiotics, and perilesional topical corticosteroids, often is helpful. *Trauma should be avoided in wound care to avoid pathergy.* Systemic antibiotics may eradicate the secondary bacterial infection. Skin grafts should be avoided because of potential pathergy. If local measures are not helpful, high-dose corticosteroids may be necessary. If ulcer expansion is not curtailed, steroids should be given as a split-dose or pulsed in an attempt to halt progression. Topical 1% sodium chromoglycate used as an adjunct to systemic steroids was recently reported to achieve good results. Intralesional steroids may be helpful. A recent report found healing in response to perilesional granulocyte-macrophage colony stimulating factor; however, another report noted the development of PG while a patient was being treated with this factor for myelodysplastic syndrome. Other systemic medications that can be helpful include dapsone, sulfapyridine, azathioprine, clofazamine, sulfasalazine, rifampin, cyclophosphamide, melphalan, ARA-C, 6-MP, and daunorubicin. Chlormabucil is an effective steroid-sparing agent in certain situations in adults, but there is a risk of development of leukemia or lymphoma in those receiving a cumulative dose of 1 gram or more.

In the present patient, an incisional biopsy revealed epidermal necrosis and a dense, mixed infiltrate, but no evidence of vasculitis or granulomatous inflammation. Stains and cultures for bacteria, fungus, and mycobacteria were negative. Tissue cultures for HSV and varicella-zoster virus likewise were negative. HIV antibody was positive in her mother by Western blot analysis. The patient's ulcers were treated with wet compresses, mupiricin ointment, topical steroids around the outside, and protection from further trauma from diapers. The ulcers healed over the next month, with cribriform scarring. At 16 months of age, repeat HIV antibody tests were positive and the T4/T8 ratio had decreased further to 0.2, confirming HIV infection in the infant.

Clinical Pearls

1. Pyoderma gangrenosum is not a pyoderma, although colonizing bacteria are present. An undermined purple border surrounding an expanding ulcer is characteristic.

2. Although idiopathic in 50% of cases, associated diseases, including inflammatory bowel disease, rheumatoid arthritis, myeloproliferative disease, chronic active hepatitis, and immunodeficient states such as HIV infection, should be excluded.

3. The clinical differential diagnosis of PG includes infections, connective tissue disease, vasculitis, malignancy, halogenodermas, and factitial causes.

4. Pathergy, in which trauma produces disease, is characteristic of PG.

REFERENCES

1. Paller AS, Sahn EE, Garen PD, et al: Pyoderma gangrenosum in pediatric AIDS. J Pediatr 117:63–66, 1990.
2. Burrus JB, Farmer ER, Callen JP: Chlorambucil is an effective corticosteroid-sparing agent for recalcitrant pyoderma gangrenosum. J Am Acad Dermatol 35:720–724, 1996.
3. Landau TA, Brenner S: Topical treatment with 1% sodium cromoglycate in pyoderma gangrenosum. Dermatol 192:252–254, 1996.
4. Lewerin C, Mobacken H, Nilsson-Ehle H, et al: Bullous pyoderma gangrenosum in a patient with myelodysplastic syndrome during granulocyte colony-stimulating factor therapy. Leuk Lymphoma 26:629–632, 1997.
5. von den Driesch P: Pyoderma gangrenosum: A report of 44 cases with follow-up. Br J Dermatol 137:1000–1005, 1997.

PATIENT 79

A 3-year-old boy with skin and nail changes

A 3-year-old boy was noted to have yellow nails at the age of 6 months. Subsequently, a red, scaly rash developed on his scalp and face. The rash was diagnosed as atopic dermatitis. In the past year, his palms and soles became erythematous and hyperkeratotic. He was in excellent health otherwise, with normal developmental milestones. There was no family history of a similar condition. He was treated with topical corticosteroids, but benefits were minimal.

Physical Examination: Vital signs: normal. Skin: sharply demarcated, erythematous, hyperkeratotic plaques over palms and soles (see figure, *top*); erythematous scaly plaques on face and scalp; hair normal. Oral exam: teeth normal; no white plaques on mucosa. Nails: yellow-brown discoloration with subungual hyperkeratosis; no pitting (see figure, *bottom*).

Laboratory Findings: Skin biopsy: pending.

Question: What is the most likely diagnosis and prognosis for this child?

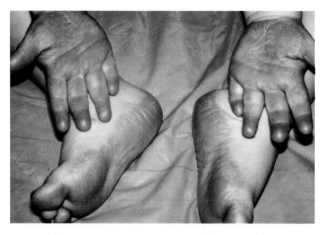

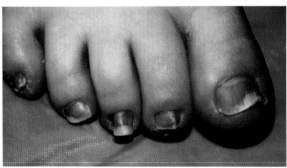

Diagnosis: Pityriasis rubra pilaris

Discussion: Pityriasis rubra pilaris (PRP) was described by Tarral in 1828 and Devergie in 1865. Besnier first used the term in 1889. It is a disease of cornification that usually begins on the scalp or face with erythema and scale and spreads in a cephalocaudal direction. Acuminate, follicular papules become confluent to produce yellow-pink, scaly plaques with sharply demarcated spared areas of normal skin (**"island-sparing"**). The rough, hyperkeratotic papules have been likened to the feel of a nutmeg grater. They characteristically are found on the dorsum of the fingers between the joints (Devergie's sign). The scales are fine and white. The salmon-yellow color of the palmoplantar keratoderma is said to resemble carnauba wax. Because of the sharp demarcation and appearance on the soles, the term "keratodermic sandle" has been applied.

PRP is classified into five types. The classic adult type has its onset during the 5th and 6th decades, clears in 80% of patients within 3 years, and is responsible for at least 50% of cases. The atypical adult form, present in 5% of patients, is characterized by alopecia and ichthyosiform changes. The classic juvenile form occurs in 10% of patients and has a good prognosis, with the majority resolved within 2 years. The circumscribed juvenile form occurs in 25% and is characterized by localized follicular papules, particularly of the elbows and knees. This form tends to be chronic, with only 30% clearing within 3 years. The atypical juvenile form is rare, occurring in 5% of patients, and shows scleroderma-like changes of the palms and soles and ichthyosiform skin lesions. Most of these cases are said to be familial and have a poor prognosis. Some authors think that this latter type may represent a follicular form of ichthyosis.

Nail changes of PRP include yellow-brown discoloration, which may be seen during the first year of life, subungual hyperkeratosis, nail plate thickening, splinter hemorrhages, and longitudinal ridging. Pitting, as seen in psoriasis, is *not* present.

On histologic examination, there may be an increased granular layer, hyperkeratosis, follicular plugging, acanthosis, and papillomatosis (psoriasiform hyperplasia). There is a sparse lymphohistiocytic infiltrate in the dermis. A characteristic finding is **"stuttering parakeratosis,"** in which there is focal parakeratosis at the follicular ostia, with orthohyperkeratosis of the interfollicular epidermis. There have been several recent reports of acantholysis and even focal acantholytic dyskeratosis (as in Grover's disease) on histopathologic examination of PRP.

The *differential diagnosis* includes severe seborrheic dermatitis (particularly early, when the face and scalp are mainly involved), psoriasis (no nail pits or neutrophils on histologic examination in PRP), pachyonychia congenita, tinea palmaris et plantaris, lichen planus (may be similar oral mucosa changes), keratosis pilaris (follicular plugging is similar), and cutaneous T-cell lymphoma (with island sparing). Other diseases to consider include atopic dermatitis, contact dermatitis, localized forms of ichthyosis, and drug eruption.

The cutaneous abnormality of PRP is not completely understood. In one recent study of four patients with familial pityriasis rubra pilaris, immunoblot analysis revealed abnormal keratins K6/16 as well as possibly abnormal K14. Epidermal proliferation and altered keratinization play a large part in the pathogenesis.

Complications seen in PRP, in addition to severe pruritus, include pain and disability secondary to the thickening and fissures of the palmoplantar keratoderma. Ectropion may be seen secondary to lower eyelid involvement. The disease may progress to an exfoliative erythroderma. Infection and bacteremia may be seen. There have been several reports of HIV infection in association with severe and refractory PRP. There also have been several case reports of PRP followed by various types of malignancy, including hepatocellular carcinoma and squamous cell carcinoma.

Treatment options include local measures, which should be tried in children for whom the prognosis is excellent and the disease is self-limited. These include keratolytics (urea, salicylate, and alpha-hydroxy acids such as lactate and pyruvate), topical steroids, and topical tretinoin, although the latter may be too irritating. Wet compresses may be helpful. Oral vitamin A has proved successful in the past, but currently when systemic therapy is needed, oral retinoids are used with good results. When oral retinoids are unsuccessful, low-dose methotrexate may be effective. Phototherapy alone has not been effective, but in combination with systemic retinoids it can be helpful. Since vitamin A is thought to play a role in PRP, some have prescribed stanozolol to increase a low retinol-binding protein level.

In the present patient, skin biopsy revealed findings characteristic of PRP. The yellow nails at 6 months of age and island sparing of the current plaques also were indicative. He was treated with topical urea cream and corticosteroids in conjunction with wet compresses. Symptoms were controlled, with almost complete resolution by the age of 5 years.

Clinical Pearls

1. Pityriasis rubra pilaris is a disorder of keratinization, as in ichthyosis, and a disorder of increased epidermal proliferation, as in psoriasis.

2. Devergie's sign and island sparing are classic clinical findings in PRP.

3. The nail changes of PRP can resemble those of psoriasis, except that pitting is not seen in PRP.

4. Childhood or juvenile PRP has a better prognosis than with onset in adulthood, with more than 50% of patients clearing within 2 years.

REFERENCES

1. Vanderhooft SL, Francis JS, Holbrook KA, et al: Familial pityriasis rubra pilaris. Arch Dermatol 131:448–453, 1995.
2. Howe K, Foresman P, Griffin T, et al: Pityriasis rubra pilaris with acantholysis. J Cutan Pathol 23:270–274, 1996.
3. Bonomo RA, Korman N, Nagashima-Whalen L, et al: Pityriasis rubra pilaris: An unusual cutaneous complication of AIDS. Am J Med Sci 314:118–121, 1997.
4. Clayton BD, Jorizzo JL, Hitchcock MG, et al: Adult pityriasis rubra pilaris: A 10-year case series. J Am Acad Dermatol 36:959–964, 1997.
5. Magro CM, Crowson AN: The clinical and histomorphological features of pityriasis rubra pilaris: A comparative analysis with psoriasis. J Cutan Pathol 24:416–424, 1997.

PATIENT 80

A 2-day-old infant with numerous polyps on the face

A 2-day-old boy was the product of a nonconsanguineous union and an uncomplicated gestation and delivery. His mother had not used alcohol, cigarettes, medications, or illicit drugs during the pregnancy. There was no family history of similar lesions.

Physical Examination: Weight, head circumference, and length: normal. General appearance: low-set ears. Neurologic: normal. Skin: numerous polyps over periorbital and preauricular areas bilaterally, each approximately 3 cm in length; some finger-like, others branched or globular (see figure); spontaneous and independent movement of elongated polyps, particularly during feedings; bilateral preauricular pits.

Laboratory Findings: Excisional biopsies of all polyps, orbital ultrasonograms, brain auditory evoked response (BAER), computed tomography (CT) scan of head and orbits, and chromosomal analysis of peripheral blood lymphocytes and skin fibroblasts: pending.

Questions: What is your diagnosis? What entities should be considered in the differential diagnosis?

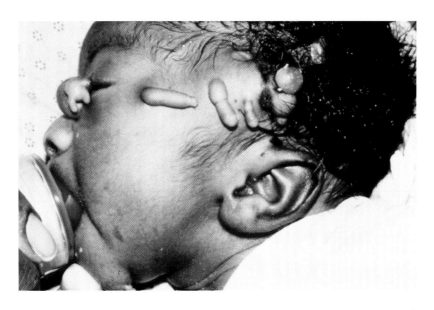

Diagnosis: Multiple rhabdomyomatous mesenchymal hamartomas of skin

Discussion: Rhabdomyomatous mesenchymal hamartomas of the skin were first described in 1986 and are characterized by polypoid, finger-like or globular projections containing **functional skeletal muscle**. The muscle allows the polyps to move spontaneously and independently. There may be associated congenital anomalies, such as orbital cysts, low-set ears, and preauricular sinuses (as in the present patient). The cause of this disorder is unknown.

Histopathologic examination of both the finger-like and the globular papules in this child showed the same features. The papules were covered by mature squamous epithelium containing follicular units. Fascicles of skeletal muscle were seen within the subcutaneous fat and extending into the reticular dermis, but not involving the papillary dermis. In some specimens, the muscle bundles formed a solid central core, which occasionally was accompanied by a large vessel and nerve. Mature fat was present. Electron microscopic examination of the muscle fibers revealed the characteristic banding pattern of normal skeletal muscle. Special stains indicated the presence of both type 1 and 2 muscle fibers. A few specimens showed foci of calcification, and one displayed a focus of ossification.

The clinical *differential diagnosis* is extensive, but the diagnosis is established on histopathologic examination. Acrochordons can be present at birth, but they are composed of loose collagen fibers, blood vessels, and mature fat—not skeletal muscle.

Fetal rhabdomyoma shows subcutaneous mesenchymal cells with embryonic skeletal muscle differentiation. However, the dermis is not involved, and there is no mature skeletal muscle. In nevus lipomatosis cutaneous superficialis of Hoffman-Zurhelle, there is ectopic fat in the reticular dermis, but no skeletal muscle. Fibrous hamartoma of infancy contains mature fat cells, fibrocollagenous bundles, and cellular areas with mixoid stroma—but no skeletal muscle. Benign Triton tumors (neuromuscular hamartomas) are found in association with peripheral nerves. They consist of collections of skeletal muscle admixed with neural elements, but are located subcutaneously and do not involve dermis. The oculocerebrocutaneous syndrome consists of orbital cysts, periorbital cutaneous appendages, focal dermal hypoplasia and aplasia, and multiple cerebral cysts. The cutaneous appendages in these patients have been termed "facial skin tags," with one case noted to show multiple periocular trichofolliculomata.

In the present patient, the ultrasonogram revealed an orbital cyst. The BAER was normal. CT scan of the head and orbits was normal, with the exception of the orbital cyst. Chromosomal analysis revealed a normal male karyotype. All of the lesions on the face were excised under general anesthesia on the 10th day of life, and they healed well. The infant was blind in the eye containing the cyst. At 2 years of age, the child showed mild developmental delay.

Clinical Pearls

1. Rhabdomyomatous mesenchymal hamartomas appear as finger-like or globular projections on the face of newborns.

2. The clinical hallmark of rhabdomyomatous mesenchymal hamartomas is independent and spontaneous movement of the polyps.

3. The characteristic histopathology of rhabdomyomatous mesenchymal hamartomas is the presence of a skeletal muscle core within the polypoid projection.

REFERENCES

1. Delleman JW, Oorthuys JWE, Bleeker-Wagemakers EM, et al: Orbital cyst in addition to congenital cerebral and focal dermal malformations: A new entity. Clin Genet 24:470–472, 1984.
2. Hendrick SJ, Sanchez RL, Blackwell SJ, et al: Striated muscle hamartoma—description of two cases. Pediatr Dermatol 3:153–157, 1986.
3. Giorgi PL, Gabrielli O, Catassi C, et al: Oculocerebrocutaneous syndrome: Description of a new case. Eur J Pediatr 148: 325–326, 1989.
4. Mills AE: Rhabdomyomatous mesenchymal hamartoma of skin. Am J Dermatopathol 11:58–63, 1989.
5. Sahn EE, Garen PD, Pai GS, et al: Multiple rhabdomyomatous mesenchymal hamartomas of skin. Am J Dermatol 12:485–491, 1990.

PATIENT 81

A 3-year-old girl with multiple bullae

A 3-year-old girl experienced pruritic bullae in the perineal area after recovering from an upper respiratory tract infection. She received several courses of oral antibiotics without benefit. As the bullae healed, new ones formed, leaving a hypopigmented background. New lesions began to appear on the thighs and legs, as well as the face. She was in good health otherwise and was receiving no other medications.

Physical Examination: Vital signs: normal. Skin: numerous tense bullae with erosions, crusts, and hypopigmentation in perineal and inguinal areas; tense blisters on legs, some forming annular shapes around healing crusted lesions in rosette configuration; scattered blisters on face (see figures). Eyes: no conjunctivitis or conjunctival scars. Mouth: two 5-mm erosions on tongue. Lymph nodes: no lymphadenopathy. Abdomen: no hepatosplenomegaly or masses palpable.

Laboratory Findings: CBC with differential and liver function tests: normal. Bacterial and viral cultures of blister fluid: no growth. Skin biopsy of perilesional skin: pending.

Question: What is the most appropriate treatment of this patient?

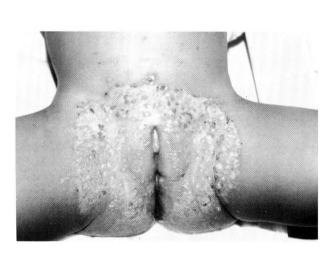

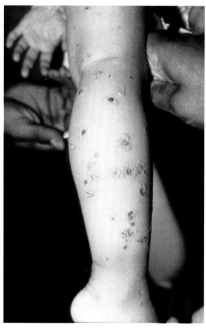

Diagnosis: Chronic bullous dermatosis of childhood

Discussion: Chronic bullous dermatosis of childhood (CBDC), or linear IgA disease, is one of the autoimmune blistering diseases, first described by Bowen in 1901. It is characterized by the sudden appearance of tense bullae on the face, buttocks, perineum, thighs, and legs. In some cases, there is a history of a previous illness, most commonly a viral upper respiratory tract infection. In a recent report, the disease followed Epstein-Barr viral conversion after infectious mononucleosis. A hallmark of this blistering disease is the formation of rosettes or "clusters of jewels." These terms refer to large, sausage-shaped bullae that curve around to form arciform or annular shapes surrounding a crusted, healing lesion. The blisters may appear on normal or erythematous skin, and other bizarre, grouped formations may appear in addition to the rosettes. The bullae appear in crops and may be pruritic, sometimes severely.

Histopathologic examination reveals a subepidermal vesicle containing neutrophils and some eosinophils, indistinguishable from the findings of bullous pemphigoid and dermatitis herpetiformis. Direct immunofluorescence of perilesional skin reveals linear deposits of IgA in the basement membrane zone, which is diagnostic. There are no granular deposits as occur in dermatitis herpetiformis. Transmission electron microscopy confirms that the blister site is within the lamina lucida. Immunoelectron microscopy reveals that the IgA is bound on one of two sites: it is either intralamina lucida or sublamina densa. Some investigators believe that double localization of the IgA, producing a "mirror image" pattern, is characteristic of CBDC. On indirect immunofluorescence examination, circulating IgA is present in up to 80% of cases, which is more common than that of adult linear IgA disease. This circulating IgA antibody is directed against the basilar surface of hemidesmosomes. The antigen recognized by the circulating autoantibodies in CBDC is a 97-kDa protein identical to that seen in adult linear IgA disease, confirming that CBDC is the childhood counterpart of adult linear IgA disease.

CBDC begins between 6 months and 10 years, with a course of 1–5 years. It is self-limited and usually heals with postinflammatory pigmentary alteration, either hyperpigmentation or hypopigmentation.

Despite the excellent prognosis, several complications may develop. There may be a prolonged or recurrent course: a third of the cases persist beyond 5 years, and relapses often occur years after remission. There appears to be an association with malignant neoplasm in about 5% of all linear IgA disease. Because of this low association, it is not considered a paraneoplastic syndrome. There have been occasional reports of the appearance of CBDC following certain drugs. Half of the children may have intraoral erosions, but severe eye or laryngeal involvement is rare. Mucosal lesions in children are less common than in adult linear IgA disease.

The *differential diagnosis* includes bullous impetigo, varicella, bullous pemphigoid (IgG deposits at basement membrane zone), cicatricial pemphigoid (oral lesions predominate), dermatitis herpetiformis, pemphigus vulgaris, bullous erythema multiforme, epidermolysis bullosa, sexual abuse, bullous urticaria pigmentosa, bullous lichen planus, and bullous lupus erythematosus. Histopathological and immunofluorescent testing differentiates these diseases from CBDC.

The treatment of CBDC is oral diaminodiphenylsulfone (dapsone). The patient must be screened for glucose 6-phosphate dehydrogenase deficiency before starting therapy, and CBC and liver function tests should be monitored. In those who cannot use dapsone, sulfapyridine has proved helpful. Resistant or severe cases may require the addition of oral corticosteroids for control; tapering should be accomplished as rapidly as possible. Antihistamines to control severe pruritus and antibiotics to control bacterial superinfection are used as necessary. Dapsone therapy generally is continued for several years.

In the present patient, histopathologic and direct immunofluorescent examination of the biopsy specimen demonstrated findings characteristic of CBDC. The misdiagnosis of bullous impetigo allowed the disease to progress for 6 weeks prior to institution of the correct treatment. The child was begun on low-dose dapsone, which she tolerated well. Within 6 weeks, almost all bullae had resolved. Several attempts to decrease the dapsone resulted in flares of recurrent blistering. At a 2-year followup, she was on low-dose dapsone and developed 1 to 2 bullae per month.

Clinical Pearls

1. Chronic bullous disease of childhood is synonymous with childhood linear IgA disease.

2. A clinical hallmark of CBDC or linear IgA disease is the rosette or "cluster of jewels" formed by the bullae.

3. The disease usually is self-limited and can be controlled with diaminodiphenylsulfone (dapsone) or sulfapyridine.

REFERENCES

1. Hamann ID, Hepburn NC, Hunter JA: Chronic bullous dermatosis of childhood: Relapse after puberty. J R Soc Med 88:296P–297P, 1995.
2. Baldari U, Raccagni AA, Celli B, et al: Chronic bullous disease of childhood following Epstein-Barr virus seroconversion: A case report. Clin Exp Dermatol 21:123–126, 1996.
3. Capesius C, de Prost Y: Linear IgA dermatosis: A heterogeneous syndrome? Nouv Dermatol 15:24–27, 1996.
4. Zone JJ, Taylor TB, Kadunce DP, et al: IgA antibodies in chronic bullous disease of childhood react with 97 kDa basement membrane zone protein. J Invest Dermatol 106:1277–1280, 1996.
5. Coleman H, Shrubb VA: Chronic bullous disease of childhood—Another cause of potential misdiagnosis of sexual abuse? Br J Gen Pract 47:507–508, 1997.

PATIENT 82

A newborn girl with a lumbosacral mass and a dimple

A newborn girl was noted to have a nodule on the left lower back as well as a midline dimple. Pregnancy and delivery had been normal, and there was no family history of congenital lesions.

Physical Examination: Vital signs: normal. Skin: soft, 1-cm, skin-colored nodule to left of midline at top of gluteal cleft; superior midline dimple (see figure). Neurologic: no motor, sensory, or sphincter abnormalities.

Laboratory Findings: Anteroposterior and lateral spine films and lumbosacral MRI: pending.

Question: What is the most likely diagnosis?

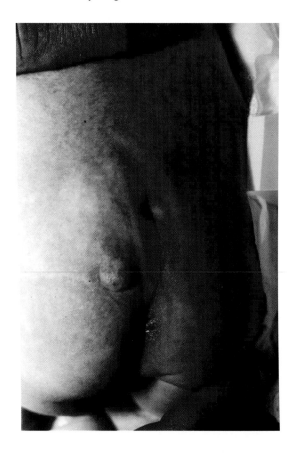

Diagnosis: Congenital lipomeningocele

Discussion: Congenital lumbosacral lipomas are rare anomalies that contain mature fat and may contain a meningocele. They range in size from 1 to 30 cm and are midline, or may be slightly lateral to the midline as in the present patient. Lumbosacral lipomas may be associated with hypertrichosis, skin tags, nevus lipomatosis cutaneous superficialis, or sinus tracts. Most cases of lumbosacral lipoma are markers for a spinal laminar defect. Fat usually extends into the defect as an intradural or extradural lipoma, and with enlargement, compresses or tethers the cord, leading to spasticity, anesthesia, and incontinence.

The term **spinal dysraphism** refers to several different congenital anomalies of the spinal cord or vertebral column. Included in this classification is diastematomyelia (split spinal cord), which produces split spinal cord malformations. These malformations contain a rigid or fibrous septum that transfixes the spinal cord and produces tethering. As the cord grows and elongates, neurologic problems are produced distally. Spinal dysraphism also includes diplomyelia, spina bifida, dermoid cysts, intraspinal lipomas, and spinal hamartomas. These defects are thought to be caused by either lack of separation or inadequate fusion of germinal layers in the developing embryo. Cutaneous markers of spinal dysraphism—hypertrichosis (faun-tail), nevus flammeus, hemangioma, melanocytic nevus, lipoma, dimple (may be ostium of sinus tract), linear depression, sinus tract (increased risk of meningitis or spinal abscess), or hypoplasia of skin—are present in at least 50% of patients.

Untreated spinal dysraphism with a tethered spinal cord can produce progressive motor and sensory dysfunction with eventual spasticity and contractures, scoliosis and low back pain, and bowel and bladder incontinence. Several recent reports of late diagnosis in adulthood have revealed a wide range of abnormalities. A 42-year-old man had back pain, sciatica, urinary retention, urgency, and severe sensory deficits in the feet, producing recurrent septic arthritis of the toes; an MRI revealed an intraspinal lipoma with a tethered spinal cord. A 24-year-old man with severe trophic ulcers of the feet was thought to have leprosy; he eventually was found to have spina bifida and lipomeningocele. A 63-year-old woman had trophic ulcers on her feet, requiring partial amputations, with sensory and motor disturbances of the lower extremities and urinary complaints for over 40 years; she had a tethered cord and lumbosacral lipoma. A tethered spinal cord undiagnosed until adulthood may present as "hereditary sensory motor neuropathy."

Children with a tethered cord frequently develop trophic foot ulcers and bladder and bowel incontinence. Even in children without clinical bladder problems, one study noted that urodynamic testing (such as bladder capacity, pressure, and sensation) revealed abnormalities in the majority of these children. These abnormalities improve after the defect is repaired surgically. A 12-year-old girl presented with polyuria and polydypsia due to hydronephrosis from a neurogenic bladder; she was found to have a tethered cord.

A newborn with any of the above-mentioned skin lesions in the lumbosacral area must *not* undergo a biopsy or excision of the lesion until after a thorough evaluation by a neurosurgeon, including an MRI to exclude a connection with the spinal cord or spinal canal.

When an underlying spinal cord abnormality is diagnosed, neurosurgical exploration and repair should be undertaken early. Several studies have reported that if release of a tethered cord is delayed until severe sensory motor deficits or bowel and bladder incontinence has occurred, reversal will not be possible. Neurosurgical repair should be performed before the age of 3 years to halt further neurologic deterioration. In some patients, modest sensory motor problems will progress after surgery as a function of the split cord or structural abnormality itself, even though tethering is not present.

In the present patient, radiographs and MRI revealed that the lipomeningocele was connected to the spinal canal. She underwent neurosurgical exploration and repair of the defect at 6 weeks of age. At age 1, the neurologic examination remained normal.

Clinical Pearls

1. Spinal dysraphism includes many congenital anomalies of the spine and spinal cord, which result from inadequate fusion or lack of separation of germinal layers in the developing embryo.

2. Cutaneous markers of an underlying spinal cord or vertebral column defect include hemangioma, lipoma, dimple, melanocytic nevus, and hypertrichosis. Any skin lesion in or near the midline of the lumbosacral area of a newborn should *not* be biopsied or excised until a thorough neurosurgical evaluation including MRI has been performed.

3. Repair of spinal dysraphism and tethered spinal cord should be done before the age of 3 to prevent irreversible neurologic deficits.

REFERENCES

1. Andar UB, Harkness WF, Hayward RD: Split cord malformations of the lumbar region. A model for the neurosurgical management of all types of "occult" spinal dysraphism? Pediatr Neurosurg 26:17–24, 1997.
2. Da Silva LF, Robin S, Guegan-Massardier E, et al: Peripheral neurological involvement as the first manifestation of spina bifida occulta. Rev Rhum Engl Ed 64:830–842, 1997.
3. Ersahin Y, Mutluer S, Kocaman S, et al: Split spinal cord malformations in children. J Neurosurg 88:57–65, 1998.
4. Fujii T, Ochi J, Miyajima T, et al: Nephrogenic diabetes insipidus and tethered cord syndrome with a lipoma of the cauda equina. Brain Dev 20:47–49, 1998.
5. Palmer LS, Richards I, Kaplan WE: Subclinical changes in bladder function in children presenting with nonurological symptoms of the tethered cord syndrome. J Urol 159:231–234, 1998.

PATIENT 83

An 8-year-old boy with pruritic, scaly feet

An 8-year-old boy endured pruritic, scaly feet during the summer while on a swim team. The symptoms improved in the fall, but recurred over the winter months. His mother reported that his feet seemed to sweat profusely. Occasionally, itchy, red, scaly spots developed on his inner arms, which she treated with nonprescription ointments. No family member had similar symptoms. The child suffered from mild asthma.

Physical Examination: Vital signs: normal. Face: Morgan-Denney folds of lower lids. Feet: shiny, brown, scaly plaques on anterior soles; instep spared; no involvement of dorsum of foot or nails; small fissures on great toes (see figure). Skin: erythematous, scaly plaques in antecubital fossae.

Laboratory Findings: KOH examination of foot scale: no hyphal elements. CBC with differential: normal. Pulmonary function tests: consistent with mild asthma.

Questions: What is your diagnosis? How would you treat this child?

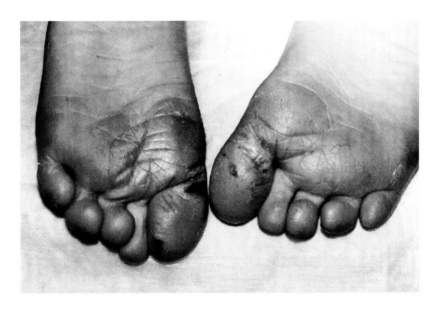

Diagnosis: Juvenile plantar dermatosis

Discussion: Juvenile plantar dermatosis (dermatitis) had been considered a variant of atopic dermatitis, but recent studies have confirmed that it frequently occurs as an isolated entity. It is characterized by erythematous or brownish, scaly plaques on the weight-bearing portions of the soles. It typically is present on the anterior part of the foot; hence the synonym "forefoot dermatitis." As the condition becomes more severe, painful fissures may develop. It is seen most commonly in children, prior to puberty. Often, the great toes are affected first.

The etiopathogenesis is thought to be repeated wetting and drying of the skin, as is seen with the use of occlusive footwear (e.g., plastic or rubber shoes and soles). The condition occasionally is termed "sneaker foot." Excessive sweating frequently is present; nylon or other synthetic socks may contribute to its severity. Because occlusive footwear is worn in winter, often in overheated classrooms, there may be worsening in the winter ("atopic winter foot"). Exacerbations also occur in the summer, when children are in and out of swimming pools ("atopic summer foot").

The *differential diagnosis* includes tinea pedis, which is uncommon in prepubertal children. The instep is spared in juvenile plantar dermatosis, while it is involved in tinea pedis. In one study of 20 children with juvenile plantar dermatosis, fungal cultures were negative in all 20. In a control group without juvenile plantar dermatosis, four cases of tinea pedis were diagnosed. Contact dermatitis of the foot usually involves primarily the dorsum of the foot rather than the sole; however, it can coexist with juvenile plantar dermatosis and, therefore, patch testing should be considered.

Switching from sneakers and rubber or plastic soles to leather shoes along with cotton socks usually produces improvement. Since xerosis is the underlying problem, continuous use of greasy emollients, such as petrolatum, often produces resolution. If fissures or severe pruritus are present, topical steroids are useful.

In the present patient, the diagnosis made by physical observation was confirmed by negative fungal cultures. Causes were discussed in detail with the parents. The boy began to apply petrolatum before and after entering the swimming pool and topical steroids twice a day, and he changed his footwear to leather sandals with cotton socks. The condition resolved over the next 4 weeks. For his atopic eczema, the parents were instructed in general skin moisturization techniques and the use of topical steroids for any outbreaks. He was prescribed a short acting β_2-agonist for his intermittent asthma.

Clinical Pearls

1. Juvenile plantar dermatosis (also called atopic summer foot, atopic winter foot, forefoot dermatitis, and sneaker foot) may be a manifestation of atopic dermatitis or may be an isolated entity.

2. Juvenile plantar dermatosis is differentiated from tinea pedis by a negative KOH examination and a distribution in which the instep is not involved.

3. Juvenile plantar dermatosis can be differentiated from contact dermatitis, which usually involves the dorsum of the foot rather than the sole.

4. Contact dermatitis may accompany juvenile plantar dermatosis, necessitating patch testing.

REFERENCES

1. Broberg A, Faergemann J: Scaly lesions on the feet in children—tinea or eczema? Acta Paediatr Scan 79:349–351, 1990.
2. Pirkl S, Tennstedt D, Eggers S, et al: Juvenile plantar dermatosis: When are epicutaneous tests indicated? Hautarzt 41:22–26, 1990.

PATIENT 84

A newborn girl with white patches on the face

A black neonate was noted to have several hypopigmented macules and patches on the side of her face. The pregnancy and delivery had been normal, and there was no family history of white or brown macules or seizures. The infant appeared in good health otherwise.

Physical Examination: Vital signs: normal. Face: hypopigmented macules and patches on right cheek (see figure); sharp margination from normal skin; no epidermal changes present; skin appearance normal other than color.

Laboratory Findings: Diascopy with glass slide at edge of lesion: blanching of surrounding normal skin and obliteration of margin between lesion and normal skin. Woods lamp examination: no accentuation of hypopigmentation.

Question: What are the diagnosis and pathogenesis of this lesion?

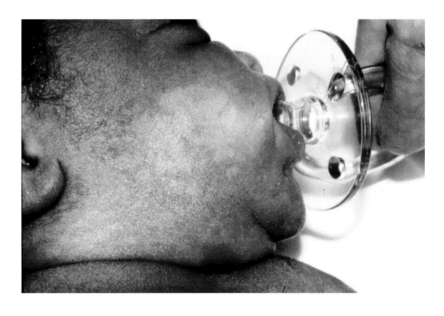

Diagnosis: Nevus anemicus

Discussion: Nevus anemicus is classified as an uncommon vascular malformation (the result of embryologic developmental anomalies) in which the blood vessel abnormality is functional rather than structural. Clinically, one or more pale or white, irregular macules or patches appear soon after birth or in infancy. Their size usually varies from 1 to 3 cm, and the borders are sharply marginated. However, the borders may be feathered or indistinct. The most common location is the trunk, but the lesions can occur on the face or extremities. Once the lesions occur, they remain fixed and unchanged throughout life.

The diagnosis is made clinically on diascopy using a glass slide. Firm pressure at the border of the nevus anemicus obliterates the margin between the lesion and normal skin. Woods lamp examination does not show accentuation of the hypopigmentation or depigmentation, as is seen in vitiligo; in contrast, it makes the lesion *less* noticeable. Firm stroking with a tongue blade across the lesion and normal skin produces a wheal, but no axon flare (redness), within the lesion and accentuates the hypopigmentation by producing redness on the adjacent skin. After application of cold or heat, there is no reflex dilatation as there is in the surrounding skin.

The pathogenesis of nevus anemicus involves a congenital hypersensitivity of blood vessels to catecholamines (vasoconstrictors) or an insensitivity to vasodilators. The patch of vasoconstriction cannot be obliterated with vasodilators, such as prostaglandins, acetylcholine, histamine, or serotonin. Histopathologic examination of a nevus anemicus reveals completely normal skin and therefore usually is not performed.

The *differential diagnosis* includes nevus depigmentosus and the ash leaf macules of tuberous sclerosis. Since some authors have noted an association with neurofibromatosis 1, the child should be examined for café au lait macules when the initial diagnosis is made. Vitiligo and tinea versicolor usually do not present diagnostic dilemmas.

Recent studies to elucidate the pathogenesis of contact dermatitis are based on the finding that in a patient with generalized contact dermatitis and a nevus anemicus, there is a lack of dermatitis both clinically and histopathologically within the nevus anemicus. Study of adhesion molecule expression found that in dermatitic skin, endothelial cells express HLA-DR, intercellular adhesion molecule-1 (ICAM-1), vascular adhesion molecule-1, and E-selectin, and keratinocytes express HLA-DR and ICAM-1. The nevus anemicus, however, lacked endothelial E-selectin and keratinocyte HLA-DR and ICAM-1 expression. In another study, interferon gamma injected into both the nevus anemicus and surrounding normal skin was found to induce endothelial and epidermal HLA-DR and ICAM-1 expression in both, but endothelial E-selectin expression only in normal skin. These authors concluded that blood vessels in nevus anemicus do not respond normally to proinflammatory cytokines (with expected E-selectin expression) and may be the explanation for a lack of dermatitis in nevus anemicus. E-selectin may be a requirement for the recruitment of circulating T-lymphocytes to skin in delayed hypersensitivity reactions.

In the present patient, diascopy and Woods lamp examinations confirmed the diagnosis. Her parents were informed that no specific treatment is yet available. They were advised that if the nevus anemicus presents a cosmetic problem, cover-up cosmetics produce a very satisfactory result.

Clinical Pearls

1. Nevus anemicus is a rare vascular malformation resulting from an embryologic developmental anomaly, which produces a functional blood vessel abnormality.

2. The clinical diagnosis of nevus anemicus is established at the bedside using diascopy with a glass slide and firm stroking with a tongue blade.

3. The skin of a nevus anemicus does not respond to injection of interferon gamma with the induction of endothelial E-selectin, as occurs in normal skin. This may be related to the lack of dermatitis within a nevus anemicus in generalized contact dermatitis.

REFERENCES

1. Mizutani H, Ohyanagi S, Umeda Y, et al: Loss of cutaneous delayed hypersensitivity reactions in nevus anemicus: Evidence of close concordance of cutaneous delayed hypersensitivity and endothelial E-selectin expression. Arch Dermatol 133:617–620, 1997.
2. Requena L, Sangueza OP: Cutaneous vascular anomalies. Part I. Hamartomas, malformations, and dilation of preexisting vessels. J Am Acad Dermatol 37:523–552, 1997.

PATIENT 85

A 10-year-old girl with tightness and change in the shape of her upper lip

A 10-year-old girl complained of tightness of her left upper lip for the past 6 months. Her parents noticed upward pulling on that side of her lip, as well as thinning of the skin on her left lateral face. An excisional biopsy had been performed on the left upper lip 1 month previously. She was in excellent health otherwise and taking no medications.

Physical Examination: Vital signs: normal. Face: asymmetry with left temporal wasting. Skin: violaceous, brown, sclerotic plaque producing elevation of left upper lip; well-healed, linear excision scar (see figures). Mouth: gingival recession over left frontal teeth. Scalp: frontoparietal, 2-cm, linear band of alopecia on left.

Laboratory Findings: CBC: mild eosinophilia. ANA: speckled positive at a titer of 1:160. Double-stranded DNA: negative. Lyme disease titer: negative. Skull series: no measurable bony asymmetry. Previous skin biopsy: requested.

Questions: What is the most likely diagnosis? What are the treatment options?

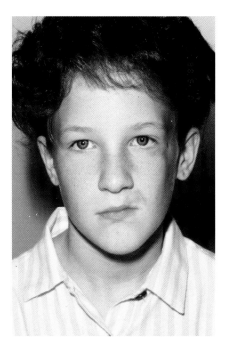
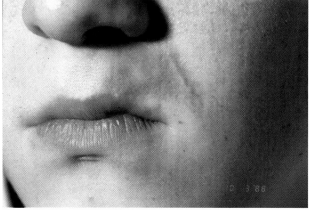

Diagnosis: Linear scleroderma (en coup de sabre)

Discussion: Linear scleroderma involving the frontoparietal areas of the face and scalp is termed "en coup de sabre" because it resembles the scar from a sabre cut of the face. Scleroderma is uncommon in children, but any of the types may be seen. Fortunately, the systemic variants of scleroderma, such as pansystemic sclerosis and CREST syndrome (calcinosis, Raynaud's phenomenon, esophageal dysfunction, sclerodactyly, and telangiectasia), are extremely rare. Localized variants of scleroderma are now divided into five types of morphea: plaque, generalized, bullous, linear, and deep. The incidence of localized scleroderma is approximately 27 new cases per million population per year.

Clinically, there is gradual appearance of an ivory-colored to violaceous, sclerotic, linear plaque with hyperpigmented borders. Linear scleroderma may be seen on any limb, most commonly the arm, and also on the frontoparietal area as in en coup de sabre. En coup de sabre scleroderma may be associated with some degree of facial hemiatrophy, but this is more superficial than that of progressive facial hemiatrophy of Parry-Romberg. A recent report of three patients with frontoparietal scleroderma (en coup de sabre) noted that the linear distribution on the face resembled Blaschko's lines, suggesting at least a partial developmental etiology.

The etiopathogenesis of scleroderma is unknown, but is probably multifactorial. Abnormalities in collagen metabolism presumably play a role. Some authors are convinced that scleroderma is related to Lyme disease.

Scleroderma in children is different from that seen in adults. A recent study noted that although children with localized scleroderma frequently have positive ANAs, as do adult patients with systemic sclerosis, they rarely have specific antibodies such as SCL-70 (topoisomerase I) and nucleolar antigens. In another study, childhood-onset scleroderma showed predominance of localized disease and lack of vascular activating markers, such as Von Willibrand's factor, angiotensin-converting enzyme, E-selectin, and endothelin-1, frequently seen in adult scleroderma. This same study noted a significant association with trauma prior to the onset of childhood localized scleroderma (mean of 3 months prior) and a lack of anticentromere antibodies in children.

Complications associated with linear scleroderma include cosmetic deformities when the face or limbs are affected; alopecia affecting scalp, brows, and lashes; and skeletal deformities. If the linear plaque extends across joint surfaces, joint function can be compromised. The tight skin can produce constriction and neurovascular compromise, which can result in diminished bone growth. Melorheostosis, defined as osteosclerosis or hyperostosis extending in a linear track through a long bone of an extremity, can be seen underlying linear scleroderma. It consists of ivory-like, new bone. Neurologic complications occur, including epilepsy and structural abnormalities in subjacent leptomeninges and brain tissue. One author suggested that linear scleroderma may represent a neurocutaneous syndrome. Restrictive ophthalmopathy can result from myopathy of ocular muscles underlying linear scleroderma. Finally, dental abnormalities including gingival recession have been noted.

The *differential diagnosis* of linear scleroderma of the en coup de sabre type includes Parry-Romberg progressive facial hemiatrophy. Many authors believe that the two are variants of the same disease; however, others think that progressive facial hemiatrophy more frequently involves the lower face and shows less cutaneous sclerosis. If the linear lesions are present at birth, congenital facial hypoplasia is in the differential diagnosis. This entity shows unilateral microdontia, as well.

The prognosis of linear scleroderma is good in that spontaneous resolution usually occurs in 3–5 years; however, there are reports of persistence for 20 years and of recurrences. The patient may be left with significant cosmetic deformities. Treatment of linear scleroderma includes emollients to decrease dryness and topical steroids to decrease itching. Some clinicians give an empiric course of antibiotics in case *Borrelia burgdorferi* plays a part. This often is done despite negative Lyme titers, since these titers may not accurately reflect Borrelia infection. If the disease is severe and progressive, systemic steroids sometimes are used for 3 months to decrease inflammation. Para-amino benzoate has been recommended by some, but found ineffective by others. Hydroxychloroquine has been found helpful in many cases. D-penicillamine decreases collagen synthesis by inhibiting collagen fiber cross-linking, and is occasionally useful, but has many severe side effects. Diphenylhydantoin and ticlopidine also have been suggested. Physical therapy is important when joint function is compromised. When the disease becomes inactive, plastic surgery procedures such as soft-tissue expansion with collagen injections, autologous bone grafting, skin grafting, and grafting from scalp to eyebrow can improve cosmesis.

In the present patient, histopathologic examination showed normal epidermis with increased normal-appearing as well as thickened collagen fibers and closely packed bundles in the dermis.

There was loss of adnexal structures, an occasional lone eccrine gland, and scant inflammatory infiltrate. Parry-Romberg progressive facial hemiatrophy was excluded by radiologic measurements. These findings confirmed the diagnosis. She received a 1-month course of antibiotics empirically and topical steroids. Because of rapid progression of gingival involvement, consultation with pediatric dentistry was obtained. The patient underwent gingival grafting to protect two teeth. She was begun on D-penicillamine therapy, which was discontinued because of leukopenia. She subsequently was treated with systemic hydroxychloroquine, with improvement. The antimalarial was tapered off over months, and at 3 years there was no further progression of the disease.

Clinical Pearls

1. Linear scleroderma of the frontoparietal areas of the face and scalp is known as en coup de sabre because it resembles the scar formed from a sabre cut.

2. This disorder may follow Blaschko's developmental lines.

3. Parry-Romberg progressive facial hemiatrophy and linear scleroderma en coup de sabre may be variants of the same disease. Both may feature underlying bony and neurologic abnormalities.

REFERENCES

1. Rosenberg AM, Uziel Y, Krafchik BR, et al: Antinuclear antibodies in children with localized scleroderma. J Rheumatol 22:2337–2343, 1995.
2. Vancheeswaran R, Black CM, David J, et al: Childhood-onset scleroderma: Is it different from adult-onset disease. Arthritis Rheum 39:1041–1049, 1996.
3. Menni S, Marzano AV, Passoni E: Neurologic abnormalities in two patients with facial hemiatrophy and sclerosis coexisting with morphea. Pediatr Dermatol 14:113–116, 1997.
4. Ortigado Matamala A, Martinez Granero MA, Pascual Castroviejo I: Scleroderma en coup de sabre with intracranial involvement: A case report. Neurologia 12:256–258, 1997.
5. Soma Y, Fujimoto M: Frontoparietal scleroderma (en coup de sabre) following Blaschko's lines. J Am Acad Dermatol 38:366–368, 1998.

PATIENT 86

A 32-year-old woman with a changing birthmark on the back

A 32-year-old white woman was born with a flat, brown patch on her back. Numerous dark macules developed within the macule during infancy. Recently, one of the spots darkened and enlarged. She was in excellent health otherwise.

Physical Examination: Skin: sharply demarcated, light-brown patch containing several small, darker macules and papules (see figure). Lymph nodes: no adenopathy. Abdomen: no hepatosplenomegaly.

Laboratory Findings: Biopsy of largest and darkest papule, including some of surrounding hyperpigmented patch: pending.

Question: What is the likely diagnosis?

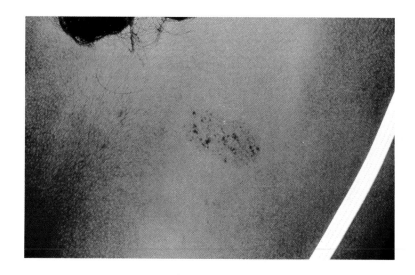

Diagnosis: Nevus spilus

Discussion: Nevus spilus (speckled lentiginous nevus) is a relatively common pigmented lesion occurring in approximately 1–3% of adults. It is hairless, solitary, and usually large, varying from 1 to 20 cm. The most common locations are face, trunk, and proximal extremities. It was considered benign until recently, when several reports surfaced of malignant melanoma developing within the lesion.

Clinically, a tan to brown macule or patch usually is present at birth, and scattered, hyperpigmented macules or papules later develop within the patch. Large lesions may have a zosteriform or dermatomal distribution. Facial lesions may be divided by the palpebral fissure.

Histopathologic examination reveals that the original patch is a lentigo simplex, with typical findings of elongation of rete ridges, increased melanocytes in the basal layer, increased melanin in both melanocytes and basal keratinocytes, and melanophages in the dermis. Some authors state that nevus cells may be found within the macular component. The speckled or dark areas of nevus spilus typically are junctional nevi, but also can be intradermal or compound nevi. Giant melanin granules, thought to represent macromelanosomes or melanolysosomes, may be present within the nevi. Giant melanin granules are not specific and can be present in many other conditions, including the café au lait macules of neurofibromatosis or Albright's syndrome, Becker melanosis, and normal nevi. Rarely, the dark component of nevus spilus represents a blue nevus. In one case, an agminated blue nevus was found; in another, a nodular neurotized nevus. This latter entity shows features of a neurofibroma, except that it lacks leu-7 staining, a marker of neurofibroma.

Malignant melanoma rarely develops within a nevus spilus. However, a recent study reported 17 patients with a nevus spilus in which a malignant melanoma developed. All of the patients were white and 35–56 years old, and the location was most often the back. Almost all lesions of nevus spilus were congenital and large (2–10 cm).

Management of nevus spilus requires followup examinations, since malignant transformation is possible. Some authors advocate laser therapy, such as the Q-switched ruby laser or liquid nitrogen cryotherapy, for cosmetic treatment. Because of the possibility of malignant transformation, these destructive methods are no longer recommended. A few clinicians advocate prophylactic excision, if practical. Since almost all melanomas have developed in large congenital lesions and are extremely rare, careful followup, as in the management of congenital melanocytic nevi, is appropriate in most cases. If a suspicious area develops within the nevus, it can be biopsied. As with all melanocytic lesions, good photoprotection should be practiced.

In the present patient, the biopsy showed a benign junction nevus on a background of lentigo simplex. She will undergo close followup.

Clinical Pearls

1. Nevus spilus (speckled lentiginous nevus) is seen in up to 3% of adults.

2. The tan patch representing the background of nevus spilus most often is found to be a lentigo simplex on histopathologic examination.

3. The darker macules or papules within a nevus spilus generally are junctional, intradermal, or compound nevi.

4. Malignant melanoma is a rare complication of nevus spilus. Destructive cosmetic procedures no longer are recommended.

REFERENCES
1. Breitkopf C, Ernst K, Hundeiker M: Neoplasms in nevus spilus. Hautarzt 47:759–762, 1996.
2. Casanova D, Bardot J, Aubert JP, et al: Management of nevus spilus. Pediatr Dermatol 13:233–238, 1996.
3. Grevelink JM, Gonzalez S, Bonoan R, et al: Treatment of nevus spilus with the Q-switched ruby laser. Dermatol Surg 23:365–369, 1997.
4. Grinspan D, Casala A, Abulafia J, et al: Melanoma in dysplastic nevus spilus. Int J Dermatol 36:499–502, 1997.
5. Hwang SM, Choi EH, Lee WS, et al: Nevus spilus (speckled lentiginous nevus) associated with a nodular neurotized nevus. Am J Dermatopathol 19:308–311, 1997.
6. Weinberg JM, Schutzer PJ, Harris RM, et al: Melanoma arising in nevus spilus. Cutis 61:287–289, 1998.

PATIENT 87

A 27-year-old woman with pruritic, red papules after swimming in the ocean

A 27-year-old woman was vacationing in Florida and noticed the sudden onset of pruritic, red papules 5 minutes after emerging from a swim in the ocean. She showered without removing her bathing suit. The eruption became more pruritic and appeared to spread. Nausea and chills prompted her to seek medical attention. She was in excellent health otherwise, and had never had a similar experience. The emergency department where she was seen had treated several other individuals with the same symptoms on the same day.

Physical Examination: Temperature 37.1°C; pulse 82; respirations 18; blood pressure 115/78. Skin: numerous, erythematous papules clustered on skin underneath two-piece, shorts-type bathing suit; some of lesions excoriated, some follicular (see figure).

Laboratory Findings: No tests performed.

Questions: What is the diagnosis? How can this skin disorder best be prevented in the future?

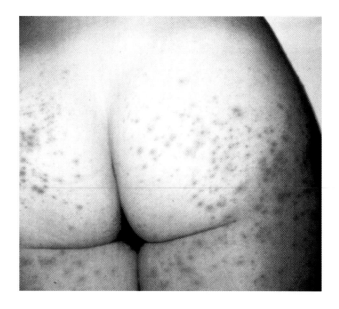

Diagnosis: Seabather's eruption

Discussion: Seabather's eruption is an inflammatory, irritant dermatitis caused by the injection of toxins into the skin from stinging nematocysts. It sometimes is incorrectly referred to as "sea lice," which actually are fish parasites particularly harmful to salmon. When larvae of the phylum Cnidaria (jellyfish, sea anemone, coral) are trapped against the skin or stimulated by friction or fresh water, their stinging nematocysts inject toxin. Each larva contains more than 200 nematocysts. The nematocyst has a coiled, barbed, hollow thread through which toxin is forcefully injected following a physical or chemical stimulus.

Cnidaria larva implicated in outbreaks of seabather's eruption include thimble jellyfish larvae (*Linuche unguiculata*) in southern Florida and the Caribbean and sea anemone larvae (*Edwardsiella lineata*) north of South Carolina. Larvae of the Portuguese man-of-war jellyfish (*Physalia physalia*) also have been implicated. *E. lineata* was responsible for an outbreak in Long Island, New York.

Clinically, pruritic macules, papules, and urticarial plaques develop within minutes to 2 hours after exposure to infected sea water. Those with a prior exposure subsequently have worse episodes, suggesting a hypersensitivity reaction. Areas covered by swimsuits, bathing caps, scuba gear, wet suits, and fins typically are involved. Friction and occlusion on the chest of surfers also has produced lesions at this site. The dermatitis is most severe where pressure from the suit is greatest, such as at the waist or shoulder. The stinging sensation is first felt as the bather leaves the water. Washing off in fresh water without removing the bathing suit immediately worsens the stinging. The lesions may progress to vesicles or pustules. Systemic symptoms such as high fever, chills, fatigue, nausea, malaise, and lymphadenopathy may be seen, particularly in children.

Outbreaks tend to occur in epidemics in localized geographic areas, perhaps related to ocean currents transporting the larvae close to shore. During epidemic years, millions of pink, round, or oval ciliated larvae, 2–3 mm long, can be found in the ocean and at the water's edge. These visible larvae are *E. lineata*; *L. unguiculata*, at only 0.5 mm long, are not visible. During nonepidemic years, arrival of the larvae at the water's edge usually has been delayed until September or October when the swimming season has ended, and few cases of seabather's eruption are reported.

The histologic picture shows a mixed perivascular and perifollicular infiltrate, with neutrophils and eosinophils. The *differential diagnosis* includes arthropod bites, varicella, syphilis, urticaria, viral exanthems, hot tub folliculitis (also occurs under bathing suits, but is seen in chlorinated water), and swimmer's itch (due to avian cercariae, a Schistosome larva that lives in fresh water and usually affects exposed, not covered, skin). The tiny hydromedusa jellyfish also can produce a pruritic stinging dermatitis under the bathing suit.

Management of seabather's eruption includes immediate removal of the bathing suit or other occlusive material and showering followed by vigorous towel drying. Prevention is especially important if prior exposure has occurred, since subsequent reactions tend to be more severe. The wearing of T-shirts while swimming and one-piece occlusive swimwear in women seem to favor the condition. Spontaneous resolution occurs within 2 weeks, usually 7–10 days. Topical corticosteroids and oral antihistamines generally are sufficient. In rare severe cases, a short course of oral corticosteroids may be given. The involved swimsuit must be destroyed, because nematocysts can remain active and discharge toxin even after their larvae are dead and the swimsuit has been thoroughly dried.

The present patient discarded her bathing suit and showered again. Oral antihistamines and topical steroids were provided for 5 days, with complete resolution of all symptoms.

Clinical Pearls

1. Seabather's eruption is an irritant dermatitis caused by toxins of Cnidarian larvae.

2. Seabather's eruption affects covered areas of skin where the larvae have been trapped, allowing the stinging nematocysts to inject their toxin.

3. Those at greatest risk of seabather's eruption are surfers, children, and individuals with a prior history of the disease. Length of time in the water does not appear to increase the risk.

REFERENCES

1. Freudenthal AR, Joseph PR: Seabather's eruption. N Engl J Med 329:542–544, 1993.
2. Tomchik RS, Russell MT, Szmant AM, et al: Clinical perspectives on seabather's eruption, also known as "sea lice." JAMA 269:1669–1672, 1993.
3. Kumar S, Hlady WG, Malecki JM: Risk factors for seabather's eruption: A prospective cohort study. Public Health Rep 112:59–62, 1997.

PATIENT 88

An 11-day-old girl with blistering

An 11-day-old girl was noted at birth to have erosions on her buttocks (attributed to breech delivery) and blisters around one thumbnail. When blistering spread, she was treated with oral antibiotics, without benefit. She eventually was readmitted to the hospital. The baby had done well at home. There was no family history of a blistering disease.

Physical Examination: Temperature 38.5°C; height and weight 60% percentile. General: hoarse cry noted. Skin: scattered, large erosions on extremities and trunk with several intact bullae; partially healed erosions containing newly formed blisters on buttocks (see figure). Nails: periungual blisters around thumbs, with dystrophic changes of nail plates.

Laboratory Findings: CBC with differential: normal. Blood cultures: no growth at 48 hours. Skin biopsies obtained for routine, electron microscopic, and immunofluorescent examination: pending.

Question: What is your most immediate concern?

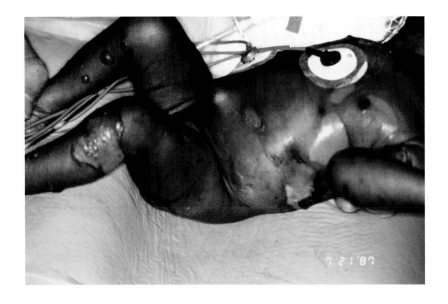

Diagnosis: Junctional epidermolysis bullosa, Herlitz subtype

Discussion: The Herlitz or letalis subtype of junctional epidermolysis bullosa (EB) is an autosomal recessive, severe, blistering disease of skin and mucous membranes, with death occurring in infancy usually within the first year of life. Any internal organ with an epithelial surface may be affected, including the gastrointestinal tract, the genitourinary tract, and the tracheobronchial tree. Tracheal stenosis develops uncommonly, with a hoarse cry often being the first clinical sign of its presence. Blistering develops in areas of pressure or friction, followed by atrophic scarring and further blistering within the scarred areas. A hallmark of Herlitz junctional EB is the presence of perioral and perinasal granulation tissue. This tissue often is heaped up, sometimes severely enough to occlude the nares.

The pathogenesis of Herlitz junctional EB is related to an abnormal expression of the anchoring filament laminin-5 (kalinin/nicein). Laminin-5 is a basement membrane macromolecule synthesized by basal cells that mediates keratinocyte attachment and dermoepidermal adhesion and cohesion. The genetic defects leading to abnormalities in laminin-5 involve mutations in one of the three genes (LAMA3, LAMB3, or LAMC2) that encode for the three polypeptide chains (subunits) of laminin-5 (alpha 3, beta 3, and gamma 2). The LAMB3 gene has been mapped to chromosome 1q32. Various authors have identified specific mutations. In one child with Herlitz junctional EB, there was a nonsense mutation in LAMA3 involving a homozygous C-to-T transition. Both parents were heterozygous carriers of the same mutation. In another report, nonsense mutations in LAMB3 were identified (termed Q936X). One particular mutation in the LAMB3 gene (termed R635X) is present in about 40% of all junctional EB laminin-5 mutations. Because it is noted so frequently in Herlitz junctional EB, it is thought to represent a mutational hotspot rather than propagation of a common ancestral allele. The R635X mutation and another mutational hotspot, R642X, are thought to account for over 50% of mutant LAMB3 alleles. The R635X hotspot mutation has been reported from many different areas of the world. Two heterozygous parental carriers usually are required to produce a homozygous child. However, in one recent report, a heterozygous carrier mother and normal father produced a child homozygous for Herlitz junctional EB. The authors suggest that the maternal LAMB3 heterozygous mutation on chromosome 1q32 was reduced to homozygosity, resulting in disease in the affected child.

Differentiating Herlitz junctional EB from the nonHerlitz, nonlethal variety of junctional EB is the focus of many investigations. One study found that nonlethal junctional EB in two patients also involved abnormalities of laminin-5. Both patients had combinations of a nonsense and a missense mutation in the LAMB3 gene, so that both patients were compound heterozygotes, rather than homozygotes as in Herlitz junctional EB. Compound heterozygosity may produce a milder form of junctional EB according to these authors. The best characterized type of nonlethal junctional EB is generalized atrophic benign EB, which shows a decreased expression of type 7 collagen and mutations in its gene, COL17A1.

An association between junctional EB and pyloric atresia now is considered a syndrome separate from Herlitz junctional EB. One study noted the absence of alpha 6 integrin in two patients with the syndrome, but normal levels in all other EB subtypes used as controls. In contrast to the patients with Herlitz junctional EB, the patients with the syndrome all had normal expression of laminin-5 in the basement membrane zone. Other differences from Herlitz junctional EB that are seen in the junctional EB–pyloric atresia syndrome include lack of prominent granulation tissue, increased frequency of genitourinary and ear abnormalities, and the occasional occurrence of aplasia cutis congenita or esophageal atresia.

Prenatal diagnosis of Herlitz junctional EB is now possible. Fetal skin biopsy with electron microscopy can be performed. Laminin-5 is a normal component of amniotic fluid, but is absent when the fetus has Herlitz junctional EB. One study of 49 pregnancies compared the results of amniocentesis with Western blot analysis to detect laminin-5. In the four fetuses with Herlitz junctional EB, none had laminin-5 in the amniotic fluid, and subsequent skin biopsy showed no GB3 (immunofluorescent marker of nicein) reactivity. In the one fetus with generalized nonHerlitz junctional EB, laminin-5 was normal in the amniotic fluid, but the fetal skin biopsy showed GB3 reactivity. The 44 normal pregnancies all had laminin-5 in the amniotic fluid. Another method of prenatal diagnosis involves polymerase chain reaction to detect mutations in the laminin-5 genes in fetal DNA. In a study of 15 families at risk for recurrent Herlitz junction EB, the two fetuses with Herlitz junctional EB were accurately identified; the others were excluded because they were genetically normal or carried the mutation on only one allele.

In the present patient, the routine histopathologic examination revealed a subepidermal vesicle, which on electron microscopic examination showed a split in the lamina lucida. The hemidesmosomes were hypoplastic. Immunofluorescent antigenic mapping of her skin showed laminin-5 and type IV collagen localized to the blister base, BP antigen on both the roof and the base, and type VII collagen only at the base. Immunofluorescent staining for laminin-5 was negative. Of immediate concern in this child was tracheal involvement, as suggested by the hoarse cry; involvement was confirmed by bronchoscopy. A tracheostomy was performed. She continued with an unstable course and progressive blistering leading to daily fluid, electrolyte, and nutrition management as well as infection prevention problems. Although she was not septic on arrival to the hospital, four episodes of sepsis occurred. The patient died at the age of 3 months.

Clinical Pearls

1. The specific genetic defect producing Herlitz junctional epidermolysis bullosa has been identified as a mutation in one or more of the genes that encode for the subunit chains of laminin-5.

2. Herlitz junctional EB can be diagnosed or excluded prenatally using electron microscopy on fetal skin biopsy, Western blot detection of laminin-5 in amniotic fluid, or fetal DNA analysis to detect mutations in the laminin-5 genes.

3. Early clinical indicators of Herlitz junctional EB include a hoarse cry, marking tracheal involvement, and perioral and perinasal heaped-up granulation tissue.

REFERENCES

1. Marinkovich MP, Meneguzzi G, Burgeson RE, et al: Prenatal diagnosis of Herlitz junctional epidermolysis bullosa by amniocentesis. Prenat Diagn 15:1027–1034, 1995.
2. Ashton GH, Mellerio JE, Dunnill MG, et al: A recurrent laminin 5 mutation in British patients with lethal (Herlitz) junctional epidermolysis bullosa: Evidence for a mutational hotspot rather than propagation of an ancestral allele. Br J Dermatol 136:674–677, 1997.
3. Christiano AM, Pulkkinen L, McGrath JA, et al: Mutation-based prenatal diagnosis of Herlitz junctional epidermolysis bullosa. Prenat Diagn 17:343–354, 1997.
4. Shaw DW, Fine JD, Piacquadio DJ, et al: Gastric outlet obstruction and epidermolysis bullosa. J Am Acad Dermatol 36:304–310, 1997.
5. Takizawa Y, Pulkkinen L, Shimizu H, et al: Maternal uniparental meroisodisomy in the LAMB3 region of chromosome 1 results in lethal junctional epidermolysis bullosa. J Invest Dermatol 110:828–831, 1998.

PATIENT 89

A 24-year-old woman with sudden onset of draining facial lesions

A 24-year-old woman noted the sudden appearance of erythematous papules, nodules, and pustules 3 weeks ago. She applied numerous nonprescription, topical medications without benefit. The nodules enlarged and spread, and some drained clear fluid. She had no fever and was in good health otherwise. She was not receiving systemic medications. During adolescence, she had mild acne vulgaris controlled with topical nonprescription agents. She had always blushed easily and noted that alcohol or Mexican food produced flushing.

Physical Examination: Vital signs: normal. Face: erythematous papules and nodules concentrated around central face and chin and extending onto forehead (see figure); scattered pustules and draining sinus tracts; some fluctuant and tender nodules; no lesions on neck, back, or chest.

Laboratory Findings: Bacterial culture of sinus drainage: mixed skin flora.

Questions: What is your diagnosis? How should this patient be managed?

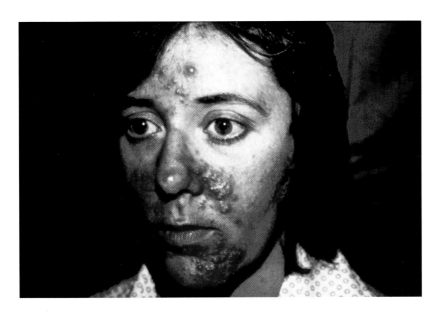

Diagnosis: Pyoderma faciale

Discussion: Pyoderma faciale was described in 1940 by O'Leary and Kierland. It is a rare disease of young women characterized by the explosive onset of inflammatory facial papules, pustules, nodules, cysts, abscesses, and draining sinuses. Nodules may be fluctuant, and they coalesce, forming grotesque cosmetic deformities. The central face is particularly susceptible. Women affected are 19–40 years old. In one study, the range was 15–46 years, with a mean of 25 years. Pyoderma faciale usually is seen after adolescence, and affected women typically do not have a history of severe acne, although many have lifelong histories of blushing and flushing. Many also have a history of seborrhea. There is rapid progression, with scarring and keloid formation, if treatment is not instituted promptly.

The etiopathogenesis is unclear. There are at least three theories leading to different classifications. Some consider pyoderma faciale a variant of the severe and explosive **acne conglobata**. Acne conglobata is seen in men, in association with the XYY genotype. It consists of comedones, papules, pustules, cysts, abscesses, draining sinuses, and scarring and is not limited to the face, but extends to the neck, trunk, and arms. In addition to these skin findings, acne fulminans also shows systemic symptoms such as fever, malaise, and arthralgias and may feature leukocytosis. Acne fulminans responds to oral steroids in association with systemic antibiotics. A second theory is that pyoderma faciale is a **folliculitis syndrome**. There is no previous history of severe acne in pyoderma faciale, and coagulase-positive staphylococcus often is present.

Moreover, no or few comedones are present, and the onset is sudden—characteristics of folliculitis and not of acne vulgaris. The authors of the third theory state that pyoderma faciale is, in fact, **rosacea fulminans**. In their study of 20 patients, all had been flushers and blushers in the past, as is characteristic of acne rosacea. Pyoderma was not present.

Histopathologic examination of pyoderma faciale reveals epithelioid granulomas; septal and lobular panniculitis; and a dense, mixed infiltrate that includes neutrophils and eosinophils and is both perivascular and periadnexal. The draining sinuses contain corneocytes, hair, serum, bacteria, inflammatory cells, and epithelioid granulomas. Draining sinuses emerge from elongated (2–5 cm), inflamed, scarred plaques; these discharge pus or clear fluid and show no spontaneous regression.

The treatment of pyoderma faciale must be prompt so that scarring is minimized. The current recommended treatment is systemic isotretinoin and systemic corticosteroids, a combination that appears to achieve a more rapid response than high-dose systemic antibiotics. Occasionally, surgical opening and drainage of sinus tracts is necessary. Rarely, total excision of the tracts may be necessary.

In the present patient, biopsy results were consistent with the typical findings of pyoderma faciale. She was started on oral isotretinoin and oral corticosteroids, and the steroids were tapered and discontinued within 6 weeks. She responded well to this treatment regimen, with marked cosmetic improvement.

Clinical Pearls

1. Pyoderma faciale is seen in post-adolescent women without a history of severe adolescent acne vulgaris, but often with a history of oily skin and easy flushing and blushing.

2. There is no consensus as to the classification of pyoderma faciale. It may represent rosacea fulminans, a variant of acne rosacea; a variant of acne conglobata; or a folliculitis syndrome.

3. Prompt diagnosis and treatment with oral isotretinoin and corticosteroids is imperative to prevent further progression and severe scarring.

REFERENCES

1. Plewig G, Jansen T, Kligman AM: Pyoderma faciale. A review and report of 20 additional cases: Is it rosacea? Arch Dermatol 128:1611–1617, 1992.
2. Jansen T, Plewig G: An historical note on pyoderma faciale. Br J Dermatol 129:594–596, 1993.
3. Jansen T, Plewig G, Kligman AM: Diagnosis and treatment of rosacea fulminans. Dermatology 188:251–254, 1994.
4. Jansen T, Lindner A, Plewig G: Draining sinus in acne and rosacea: A clinical, histopathologic and experimental study. Hautarzt 46:417–420, 1995.
5. Tan BB, Lear JT, Smith AG: Acne fulminans and erythema nodosum during isotretinoin therapy responding to dapsone. Clin Exp Dermatol 22:26–27, 1997.

PATIENT 90

A 2-year-old girl with brown patches on the arm and back

A 2-year-old girl was born with several large, irregular, brown patches on her right upper back, shoulder, arm, and forearm. The parents had been reassured that these were "normal birthmarks." In the last month, they noticed the appearance of pubic hair. Two days previously, vaginal bleeding developed. She was otherwise in good health.

Physical Examination: Vital signs: normal. Skin: large, irregular, brown patches with jagged borders on right upper back, shoulder, arm, and forearm; patch on back stops abruptly at midline (see figure, *left*). Thyroid: no nodules, enlargement, or tenderness. Abdomen: no organomegaly or masses. Genitalia: scant pubic hair; scant blood at introitus. Extremities: slightly bowed.

Laboratory Findings: CBC, serum chemistries, thyroid function studies: normal. Radiographs of legs: several areas of radiolucency (see figure, *right*). A pediatric endocrinologist was consulted.

Question: What is the diagnosis?

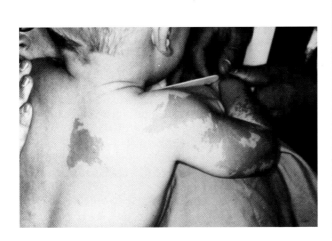
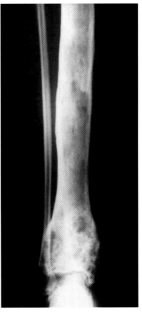

Diagnosis: McCune-Albright syndrome

Discussion: McCune-Albright syndrome (polyostotic fibrous dysplasia) consists of the triad of skin, bone, and endocrinologic abnormalities. Abnormalities of two of these three areas are required for diagnosis. Only about a third of patients have skin manifestations.

The skin manifestations consist of hyperpigmented patches that usually are large, few in number, and unilateral, respecting the midline. They often have jagged, irregular borders, described as "coast of Maine," in contrast to the "coast of California" café au lait macules of neurofibromatosis, which are smooth-bordered. McCune-Albright patches typically are darker than those of neurofibromatosis and usually are seen on the same side as the underlying bone lesions. They may be present at birth or may appear during infancy.

Bony abnormalities, most commonly seen in the long bones, consist of radiolucencies early and radiodensities later in life. The femur is the most frequent site, followed by the ilium. Lesions can occur anywhere, including the skull, clavicles, and pelvis. Symptoms and signs from the fibrous dysplasia include bowing or other deformities, pain, and fractures. Craniofacial involvement may produce impingement on neurovascular structures. Calcium and phosphorous levels typically are normal, but alkaline phosphatase may be increased. In the past, it was estimated that 1–5% of bony lesions become malignant. However, this rate may have been related to previous irradiation. Some authors think that malignant transformation of bone does not occur in McCune-Albright syndrome.

Precocious puberty is the most common endocrinopathy, occurring in a third of affected girls. Menarche may be seen in the first year of life. Precocious puberty is ovarian controlled, with normal pituitary function. Ovarian cysts frequently are present. The second most common endocrinopathy is **hyperthyroidism**, which also is under local control. Thyroid disease in McCune-Albright syndrome often is recurrent and has a high morbidity, including thyroid storm during surgery. Thyroid ablation generally is required for control. Other endocrinopathies that may be seen include Cushing's syndrome, acromegaly, adenomas, and hyperprolactinemia.

Histopathologic examination of the hyperpigmented patches reveals findings identical to the café au lait macules of neurofibromatosis. There is hyperpigmentation of the basal layer, with no elongation or clubbing of the rete ridges as seen in lentigines. There is no change in the number or size of melanocytes. Rarely, one may see giant melanin granules, which are present in many other conditions such as neurofibromatosis, lentigo simplex, multiple lentigines syndrome, speckled lentiginous nevus (nevus spilus), Becker's melanosis, melanocytic nevus, Spitz nevus, and normal skin. Electron microscopic examination demonstrates many enlarged melanosomes that are dispersed within the cytoplasm rather than within melanosome complexes; this is similar to what is observed in black skin. It is thought that this finding is due to increased melanin degradation.

The *differential diagnosis* of large, hyperpigmented patches includes neurofibromatosis 1 or segmental neurofibromatosis. Other causes of café au lait macules include tuberous sclerosis, Bloom syndrome, ataxia telangiectasia, Fanconi anemia, multiple lentigines syndrome, Maffucci syndrome, Russell Silver syndrome, Watson syndrome, and Bannayon-Riley-Ruvalcaba syndrome.

The cause of McCune-Albright syndrome has been partially elucidated. There are activating missense mutations in exon 8 of the Gs-alpha gene that cause an increase in Gs-alpha membrane-associated protein, leading to an increase in cyclic AMP activity. These are thought to represent post-zygotic (somatic) mutations of an autosomal dominant gene. The resulting individual is mosaic for both normal and mutated cells. One group applied this information to the bone abnormalities and isolated progenitor cells from McCune-Albright fibrous dysplastic marrow. Analysis of the Gs-alpha gene revealed two distinct genotypes within a single fibrous dysplasia lesion. One genotype was normal, with normal Gs-alpha alleles, and the other was abnormal, with one normal allele and one mutated allele. Clonal populations of the normal progenitor cells were transplanted into immunocompromised mice. Normal bone formed. When only the mutant cells were transplanted, no bone growth occurred. Transplantation of both the normal and mutant cells led to the production of an abnormal ossicle with fibrous dysplasia.

Others have proposed that overactivity of adenylyl cyclase and excess cyclic AMP could produce the bony abnormality. They showed that Gs-alpha expression was critically up-regulated during maturation of precursor osteogenic cells to normal osteoblastic cells in lesions of polyostotic fibrous dysplasia. This tissue subsequently contained excess preosteogenic cells, as well as abnormal osteoblasts. These abnormal osteoblasts produced a bone matrix rich in certain anti-adhesion molecules and poor in certain pro-adhesive molecules, the opposite of that seen in normal bone. This finding may be evidence of a direct link between the gene product and the histopathologic abnormality.

The Gs-alpha protein mediates thyrotropin (TSH)-induced activation of adenylyl cyclase. In one patient with McCune-Albright syndrome whose symptoms included precocious puberty, hyperthyroidism, and liver dysfunction, the somatic activating mutation of the Gs-alpha gene was identified in ovary, thyroid, and peripheral blood. The gene has been identified in ovarian cyst fluid alone.

Treatment of McCune-Albright syndrome includes reassuring the parents that lifespan is normal and fertility and stature usually are not affected. Some authors have reported short stature, secondary to premature closure of epiphyses. Orthopedic management is critical. Bone lesions *should not be irradiated* because of the risk of malignant transformation. Avoidance of bone fracture should be attempted, but fractures may heal normally if they do occur. For severe pain, deformities, and nonhealing fractures, more advanced orthopedic procedures such as curettage of symptomatic fibrous lesions, osteotomy, bone grafts, internal fixation with rods, and even amputation are used. Endocrinologic evaluation and treatment requires consultation from a pediatric endocrinologist.

In the present patient, an extensive pediatric endocrinologic evaluation revealed ovarian cysts; these were managed with hormonal therapy. The cystic bone lesions were asymptomatic. The child is being closely followed for the development of any orthopedic problems.

Clinical Pearls

1. The most common endocrinopathies seen in McCune-Albright syndrome are precocious puberty, seen in a third of affected girls, and hyperthyroidism with or without goiter.

2. McCune-Albright syndrome is caused by somatic mutations in the large Gs-alpha gene that produce increased cyclic AMP activity. This increased activity is related to the endocrinopathies and may be related to the bony changes.

3. Treatment of symptomatic bone lesions in McCune-Albright syndrome should never include irradiation because of the risk of malignant transformation.

REFERENCES

1. Mastorakos G, Mitsiades NS, Doufas AG, et al: Hyperthyroidism in McCune-Albright syndrome with a review of thyroid abnormalities 60 years after the first report. Thyroid 7:433–439, 1997.
2. Riminucci M, Fisher LW, Shenker A: Fibrous dysplasia of bone in the McCune-Albright syndrome: Abnormalities in bone formation. Am J Pathol 151:1587–1600, 1997.
3. Spiegel AM: The molecular basis of disorders caused by defects in G proteins. Horm Res 47:89–96, 1997.
4. Bianco P, Kuznetsov SA, Riminucci M, et al: Reproduction of human fibrous dysplasia of bone in immunocompromised mice by transplanted mosaics of normal and Gs-alpha-mutated skeletal progenitor cells. J Clin Invest 15:1737–1744, 1998.

PATIENT 91

A 28-year-old woman with pruritic "blackheads"

A 26-year-old woman complained of numerous "blackheads," of 13-year duration, on her cheeks, nose, and forehead. They were moderately pruritic. Despite numerous nonprescription creams and ointments, the lesions persisted. Her 23-year-old sister has similar lesions.

Physical Examination: Skin: numerous tiny, black papules within enlarged follicular openings over cheeks, nose, and forehead (see figure); no keratotic or cystic lesions elsewhere on skin.

Laboratory Findings: Epilumescent microscopy: each black papule consisted of a follicular plug containing multiple thin hairs.

Question: What treatment do you recommend for this patient?

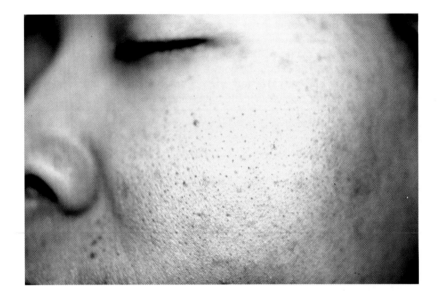

Diagnosis: Trichostasis spinulosa

Discussion: Trichostasis spinulosa is a common but underdiagnosed disorder of the pilosebaceous unit with follicular hyperkeratosis. **Vellus hairs** are not shed and become embedded in the hyperkeratotic material. It is a common disorder in the elderly after sun damage and has been reported frequently in adults and even in a 13-year-old child whose lesions began at the age of 18 months. It often is pruritic and typically is located on the face. Occasionally, however, lesions may be seen on the trunk and extremities. The clinical picture is one of noninflammatory black papules resembling open comedones or raised follicular spines.

The *differential diagnosis* includes the open comedones of acne vulgaris, which are easily differentiated on examination with a magnifying lens. Both keratosis pilaris and eruptive vellus hair cysts may coexist with trichostasis spinulosa. Again, they are easily differentiated on magnification because they do not show vellus hairs protruding from the follicular opening. A trichofolliculoma is a solitary nodule on the neck, face, or scalp with a central pore containing feathery, fine, vellus hairs resembling a white wooly or cotton tuft.

Biopsy of trichostasis spinulosa reveals a dilated vellus hair follicle containing a keratinous plug or sheath within the infundibulum. Embedded within this plug are 6–20 parallel, vellus, telogen (club) hairs. These hairs have all been produced by the same hair matrix and are retained (not shed) because of the follicular infundibular hyperkeratosis that obstructs their exit. Abnormal angulation of the isthmus relative to the infundibulum also may contribute to this hair entrapment.

Treatment of trichostasis spinulosa primarily is cosmetic; it may be symptomatic if pruritus is a complaint. Medications used with success include topical tretinoin, keratolytics, and topical corticosteroids. Pore stripper tape also works well.

In the present patient, topical tretinoin was prescribed because of the extent of involvement. She was pleased with the cosmetic outcome and continues to use the medication daily.

Clinical Pearls

1. Trichostasis spinulosa is a common, but frequently underdiagnosed, condition. Use of a magnifying lens or epilumescent microscopy simplifies the diagnosis.
2. Trichostasis spinulosa consists of 6–20 vellus hairs embedded in a follicular keratin plug.
3. Treatment is removal of the keratinous plug with tretinoin or pore stripper tape.

REFERENCES
1. Young MC, Jorizzo JL, Sanchez RL, et al: Trichostasis spinulosa. Int J Dermatol 24:575–580, 1985.
2. Lazarov A, Amichai B, Cagnano M, et al: Coexistence of trichostasis spinulosa and eruptive vellus hair cysts. Int J Dermatol 33:858–859, 1994.
3. Harford RR, Cobb MW, Miller ML: Trichostasis spinulosa: A clinical simulant of acne open comedones. Pediatr Dermatol 13:490–492, 1996.
4. Noel N, Gerstein D, Faust H: Pruritic hyperkeratotic facial papules: Trichostasis spinulosa. Arch Dermatol 133:1579, 1582, 1997.

PATIENT 92

A 35-year-old woman with a pruritic axillary rash

A 35-year-old woman sustained pruritic papules in the axillae 10 years previously. She consulted a physician 5 years ago and was diagnosed with contact dermatitis from her deodorant. Despite trying numerous different deodorants and nonprescription topical medications, she had been unable to obtain relief from the pruritus. She noted that during the pregnancy with her 3-year-old child, the pruritus was absent during the latter months. She used birth control pills until the age of 25, but was on no medications since. There was no family history of a similar eruption.

Physical Examination: Skin: axillae hyperpigmented, scant axillary hair, no odor; numerous tiny, discrete papules that are firm, follicular, and acuminate in both axillae (figure); a few similar lesions in pubic region and between breasts. Remainder of skin examination: normal.

Laboratory Findings: No tests performed.

Questions: What is the diagnosis? How would you best control the pruritus?

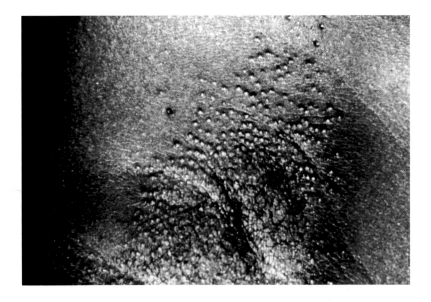

Diagnosis: Fox-Fordyce disease (apocrine miliaria)

Discussion: Fox-Fordyce disease is a disorder of apocrine sweat retention first described by Fox and Fordyce in 1902. It begins in adolescence, but may have its onset between 13 and 35 years. It is more common in females, with a predominance of 10:1. Black and white individuals are affected equally. It has been reported rarely in families, and there has been occasional onset in a post-menopausal woman.

Clinically, Fox-Fordyce disease presents with extremely pruritic papules that tend to be acuminate or round-topped and involve the axillae and pubic regions. Other areas of apocrine gland distribution, including the areolae, inframammary areas, and the midline infraumbilical area, also may be involved.

The pathogenesis of Fox-Fordyce disease involves an initial keratin plug in the infundibulum of the hair follicle that then extends into the apocrine duct. Following this complete obstruction, intraepidermal parts of the apocrine duct rupture, and microvesicles form. This **apocrine sweat retention vesicle** is pathognomonic. Periductal acanthosis, spongiosis, an inflammatory infiltrate, and dermal mucin then occur. A bedside test to confirm the diagnosis of Fox-Fordyce disease involves the injection of a small amount of epinephrine or oxytocin into the axillary skin; this normally produces apocrine sweating. In Fox-Fordyce disease, no apocrine sweat appears, although symptoms of pruritus may follow the injection.

There is a relationship between Fox-Fordyce disease and hormones, but it has not been clearly elucidated. Most women improve dramatically during the last trimester of pregnancy. However, treatment with topical or systemic estrogens (such as conjugated estrogens) has been ineffective. There is no relationship of symptoms to the menstrual cycle; however, estrogen-containing birth control pills may provide relief.

Differentiating Fox-Fordyce disease from other follicular axillary diseases usually is not difficult. The following diseases may present in similar ways: folliculitis, neurodermatitis, Hailey-Hailey disease, hidradenitis suppurativa, and lichen planus.

Topical treatments such as topical corticosteroids, retinoids, and keratolytics can produce some relief, but the results are variable. Intralesional steroids occasionally are beneficial, but they are difficult to administer. Topical antibiotics, including clindamycin, have been used successfully. Oral contraceptives containing estrogen usually are helpful. Oral isotretinoin has provided temporary relief in one man. Rarely, surgical excision with grafting is necessary. There is a recent report of surgical treatment of a patient who only had areolar involvement. In this case, the areolae were detached (preserving the nipples), the underlying apocrine glands were excised, and the areolae were reattached.

In the present patient, topical tretinoin was tried for 6 weeks, with only moderate benefit. She was then placed on an oral contraceptive, and her symptoms almost completely resolved.

Clinical Pearls

1. Fox-Fordyce disease (apocrine miliaria) is produced by a keratinous obstruction in the apocrine duct, which results in rupture of the intraepidermal portion of the duct and formation of a microvesicle containing apocrine sweat.

2. The disease causes apocrine anhidrosis, so that injections of epinephrine or oxytocin fail to produce apocrine sweating.

3. Treatment sometimes is problematic. Oral contraceptives may be helpful, particularly in women who have experienced remissions during pregnancy.

REFERENCES

1. Chavoin JP, Charasson T, Bernard JD: Surgical treatment of hidradenitis and Fox-Fordyce disease of the nipples. Ann Chir Plast Esthet 39:233–238, 1994.
2. Effendy I, Ossowski B, Happle R: Fox-Fordyce disease in a male patient—response to oral retinoid treatment. Clin Exp Dermatol 19:67–69, 1994.
3. Ranalletta M, Rositto A, Drut R: Fox-Fordyce disease in two prepubertal girls: Histopathologic demonstration of eccrine sweat gland involvement. Pediatr Dermatol 13:294–297, 1996.

PATIENT 93

A 4-year-old boy with a birthmark on the face

A 4-year-old boy was brought by his parents for treatment of a pink, facial birthmark. The lesion was light pink at birth and had gradually become slightly more erythematous. The patient had never had a seizure, appeared to be in good health, and had shown normal developmental milestones.

Physical Examination: Vital signs: normal. Skin: erythematous patch on left face extending from eyebrow to lower cheek; midline respected except for one patch extending onto right upper cheek (see figure). Eyes: pink patches on left upper and lower lids; sclera and conjunctiva clear. Fundoscopy: no abnormalities. Neurologic: normal.

Laboratory Findings: Skull x-rays: no intracranial calcifications. Ophthalmologic examination: no increased intraocular pressure or structural abnormalities. MRI: pending.

Questions: What syndrome must be considered in this child? How should cosmetic concerns be approached?

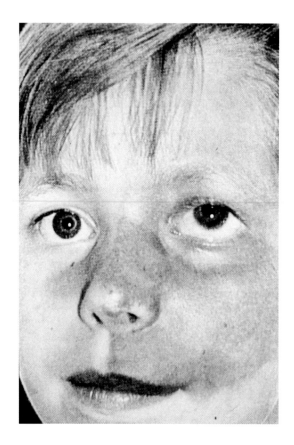

Diagnosis: Port wine stain (nevus flameus)

Discussion: A new classification system divides vascular birthmarks or anomalies into hemangiomas, in which endothelial proliferation is present, and vascular malformations, in which endothelial proliferation is absent. The port wine stain (nevus flameus) is a **vascular malformation**. The nevus simplex resembles the nevus flameus clinically, but represents ectatic vessels of persistent fetal circulation and behaves differently. The nevus simplex also is known as the "salmon patch," "stork bite," or "angel's kiss."

Port wine stains are flat, pink patches present at birth, occurring in 0.3% of newborns. The face is the most common site, but the neck, trunk, or any area may be involved. These birthmarks usually are unilateral or dermatomal, but may have areas that cross the midline. Port wine stains grow proportionate to the child and never regress spontaneously. Their color becomes darker red to purple, and eventually they thicken and develop angiomatous papules and nodules. These lesions may develop underlying soft tissue hypertrophy secondary to the increased vascular supply to the area.

There are several syndromes involving port wine stains that should be of concern to the clinician. **Sturge-Weber syndrome** (encephalotrigeminal angiomatosis) is a facial port wine stain that follows the distribution of the trigeminal nerve and is associated with vascular malformations of the leptomeninges overlying the ipsilateral cerebral cortex. Many believe that involvement of the first division of the trigeminal nerve (V_1) is necessary for the neuro-ocular syndrome to be present. Even when V_1 is involved, only about 10% of patients have the Sturge-Weber syndrome. Seizures occur in about 80%. Mental retardation is present in over a third, and other neurologic problems include focal neurologic defects; contralateral hemiplegia; and ipsilateral, intracranial, doubly-contoured, and curvilinear calcifications. These calcifications are most common in the occipital regions and are said to resemble railroad tracks or tramlines. The calcifications are not present at birth, but are seen in approximately 60% of patients with Sturge-Weber syndrome on the skull x-ray by the age of 2 years. Eye involvement occurs in 33% of patients. Choroid, conjunctival, or iris angiomas may be present, leading to retinal detachment, hemianoptic visual defects, and glaucoma.

Other syndromes that may be seen in association with port wine stains include **Klippel-Trenaunay** (angio-osteohypertrophy), in which port wine stains are associated with varicosities and hypertrophy of bone and soft tissue; **Parks-Weber**, which includes arteriovenous fistulae in addition to the findings of Klippel-Trenaunay syndrome; and **Cobb**, in which a port wine stain is associated with a spinal cord angioma.

Histopathologic examination of a port wine stain at birth reveals normal skin. Eventually, dilated mature capillaries surrounded by loosely arranged collagen fibers are seen in the upper and mid dermis. As the child ages, the capillary ectasias gradually increase and spread deeper in the dermis and even the subcutaneous tissue. There is never endothelial proliferation. Theories on the histogenesis include a congenital weakness of the capillary walls, weakness of the supporting dermal elements, or an abnormality of neural control of blood vessels.

Treatment of a port wine stain is best accomplished with the 585-nm flashlamp-pumped pulsed-dye laser. The wavelength is selectively absorbed by oxyhemoglobin, resulting in superficial destruction of blood vessels with minimal damage to surrounding tissues. The pulse duration is 450 microseconds, which approximates the thermal relaxation time for dermal blood vessels. Many clinicians believe that early treatment in infancy is best because fewer total treatments are needed. One recent study found no evidence that it is necessary to treat in early childhood as opposed to later; however, the thickness of the port wine stains in each group was not controlled for and was not equal. The rationale for treatment includes prevention of psychological harm from feelings of stigmatization, which are thought to begin when the child starts school. Also, port wine stains are known to become thicker and more nodular with age, and these changes can be prevented with early treatment. Finally, soft tissue hypertrophy may appear late, and early treatment is preventative.

Complications of laser therapy are many. The degree of fading of a port wine stain is variable and unpredictable at the outset. Treatment outcomes have not been objectified, although one group has attempted measurement using skin reflectants, ultrasonography, and surface contour analysis. Most results are said to be good, but incomplete. Moreover, the laser is painful. Pigmentary changes may occur in some individuals, and scarring has been reported, including hypertrophic facial scarring. Finally, one recent study reported recurrences of port wine stains within 3–4 years in 50% of treated patients.

Central facial and port wine stains in the V_2 distribution of the trigeminal nerve are more difficult to treat. Patches over bony prominences may require fewer treatments. When used, anesthesia in laser treatment of port wine stains has included a eutectic mixture of local anesthesia (EMLA), sedatives, iontophoresis of 5% lidocaine plus epinephrine (one study of 36 patients, good results), and general anesthesia. Treatments are given every 2 or 3 months.

In the present patient, the MRI was normal, with no calcifications and no brain or blood vessel abnormalities noted. He underwent seven treatments with the pulse-dye laser over 2 years and obtained a 75% lightening of his port wine stain. General anesthesia was necessary in this child. The parents were satisfied with the cosmetic results.

Clinical Pearls

1. A port wine stain (nevus flameus) is a vascular malformation in which endothelial proliferation does *not* occur.

2. A port wine stain in the distribution of the first division of the trigeminal nerve (V_1) raises the possibility of Sturge-Weber syndrome, which includes vascular malformations of the underlying leptomeninges and brain and possibly eye involvement, such as glaucoma.

3. The treatment of choice for port wine stains is the 585-nm flashlamp-pumped pulsed-dye laser.

REFERENCES

1. Orten SS, Waner M, Flock S, et al: Port-wine stains. Arch Otolaryngol Head Neck Surg 122:1174–1179, 1996.
2. Nunez M, Miralles ES, Boixeda P, et al: Iontophoresis for anesthesia during pulsed-dye laser treatment of port-wine stains. Pediatr Dermatol 14:397–400, 1997.
3. Gaston DA, Clark DP: Facial hypertrophic scarring from pulsed-dye laser. Dermatol Surg 24:523–525, 1998.
4. Haedersdal M, Efsen J, Gniadecka M, et al: Changes in skin redness, pigmentation, echostructure, thickness, and surface contour after one pulsed-dye laser treatment of port-wine stains in children. Arch Dermatol 134:175–181, 1998.
5. Van der horst CM, Koster PH, de Borgie CA: Effect of the timing of treatment of port-wine stains with the flash lamp-pumped pulsed-dye laser. N Engl J Med 338:1028–1033, 1998.

PATIENT 94

A 2½-month-old girl with multiple red papules and right-sided abdominal fullness

A 2½-month-old infant was referred with increasing numbers of erythematous papules and suspected liver enlargement. She was born, following a normal pregnancy and delivery, with three small hemangiomas on her skin. Since that time, 21 additional small hemangiomas had appeared over her back, scalp, extremities, hands, and feet. She appeared to be in good health otherwise, with no dyspnea, change in behavior, or disruption of feeding patterns.

Physical Examination: Vital signs: normal. Skin: more than 25 erythematous, blanchable, purplish papules, 2 to 6 mm in size, scattered over abdomen, scalp, back, buttocks, extremities, and fingers (see figure). Abdomen: right-sided fullness with hepatomegaly; no bruit or splenomegaly. Chest: clear. Cardiac: no murmurs. Neurologic: normal; no cranial bruits. Eyes: no hemangiomas.

Laboratory Findings: Stool hematest: negative. Urinalysis: no blood. CBC, platelet count, coagulation profile, liver function tests: normal. EKG and chest radiograph: no congestive heart failure or abnormalities. Liver ultrasound: pending.

Questions: What is the most likely diagnosis? The best treatment plan?

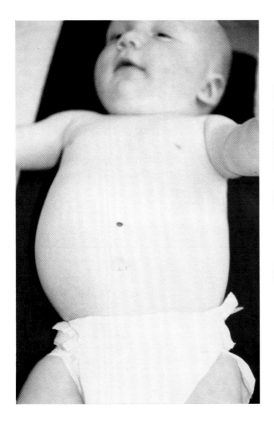

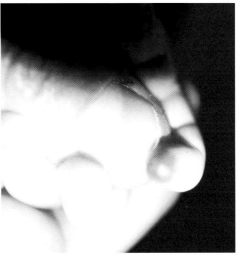

Diagnosis: Diffuse neonatal hemangiomatosis

Discussion: Diffuse neonatal hemangiomatosis refers to the association of numerous cutaneous hemangiomas with internal organ hemangiomas. It is a rare disease that frequently was fatal in the past. Vascular birthmarks or anomalies currently are classified into tumors that proliferate, such as hemangiomas, and vascular malformations that do not proliferate and are structural.

The organs most commonly involved in diffuse neonatal hemangiomatosis include the liver, gastrointestinal tract, lungs, and central nervous system. Life-threatening complications, when they occur, usually present within the first 2 months of life and include congestive heart failure, hemorrhage, hepatic complications, central nervous system compression or hemorrhage, and anemia. Liver hemangiomas are either solitary or multiple and show the same histopathology as those seen on the skin. They also show the same biologic behavior as the skin tumors, regressing over time if the child survives. In the past, the liver lesions were thought to be arteriovenous malformations or "hemangioendothelioma." Hepatic arteriovenous malformations have an extremely high mortality rate and may present with the same triad of symptoms at birth as both solitary and multiple hepatic hemangiomas: hepatomegaly, congestive heart failure, and anemia. In one study, 90% of hepatic vascular anomalies were hemangiomas, and only 10% were arteriovenous malformations. The differentiation can be made on ultrasound or MRI.

In addition to the gastrointestinal tract, lungs, and central nervous system, the eye also may be involved in diffuse neonatal hemangiomatosis. Recently, a neonate suffered involvement of the lid, conjunctiva, iris, ciliary body, and ciliary processes, as well as hyphema and vitreous hemorrhage. Another child had dermal hematopoiesis, presenting as bluish, subcutaneous nodules, in association with diffuse neonatal hemangiomatosis—leading to the first report of this association.

The only way to differentiate diffuse neonatal hemangiomatosis, in which internal organs are involved, from benign neonatal hemangiomatosis, which requires no treatment and spontaneously resolves, is to carefully search for internal involvement on physical exam, perform indicated screening tests, and carefully follow the child.

Treatment of diffuse neonatal hemangiomatosis with life-threatening or extensive involvement primarily involves systemic corticosteroids. If unsuccessful, interferon alpha-2a may be used subsequently or in addition. Spastic diplegia is a recently noted complication of interferon alpha-2a therapy. Interferon alpha-2b has been used, as well. If liver hemangiomas are extensive or symptomatic, and the above medications do not work, embolization or surgical resection often is attempted. Of course, angiography should be performed prior to these procedures. Extensive cutaneous hemangiomas can be successfully treated with the tuneable pulsed-dye laser to prevent hemorrhage or ulceration and to decrease the extent of the cosmetic abnormality.

In the present patient, the liver ultrasound revealed multiple small hepatic hemangiomas. This finding was confirmed on MRI. The child was treated with prednisone and followed carefully by clinical examination as well as repeat MRI studies. Congestive heart failure never developed, and the size of all hemangiomas gradually diminished. By the age of 2 years, hemangiomas on the skin and liver had resolved.

Clinical Pearls

1. Diffuse neonatal hemangiomatosis cannot be differentiated from benign neonatal hemangiomatosis from the skin presentation alone.

2. Diffuse neonatal hemangiomatosis can involve the liver, gastrointestinal tract, lungs, central nervous system, and eye.

3. Treatment of liver hemangiomas seen in diffuse neonatal hemangiomatosis involves systemic corticosteroids, interferon alpha-2a or alpha-2b, embolization, or surgical resection.

REFERENCES

1. Stratte EG, Tope WD, Johnson CL, et al: Multimodal management of diffuse neonatal hemangiomatosis. J Am Acad Dermatol 34:337–342, 1996.
2. Evolve-Buselli M, Hernandez-Marti MJ, Gasco-Lacalle B, et al: Neonatal dermal hematopoiesis associated with diffuse neonatal hemangiomatosis. Pediatr Dermatol 14:383–386, 1997.
3. Chang CW, Rao NA, Stout JT: Histopathology of the eye in diffuse neonatal hemangiomatosis. Am J Ophthalmol 125:868–870, 1998.
4. Enjolras O, Mulliken JB: Vascular tumors and vascular malformations (new issues). Adv Dermatol 13:375–423, 1998.

PATIENT 95

A 38-year-old man with an erythematous eruption and flaccid blisters

A 38-year-old man was diagnosed with acute myelogenous leukemia and underwent two courses of chemotherapy. He then received an allogeneic bone marrow transplant from his son. He had a difficult postoperative course, with fever, neutropenia, and liver, pulmonary, and kidney abnormalities. A widespread, macular and papular, erythematous eruption occurred 2 weeks after the transplant and was followed by skin necrosis, flaccid bullae formation, and skin sloughing.

Physical Examination: Skin: widely disseminated, brightly erythematous macules and papules, confluent into patches of erythema on trunk and ears; vesicles and bullae with positive Nikolsky sign and areas of skin sloughing in acral areas (see figure). Abdomen: no hepatomegaly. Eyes: no scleral icterus.

Laboratory Findings: Skin biopsy: pending.

Question: What is the differential diagnosis of this clinical presentation?

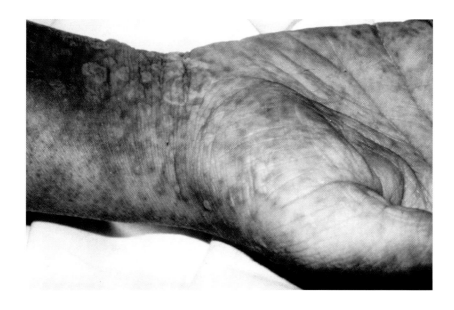

Diagnosis: Acute graft-versus-host disease

Discussion: Graft-versus-host disease (GVHD) is a frequent complication of bone marrow transplants and is the cause of death in 12–20% of graft recipients. The cause of GVHD is unknown, but three factors are necessary: (1) the transplanted organ must contain immune-competent T-cells; (2) there must be a difference in tissue antigens between the donor and recipient; (3) the recipient (host) must be immunocompromised.

Acute GVHD occurs within 3 months or 100 days of the transplant. It involves only epithelium; the main target organ is the skin. Its incidence has been estimated at 6–90%, depending on many factors, most importantly the age of the patient. Skin involvement typically begins 7–21 days after bone marrow transplant. A morbilliform appearance, with erythematous macules and papules, is typical. There may be pain or itching, and lesions are said to be characteristically perifollicular in distribution. An acral distribution also is common, with palms, soles, and ears usually affected. There may be a scarlatiniform presentation, with confluent erythema followed by sheets of desquamation, or there may be a varicelliform eruption. A generalized erythema develops as the disease progresses, and epidermal necrosis, flaccid blisters as in toxic epidermal necrolysis (TEN), and eventual skin sloughing may result. Gastrointestinal tract involvement leads to nausea, vomiting, diarrhea, and abdominal pain. Liver changes most often manifest as increased hepatic enzymes, hepatomegaly, and jaundice.

Histopathologic findings in acute GVHD are divided into four grades. **Grade I** reveals vacuolar degeneration of the basal cells and lymphocytic infiltrate. **Grade II** reveals Grade I changes plus keratinocyte necrosis. The finding of lymphocytes clustered around a dead keratinocyte is termed "satellite cell necrosis" and is highly suggestive of graft-versus-host disease. **Grade III** shows Grade II plus blister formation. **Grade IV** shows Grade III plus full thickness epidermal necrosis.

Chronic GVHD follows acute GVHD in two-thirds of cases and occurs de novo in a third. Some suggest that it can be triggered by herpes zoster, ultraviolet irradiation, physical trauma, or even Borrelia infection. The mouth is involved in 90% of patients, with salivary gland dysfunction, atrophic and ulcerative lesions, and frequent candida superinfection. Two types of skin lesions are seen, lichenoid and sclerodermoid. There can be severe systemic involvement. The risk factors for chronic GVHD include previous acute GVHD, increased age, non-T-cell–depleted bone marrow,

and a female donor to male host if the female had previous pregnancy or transfusion.

The *differential diagnosis* of acute GVHD includes drug reactions, particularly to the conditioning chemotherapeutic regimen, a viral illness, or reaction to irradiation.

The development of GVHD in patients who have undergone allogeneic bone marrow transplant for leukemia and lymphomas is associated with a decreased rate of relapse. This is thought secondary to an anti-tumor effect, termed "graft-versus-leukemia," of the adoptively transferred cells. The transfused donor T-cells can eradicate residual leukemia or decrease the rate of relapse. This graft-versus-leukemia effect is associated with GVHD. If the donor T-cells are depleted from the donor bone marrow through aggressive conditioning with chemotherapy and irradiation, the incidence of GVHD is decreased, but the relapse rate is increased. In addition to the role of donor T-cells in the pathogenesis of GVHD, recipient keratinocyte cytokines, including tumor necrosis factor-alpha and interleukin-1, are important. Interestingly, cyclosporin A is known to induce a mild, usually self-limited skin GVHD.

Treatment depends on the type and severity of disease. The mainstay of treatment for acute GVHD is high-dose systemic corticosteroids. Grade IV acute GVHD, which resembles TEN, has a mortality rate of 80–100% (30% in TEN). Treatment of the lichenoid-type of chronic GVHD involves corticosteroids and immunosuppressives, most often cyclosporin A. Other therapies include methotrexate, azathioprine, cyclophosphamide, thalidomide, and psoralen plus UV radiation. Recombinant granulocyte-colony stimulating factor may decrease the incidence of chronic GVHD in allogeneic bone marrow transplant recipients. In another study, the antimalarials chloroquin and hydroxychloroquine (which inhibit major histocompatibility Class II antigen presentation) inhibited the development of chronic disease. Positive results have been reported recently with extracorporeal photochemotherapy.

In the present patient, the biopsy showed Grade III acute GVHD and an additional finding of Bowenoid changes, which were thought to be secondary to cyclosporin A toxicity. He was treated with high-dose systemic corticosteroids, and meticulous attention was paid to fluid and electrolyte balance as well as infection prevention and treatment. Despite these measures, his condition progressively deteriorated, and he died 8 weeks after the bone marrow transplant.

Clinical Pearls

1. The mean frequency of acute graft-versus-host disease in adults receiving an HLA-matched graft is approximately 35%.

2. Acute GVHD is staged according to clinical findings and graded according to histopathologic features.

3. Patients who develop GVHD following an allogeneic bone marrow transplant for leukemia or lymphoma have a lower rate of disease relapse. This lower relapse rate is obliterated if T-cells are first depleted from donor marrow.

REFERENCES

1. Bulengo-Ransby SM, Sahn EE, Metcalf JS, et al: Bowenoid change in association with graft-versus-host disease: A cyclosporine toxicity? J Am Acad Dermatol 31:1052–1054, 1994.
2. Appelbaum FR: Graft versus leukemia (GVL) in the therapy of acute lymphoblastic leukemia (ALL). Leukemia 11 Suppl 4:S15–S17, 1997.
3. Schultz KR, Gilman AL: The lysosomotropic amines, cloroquine and hydroxychloroquine: A potentially novel therapy for graft-versus-host disease. Leuk Lymphoma 24:201–210, 1997.
4. Aractingi S, Chosidow O: Cutaneous graft-versus-host disease. Arch Dermatol 134:602–612, 1998.
5. Ikehara S: Bone marrow transplantation for autoimmune diseases. Acta Haematol 99:116–132, 1998.

PATIENT 96

A 61-year-old woman with recurrent epistaxis and dyspnea

A 61-year-old woman had recurrent epistaxis since late childhood. Over the past 5 years, she had become increasingly breathless, with severe dyspnea on walking 50 yards. Her younger brother had a history of recurrent epistaxis and died at the age of 42 of a "brain hemorrhage." Her mother had recurrent epistaxis and died of a "bleeding ulcer" at the age of 48.

Physical Examination: Temperature 37°C; pulse 106; respirations 42, blood pressure 118/78. Skin: blanchable, purple-red spider telangiectasias on lips, tongue, buccal mucosa, face, fingers, and toes (see figure). Nasal mucosa: numerous telangiectasias easily visualized. Chest: bruit over right lower lobe increased with inspiration. Cardiac: tachycardia. Abdomen: moderate hepatomegaly and mild splenomegaly. Nails: cyanotic; Lovibond's angle > 180 degrees, diagnostic of clubbing.

Laboratory Findings: Chest radiograph: 2-cm nodule in right lower lobe. Arterial blood gas (room air): pH 7.43, PCO_2 32 mmHg, PO_2 50 mmHg. CBC: hematocrit 50%. Stool hematest: negative. MRI studies of lungs, brain, and liver: pending.

Question: What is the underlying diagnosis?

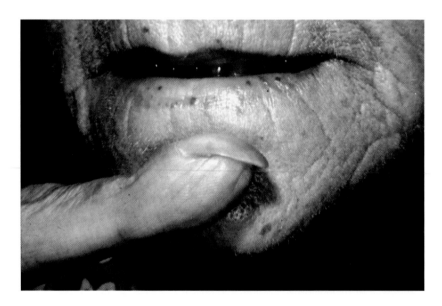

Diagnosis: Hereditary hemorrhagic telangiectasia (Rendu-Osler-Weber disease)

Discussion: Hereditary hemorrhagic telangiectasia (HHT) is a multisystem vascular dysplasia characterized by mucocutaneous and visceral telangiectasias, recurrent epistaxis, gastrointestinal hemorrhage, and pulmonary, cerebral, and hepatic arteriovenous malformations (AVMs). The incidence is estimated at 1/50,000, but in one recent study in Cantabria, Spain, 1/12,000 people were affected. The telangiectasias most commonly involve the face (35%) and fingers, toes, and nail beds (40%). Mucous membranes are always involved, particularly the lips, tongue, nasal septum, and buccal mucosa. Telangiectasias usually do not develop until the third or fourth decade, but the most common presentation, epistaxis, usually appears during childhood, typically between the ages of 8 and 10. Recurrent and severe epistaxis with resultant anemia occurs in 50–90% of patients with HHT. Cutaneous telangiectasias are punctate, spidery, or linear, with a papular component, and are seen on the palms, soles, distal fingers, and nail beds. They may present as subungual flame hemorrhages.

Both upper and lower gastrointestinal bleeding occurs in 40–44% of patients with HHT. Hematemesis and melena occur in 20%. Often the source is not visualized on barium studies, but requires endoscopy, arteriography, or laparotomy for diagnosis and localization. Hepatomegaly or abnormal liver function tests occur in 30% of patients, possibly due to dilated hepatic arteries, multiple AVMs, or patchy hepatic fibrosis. Rarely, hepatic failure follows.

Pulmonary arterial venous fistulae occur in about 20% of patients with HHT, with a third being multiple. Of all patients with pulmonary AV shunts, 40% have HHT. Symptoms and signs include dyspnea, cyanosis, clubbing, polycythemia, hemoptysis, and bruit, as well as the findings of a nodule on chest radiograph and hypoxemia on arterial blood gas analysis. Pulmonary AVMs may become infected, producing a lung abscess. Septic emboli from the lungs produce brain abscesses in 1% of patients with HHT. There also is a high incidence of AVMs in the brain; one recent study using magnetic resonance imaging reported a 23% incidence. Central nervous system hemorrhage is thought to occur in 2–3% of patients with HHT. Other CNS symptoms are seizures, hemiparesis, and visual disturbances.

The *differential diagnosis* includes generalized essential telangiectasia, and when mats of telangiectasia are present, the CREST variety of scleroderma (calcinosis cutis, Raynaud's, esophageal motility problems, sclerodactyly, telangiectasia) and the telangiectasia macularis eruptiva perstans variety of mastocytosis should be included in the differential. Primary biliary cirrhosis also shows matted telangiectasia without a hemorrhagic tendency.

Histopathologic examination reveals thin-walled, dilated, papillary and subpapillary dermal vessels lined by one layer of flattened endothelial cells.

HHT is an autosomal dominant disease with genetic heterogeneity: different mutations produce a similar phenotype. Two genes have been identified for HHT. The gene for HHT1 is the endoglin gene, which encodes an endothelial membrane glycoprotein (a receptor) that binds transforming growth factor-beta (TGF-β). The locus of this gene has been mapped to chromosome 9q33-34. Endoglin normally is expressed in high levels in vascular endothelium. TGF-β is an angiogenic factor and mediator of vascular remodeling. The gene for HHT2 is activin receptor-like kinase 1 gene of endothelium (ALK1). This gene maps to chromosome 12q. Both gene products are thought to be involved in vascular remodeling in association with TGF-β, but the exact pathogenesis remains unclear.

Management and treatment of HHT begins with a prompt diagnosis. Any child with recurrent epistaxis, particularly when there is a family history of the same, must be examined carefully to exclude HHT. If the epistaxis is severe, as it often is, long-term management with electrocautery, tamponade, systemic or topical estrogen therapy, and, eventually, laser photocoagulation is necessary. Good results have been obtained with septodermoplasty in severe cases. The pulse-dye laser treats telangiectasia in the anterior nasal cavity, but there is some evidence that these lesions recur. Iron supplementation and transfusions often are needed. Management of the AVMs in the lungs, liver, and brain often includes embolization. Surgical resection also is an option. Treatment of pulmonary AVMs should be prompt because of the risk of abscess formation and septic embolus to the brain. Gastrointestinal bleeding may be difficult to manage because of multiple bleeding sites.

In the present patient, the MRI of the brain and liver revealed no AVMs. The MRI study of the chest showed an AVM in the right lower lobe, and the 100% oxygen study confirmed a right to left shunt. Pulmonary angiography demonstrated only one AVM; therefore, she underwent an embolization procedure. Over the following weeks, her hypoxemia and dyspnea improved markedly. She is being closely followed for further cerebral, pulmonary, hepatic, and gastrointestinal symptoms.

Clinical Pearls

1. Hereditary hemorrhagic telangiectasia (Rendu-Osler-Weber disease) is an autosomal dominant genodermatosis. Two genes mapping to chromosomes 9 and 12 have been identified. Any one of several different mutations in either of these genes may result in the HHT phenotype.

2. A patient who presents with a pulmonary arteriovenous malformation likely has HHT. The skin, central nervous system, liver, and gastrointestinal tract also may show vascular anomalies, including telangiectasias and AVMs.

3. It is important to make the diagnosis of HHT early, so that some of its complications can be anticipated and prevented. A child with recurrent or severe epistaxis and a family history of the same should be examined carefully for mucocutaneous telangiectasias and followed closely.

REFERENCES

1. Harries PG, Brockbank MJ, Shakespeare PG, et al: Treatment of hereditary haemorrhagic telangiectasia by the pulsed-dye laser. J Laryngol Otol 111:1038–1041, 1997.
2. Morales Angulo C, Megia Lopez R, del Valle Zapico A, et al: Rendu-Osler-Weber disease (hereditary hemorrhagic telangiectasia): Report of 30 cases. Acta Otorrinolaringol Esp 48:625–629, 1997.
3. Caselitz M, Wagner S, Chavan A, et al: Clinical outcome of transfemoral embolisation in patients with arteriovenous malformations of the liver in hereditary haemorrhagic telangiectasia (Weber-Rendu-Osler disease). Gut 42:123–126, 1998.
4. Fulbright RK, Chaloupka JC, Putman CM, et al: MRI of hereditary hemorrhagic telangiectasia: Prevalence and spectrum of cerebrovascular malformations. Am J Neuroradiol 19:477–484, 1998.
5. Callione CJ, Klaus DJ, Yeh EY, et al: Mutation and expression analysis of the endoglin gene in hereditary hemorrhagic telangiectasia reveals null alleles. Hum Mutat 11:286–294, 1998.
6. Mukasa C, Nakamura K, Chijiiwa Y, et al: Liver failure caused by hepatic angiodysplasia in hereditary hemorrhagic telangiectasia. Am J Gastroenterol 93:471–473, 1998.

PATIENT 97

A 74-year-old man with gingival bleeding and "palpable purpura" on the legs

A 74-year-old chronic alcoholic was treated in the emergency department for a scalp laceration. The dermatology service was consulted when numerous palpable, purpuric lesions on his legs and hypertrophied, bleeding gingivae were noted. His oral intake over the past 4 months consisted of whole milk, white bread, bologna, and whiskey.

Physical Examination: Temperature 37.3°C. Skin: hemorrhagic, follicular hyperkeratoses on arms, legs, and abdomen (see figure); broken, curly, "corkscrew" hairs protruding from many hyperkeratoses; ecchymoses on legs, buttocks, and thighs. Mouth: gingival hypertrophy with bluish discoloration, friability with easy bleeding, and absence of several teeth.

Laboratory Findings: Hematocrit 34%. Liver function tests: changes consistent with acute and chronic alcoholism.

Questions: What is your diagnosis? What is the pathogenesis of this entity?

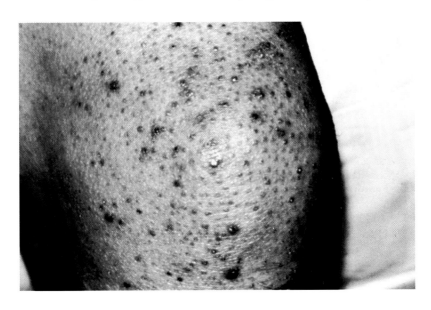

Diagnosis: Scurvy

Discussion: Scurvy refers to the clinical and metabolic abnormalities that result from inadequate vitamin C intake. It is rare in the United States, but during the 16th and 17th centuries, scurvy sometimes decimated whole populations in rural areas or at sea. Before vitamin C was discovered, the British navy in the 1700s recognized the relationship between scurvy and citrus fruits and required a daily ration of limes or lemons for all of its sailors (hence the term "limey"). Many mammals synthesize their required ascorbic acid, but humans are unable to do so and must rely on daily intake.

Currently, scurvy is seen most often among elderly, institutionalized patients and those consuming excessive amounts of alcohol. Inadequate intake of fresh fruits and vegetables occurs rarely in other situations, such as food fads, special diets, and anorexia nervosa. Infants who are not breast-fed (breast milk is a source of vitamin C) occasionally are diagnosed with scurvy, most often between the ages of 6 and 24 months. Affected infants are fed formula or diets that are not adequately supplemented with vitamin C. Situations that increase the requirement for vitamin C include infection accompanied by fever and diarrhea, iron deficiency, or protein malnutrition. It is well documented that cigarette smokers have significantly depressed levels of vitamin C.

Vitamin C is a cofactor for normal collagen metabolism. Without vitamin C, hydroxylation of procollagen, proline, and lysine does not occur, resulting in abnormal collagen production. Abnormal collagen causes abnormalities of teeth, bones, and blood vessel supporting tissue. Vitamin C also is required for normal leukocyte function, immune responses, wound healing, allergic reactions, and pulmonary function. It may play a role in the prevention of coronary heart disease, cancer, and cataracts.

After 2 months of a diet severely restricted in or devoid of vitamin C, the characteristic clinical findings in the skin are produced. One of the most distinctive and early signs of scurvy is **hemorrhagic follicular hyperkeratoses with corkscrew hairs**, most commonly seen over the knees. There may be enlarged red follicles with petechiae. Distribution tends to be seborrheic, and purpura and ecchymoses are common. The gingivae become friable, erythematous, and swollen, with hemorrhages at the tips of the interdental papillae. Eventually the gingivae become blue and spongiotic, with loss of periodontal bone and, finally, tooth loss. Bone changes include fractures of cartilaginous matrix, decreased osteoid formation, and subperiosteal or bone marrow hemorrhages. The tibia and fibula are the bones most commonly affected. Infants with these findings may assume a "frogleg" position, with the hips flexed and the knees and feet rotated outward. Systemic findings from vitamin C deficiency include low-grade fever, anemia, lethargy, apathy, poor wound healing, cardiac hypertrophy, bone marrow depression, adrenal atrophy, skeletal muscle degeneration, and generalized hemorrhaging including epistaxis, hematuria, melena, and bleeding into the subcutaneous tissue and muscles (producing "woody" edema of the legs).

The *differential diagnosis* includes leukemia, meningococcemia, thrombocytopenic purpura, osteomyelitis (can resemble the periosteal hemorrhage of scurvy), other vitamin deficiencies, periodontal disease (both can present with bleeding gums, but periodontal disease is caused by oral plaque micro-organisms), and leukocytoclastic vasculitis (can resemble the hemorrhagic follicular hyperkeratoses of scurvy).

Histologic examination reveals only red blood cell extravasation around hair follicles, without capillary changes or inflammation. There may be hemosiderin deposition. The intrafollicular keratotic plugs may show sections of coiled hairs.

Current research efforts make use of the scorbutic guinea pig model. Like humans, guinea pigs cannot synthesize ascorbic acid. Studies using this model have documented decreased bone mass, decreased collagen synthesis, and decreased serum and bone alkaline phosphatase activity during vitamin C deficiency. Another study of vitamin C–deficient individuals found that metabolic changes independent of collagen metabolism occur prior to the clinical signs of scurvy. Other researchers found that both blood histamine and plasma-free carnitine were inversely related to vitamin C levels as they fell. Finally, a very low (scurvy range) level of ascorbic acid was detected in 20 subjects in a study of elderly institutionalized persons. These individuals had a concomitant low beta-carotene, but normal alpha-tocopherol levels.

In the present patient, a serum ascorbic acid assay was less than 0.1 mg/dl, and a leukocyte ascorbic acid assay was less than 7 mg/dl. He was treated with supplemental ascorbic acid 300 mg per day, with rapid improvement in the follicular and gingival hemorrhages. He was provided nutritional counseling and offered treatment of his alcoholism.

Clinical Pearls

1. Scurvy continues to be seen in current practice, most often in alcoholics, the institutionalized elderly, and infants aged 6–24 months.

2. The distinctive dermatologic signs of scurvy include hemorrhagic follicular hyperkeratoses with corkscrew hairs.

3. Only 2 months of severe vitamin C deficiency are required to produce the characteristic dermatologic findings of scurvy.

REFERENCES

1. Birlouez-Aragon I, Girard F, Ravelontseheno L, et al: Comparison of two levels of vitamin C supplementation on antioxidant vitamin status in elderly institutionalized subjects. Int J Vitam Nutr Res 65:261–266, 1995.
2. Johnston CS, Solomon RE, Corte C: Vitamin C depletion is associated with alterations in blood histamine and plasma free carnitine in adults. J Am Coll Nutr 15:586–591, 1996.
3. Weber P, Bendich A, Schalch W: Vitamin C and human health: A review of recent data relevant to human requirements. Int J Vitam Nutr Res 66:19–30, 1996.
4. Leone J, Delhinger V, Maes D, et al: Rheumatic manifestations of scurvy: A report of two cases. Rev Rhum Engl Ed 64:428–431, 1997.
5. Touyz LZ: Oral scurvy and periodontal disease. J Can Dent Assoc 63:837–845, 1997.

PATIENT 98

An 8-month-old girl with numerous brown macules

An 8-month-old infant was noted to have brown macules on her trunk at the age of 2 months. These macules gradually increased in number. The parents reported that after a bath and towel drying, some of the lesions became red and raised and developed small blisters. The child occasionally scratched the lesions. The child was in excellent health otherwise. She was on no medications.

Physical Examination: Vital signs: normal. Skin: numerous 5- to 15-mm, pale brown macules scattered over trunk (see figure); vigorous stroking of lesion with tongue blade produced red, raised plaque. Abdomen: no hepatosplenomegaly or masses. Lymph nodes: no lymphadenopathy. Musculo-skeletal: no bone pain on palpation.

Laboratory Findings: CBC with differential and chemistry profile: normal. 24-hour urine: pending.

Question: What is your diagnosis?

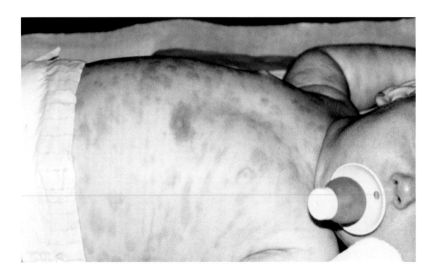

Diagnosis: Urticaria pigmentosa

Discussion: Urticaria pigmentosa is the most common type of mastocytosis (mast cell hyperplasia) seen in children. Mast cells are derived from a CD34+ bone marrow stem cell. They express a receptor on their surface to which an IgE antibody binds. When this IgE antibody recognizes a specific antigen, it causes the mast cell to degranulate and release biologic mediators, including histamine, heparin, triptase, prostaglandin D2, leukotreines, and platelet activating factor. Mast cell degranulation can be precipitated by drugs (e.g., codeine, morphine, dextromethorphan, aspirin, atropine, procaine, polymyxin B, radiographic dyes, and nonsteroidal anti-inflammatory medications), hot baths, cold water swimming, exercise, stress, and vigorous trauma or rubbing, such as in towel drying.

Urticaria pigmentosa typically arises between birth and 9 months, but may occur in adults as well. There are multiple (typically 25–100) red-brown, hyperpigmented macules and papules, with occasional nodules and plaques, scattered symmetrically over the trunk. The head, neck, and extremities also may be involved, but palms and soles are spared, and mucous membranes are rarely involved. **Darier's sign** is pathognomonic for mastocytosis: stroking of a lesion produces mast cell degranulation with resultant urtication. Occasionally, the lesions appear purpuric secondary to the release of heparin; in such cases, child abuse has been erroneously suspected.

Symptoms in mastocytosis are due to either mast cell mediator release or mast cell infiltration of an organ. Urticaria pigmentosa frequently is asymptomatic or may show mild pruritus or flushing. Occasionally, vomiting, diarrhea, abdominal pain, and headache occur. Bronchospasm and hypotension are rare.

Urinary histamine metabolites, including N-methylhistamine and N-methylimidazole acetic acid, may give an estimate of the total mast cell load in an individual. Systemic mastocytosis, in which mast cells infiltrate other organs, can produce additional laboratory abnormalities, including anemia with eosinophilia, radiographic bone abnormalities (cystic or lytic lesions, osteoporosis or osteosclerosis), gastrointestinal findings (peptic ulcer disease, hepatosplenomegaly with attendant laboratory abnormalities, or thickening of the gastrointestinal mucosa), hypocholesterolemia, (secondary to heparin release), and, occasionally, hematologic malignancies.

Histologic examination of a lesion reveals a sparse mast cell infiltrate in the perivascular areas of the upper third of the dermis. There is associated epidermal hyperpigmentation. If bullae are present, the split is subepidermal. Giemsa and toluidine blue stains often are necessary to demonstrate the increased mast cells. If a lesion is urticated just before or during biopsy, the increased mast cells may not be seen.

The *differential diagnosis* of urticaria pigmentosa includes multiple lentigines, neurofibromatosis, nevi, eruptive xanthomas, other causes of eosinophilia if this is prominent, and carcinoid syndrome if systemic symptoms such as flushing, tachycardia, and syncope are prominent (carcinoid syndrome shows increased urinary 5-hydroxyimidazole acetic acid).

Research has determined that, in addition to mediators, mast cells release cytokines and participate in chronic inflammatory events. The c-kit protooncogene encodes a tyrosine kinase receptor that plays a crucial role in hematopoiesis. An activating mutation in this oncogene has been found in patients with mastocytosis and an associated hematologic disorder. It may play a role in other types of mastocytosis as well. Mast cell growth factors and their receptors also appear to be important in mast cell proliferation.

Urticaria pigmentosa with onset in childhood disappears by adolescence in 50% of patients. However, it persists into adulthood in the other 50%, at which time it features the same incidence of complications as adult-onset cases, particularly the 10% incidence of systemic involvement. In an infant with newly diagnosed urticaria pigmentosa, systemic organ involvement must be considered. A CBC with differential and a chemistry profile are good screening tests, and a 24-hour urine for N-methylhistamine or N-methylimidazole acetic acid provides an estimate of mast cell load. Radiographic examinations of bones are not indicated unless bone pain or other evidence of bony involvement is present. A bone marrow aspirate or gastrointestinal examination is not indicated unless symptoms or signs suggest specific involvement.

Management begins with educating the parents and the pediatrician to avoid mast cell degranulators in these children. Mild symptoms such as pruritus, flushing, and gastrointestinal symptoms often can be controlled with H1- and H2-blocking antihistamines. Strong topical corticosteroids, particularly under occlusion, have been shown to decrease cutaneous mast cell infiltrates and lessen symptoms. Disodium chromoglycate (chromolyn sodium) and nifedipine both stabilize the mast cell membrane, thereby inhibiting degranulation and activation. Aspirin inhibits prostaglandin production and occasionally has been used in a hospital setting with careful monitoring, since aspirin itself is a mast cell degranulator. Ketotifen is thought to block histamine receptors and to inhibit mast cell degranulation. It has proved helpful in some cases. Oral psoralen with UVA (PUVA) therapy has been found to inhibit histamine release, but caution must be used initially to prevent massive mast cell degranulation. In one study of 20 patients with urticaria pigmentosa, 70% were improved on PUVA, and in 25% who were followed for more than 5 years, this improvement continued. When vesicles or bullae occur, mupirocin ointment can be used to treat the erosions, since nonprescription antibiotic ointments often contain polymyxin B, which is a mast cell degranulator. Some adults with mastocytosis have reacted with severe anaphylaxis to insect stings; therefore, the clinician may recommend that the patient carry an epinephrine injection kit and wear a medical alert bracelet.

In the present patient, the 24-hour urine levels of histamine metabolites were slightly elevated. Low-dose oral antihistamines provided relief from pruritus. The parents and pediatrician were provided with educational materials, including a list of mast cell degranulators to be avoided in this child. At 2 years of age no new macular lesions were appearing. A repeat of her 24-hour urine histamine metabolites showed that they had fallen to within normal range.

Clinical Pearls

1. Urticaria pigmentosa developing in early childhood has a good prognosis, with resolution in 50% of patients by adolescence. However, the other 50% experience adult mastocytosis, sometimes with systemic involvement and attendant complications.

2. The evaluation for most infants and young children includes screening blood work and a 24-hour urinary measurement of histamine metabolites, either N-methylhistamine or N-methylimidazole acetic acid.

3. The most important aspect of management is education of the parents and pediatrician. Nonprescription medications such as synthetic opioids can produce marked degranulation and severe bullous reactions.

4. Do not use nonprescription antibiotic ointments containing polymyxin B to treat eroded vesicles and bullae in urticaria pigmentosa, because polymyxin B is a mast cell degranulator.

5. Psoralen plus UVA has produced good results in urticaria pigmentosa.

REFERENCES

1. Cook J, Stith M, Sahn EE: Bullous mastocytosis in an infant associated with the use of a nonprescription cough suppressant. Pediatr Dermatol 13:410–414, 1996.
2. Godt O, Proksch E, Streit V, et al: Short- and long-term effectiveness of oral and bath PUVA therapy in urticaria pigmentosa and systemic mastocytosis. Dermatology 195:35–39, 1997.
3. Pignon JM: C-kit mutations and mast cell disorders: A model of activating mutations of growth factor receptors. Hematol Cell Ther 39:114–116, 1997.
4. Miyachi Y, Kurosawa M: Mast cells in clinical dermatology. Australas J Dermatol 39:14–18, 1998.

PATIENT 99

A 2-day-old girl born with tight, red skin

A 2-day-old girl was born with a yellowish-brown, tight, shiny membrane encasing most of her skin. The membrane rapidly cracked and fissured, and subsequent peeling revealed red, moist skin underneath. She had difficulty with temperature regulation and feeding and was transferred to a large teaching hospital. There was no family history of congenital abnormalities.

Physical Examination: Vital signs: normal. Skin: large areas of moist, erythematous skin on face, with peeling keratinous membrane at edges (see figure); large, shiny, yellowish scales over back, scalp, and extremities, some with fissures and large cracks. HEENT: ectropion, eclabion, and flattened ears.

Laboratory Findings: CBC, differential, and biochemical survey: normal. Skin biopsy for routine histopathologic examination and electron microscopy: pending.

Question: What is your diagnosis?

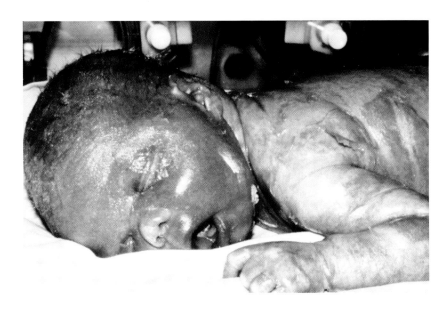

Diagnosis: Collodion baby

Discussion: "Collodion baby" refers to a phenotype in which the newborn is encased in a keratin cast that resembles oiled parchment or plastic wrap with a brownish-yellow discoloration. There may be fissures and cracking of this membrane at birth. There may be ectropion (inverted eyelids), eclabion ("fish mouth"), "crumpled" pinnae, tapered and flexed fingers, and dystrophic nails. The membrane peels, revealing normal skin, mild scaling, or severe ichthyosis.

The management of these babies until the membrane is shed, usually by 10–14 days of age, can be problematic. Secondary infection with bacteria or candida is frequent, and septicemia may result. Temperature instability must be carefully managed. Fluid and electrolyte balance is challenging, with large areas of denuded skin. Occasionally, the keratin cast is so thick that respiratory motion of the chest is restricted, and respiratory failure may ensue. Areas of deep fissuring or cracking may result in scarring.

Histopathologic examination of the collodion membrane shows compact orthohyperkeratosis with plugged hair follicles. A biopsy often is required after the membrane is shed to clarify the underlying disease. Electron microscopic examination shows a normal proximal stratum corneum, but a distal stratum corneum with irregular, convoluted keratinocytes containing numerous intracellular lamellar granules (Odlin bodies) and nuclear debris; desmosomes are normal.

The *differential diagnosis* of the collodion baby is extensive. When shedding of the collodion membrane results in normal skin, the diagnosis is lamellar exfoliation of the newborn. Commonly, a recessive ichthyosis, either lamellar ichthyosis or nonbullous congenital ichythosiform erythroderma, follows shedding. A **harlequin fetus** is encased in thick plates of scale, more severe than that of a collodion baby, and the survival rate is lower. Other diseases that can present as a collodion baby include the Hay-Wells syndrome (ankyloblepharon-ectodermal dysplasia-clefting syndrome), chondrodysplasia punctata (Conradi-Hunermann disease), Netherton syndrome, Tay syndrome, Sjogren-Larsson syndrome, ectodermal dysplasia (especially the hypohidrotic variety), neutral lipid storage disease with ichthyosis, trichothyodystrophy (IBIDS), recessive X-linked ichthyosis (sterol sulfatase deficiency), and Gaucher disease.

It may be difficult to differentiate a collodion baby from a harlequin fetus at birth. One group found that the **marginal band** was absent in early lamellar ichthyosis, but present in the harlequin fetus. The marginal band is the cellular envelope of cornified cells, produced in the upper spinous or granular layers as keratinization progresses. It is formed from precursor proteins such as loricrin and envolucrin, with the aid of keratinocyte transglutaminase. The gene for keratinocyte transglutaminase has been located on chromosome 14q11, and mutations in this gene have been identified in patients with autosomal recessive congenital ichthyosis. The harlequin fetus also shows the ultrastructural features of giant mitochondria, abnormal lamellar granules, and excess lipid inclusions in the stratum corneum.

In another case, a patient with collodion membrane (which later progressed to lamellar ichthyosis) showed the changes of a harlequin fetus, including lipid inclusions in corneocytes and abnormal lamellar granules in the granular layer. Further ultrastructural studies are necessary on both collodion baby and harlequin fetus to substantiate these findings.

A rapid in situ test for transglutaminase activity, to provide prognostic information on a collodion baby, has been described. Recessive ichthyosis was found to develop in those with markedly decreased transglutaminase activity. Mutations in the gene for keratinocyte transglutaminase are one cause of autosomal recessive congenital ichthyosis, and about 50% of these patients show markedly decreased keratinocyte transglutaminase activity. The older method of assaying transglutaminase was an in vitro method that required culturing of keratinocytes.

Management of the collodion baby includes temperature monitoring, fluid and electrolyte balance, and surveillance cultures for infection. Prophylactic antibiotics are not indicated. Emollients should be thin, such as petrolatum-based ointments. No lactate or urea products should be used, since these can be absorbed.

In the present patient, the above supportive measures resulted in complete shedding of the membrane within 2 weeks. Mild erythema and scale remained. The clinical diagnosis of nonbullous congenital ichthyosiform erythroderma was supported by the repeat skin biopsy at 3 months of age.

Clinical Pearls

1. The collodion baby refers to a phenotype in which the newborn is encased in a yellow-brown keratin cast. It may evolve into one of many different ichthyoses or genodermatoses, or may resolve, leaving normal skin.

2. Severe collodion baby often resembles harlequin fetus. Ultrastructural studies suggest that there may be findings specific to one that are not seen in the other.

3. Major management problems of collodion baby involve fluid and electrolyte balance, infection, temperature instability, and respiratory compromise.

REFERENCES

1. Akiyama M, Shimizu H, Yoneda K, et al: Collodion baby: Ultrastructure and distribution of cornified cell envelope proteins and keratins. Dermatology 195:164–168, 1997.
2. Hohl D, Aeschlimann D, Huber M: In vitro and rapid in situ transglutaminase assays for congenital ichthyoses: A comparative study. J Invest Dermatol 110:268–271, 1998.
3. Sandler B, Hashimoto K: Collodion baby and lamellar ichthyosis. J Cutan Pathol 25:116–121, 1998.

PATIENT 100

A 55-year-old man with blisters and crusts in the axillae

A 55-year-old man suffered pruritic blisters and erosions in the axillary and inguinal areas at the age of 25. Despite numerous treatments with systemic and topical antibiotics and corticosteroids, the lesions recurred. His two older brothers were unaffected, but his 53-year-old sister and his mother had similar complaints.

Physical Examination: Vital signs: normal. Skin: erythematous, crusted, eroded plaques in axillae and groin, with malodor (see figure). Hair: normal in these areas. Conjunctiva: normal. Mouth: normal.

Laboratory Findings: Skin biopsy: pending.

Question: What is your diagnosis?

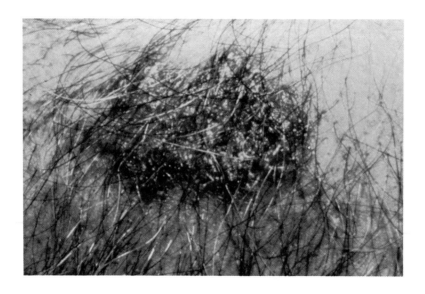

Diagnosis: Hailey-Hailey disease

Discussion: Hailey-Hailey disease (benign familial pemphigus) is an autosomal dominant, nonimmune-mediated, acantholytic disease described by the Hailey brothers in 1939. The gene has been mapped to 3q21-q24, and a positive family history is present in two-thirds of cases. Onset is between puberty and the late 30s. The primary lesion is a small, flaccid vesicle on a red base, which is easily eroded. Crusts become thick and heaped-up, producing vegetating lesions. There is an advancing serpiginous border, and lesions may be circinate. The sites of involvement mainly are intertriginous areas, particularly the axilla and groin. Other areas that may be affected include the sides and nape of the neck, the antecubital fossae, the scalp, and the inframammary or perianal areas. Mucous membrane involvement is rare, but mouth, esophagus, conjunctiva, and labia majora involvement have been reported. The lesions heal with hyperpigmentation. Nails may show broad white bands, but no notching or red bands as in Darier-White disease.

Symptoms of Hailey-Hailey disease include pain, pruritus, and burning. The disease often is worse in warm weather and may be exacerbated by secondary infections. Secondary bacterial infection is common, as is candidiasis, and both contribute to the malodor. Herpes simplex infection was identified in one patient on polymerase chain reaction, when there was no response to high-dose oral corticosteroids. There are no reported extracutaneous manifestations of Hailey-Hailey disease.

Histopathologic examination typically reveals three characteristics. First is suprabasal separation of the epidermis, which is caused by acantholysis and produces lacunae, vesicles, and bullae. The acantholysis extends throughout the epidermis, resulting in individual and clumps of keratinocytes, giving the characteristic "**dilapidated brick wall**" appearance. Second, villi (elongated papillae lined by a single layer of basal cells) proliferate upward into these lacunar spaces or vesicles. Third, acantholytic cells demonstrate faulty keratinization ("corps ronds" or "grains"), as is characteristic of Darier-White disease. Both direct and indirect immunofluorescence are negative.

Attempts are underway to define the primary defect in cell adhesion in Hailey-Hailey disease and the other nonimmune acantholytic diseases, Darier-White disease, and transient acantholytic dermolysis (Grover disease). The first event in Hailey-Hailey disease appears to be the disruption and internalization of desmosomes. *Intra*cellular desmosomal proteins are desmoplakin I, II, and plakoglobin. *Inter*cellular desmosomal proteins are desmoglein and CD44. One study used immunostaining to demonstrate loss of desmoplakin I, II, and plakoglobin from desmosomes and diffuse staining in the cytoplasm in Hailey-Hailey, Grover, and Darier-White diseases. Another study determined that diffuse cytoplasmic staining is not due to internalization of desmosomes, but rather to trapping within tonofilament aggregates and attachment to cell membranes. Immunogold techniques also have shown absence of the desmosomal attachment plaques in these three acantholytic diseases. Studies of the adherens junction protein vinculin showed that it remains intact in Hailey-Hailey, Darier-White and Grover diseases, but is damaged in pemphigus vulgaris. This may help to explain why clumps of cells remain together in Hailey-Hailey disease.

The *differential diagnosis* of Hailey-Hailey disease includes Darier-White disease, which features a similar bullous variety; however, nail changes and distribution are different. Transient acantholytic dermatosis, pemphigus vulgaris, and pemphigus vegetans occasionally mimic Hailey-Hailey disease, but they can be differentiated by histology. Diseases less likely to produce confusion include acrodermatitis enteropathica, Fox-Fordyce disease, hidradenitis suppurativa, impetigo, fungal infection, herpes simplex virus, eczematous dermatitis, seborrheic dermatitis, intertrigo, and necrolytic migratory erythema.

Treatment of Hailey-Hailey disease often is unsatisfactory. In this chronic, recurrent disease, topical and systemic antibiotics for malodor and impetigo may be helpful. Treatment of viral and fungal infections should be prompt. Aluminum chloride to decrease sweating occasionally may decrease blistering, as well. Strong topical corticosteroids, cryotherapy, CO_2 laser therapy, dermabrasion, and even excision and split-thickness grafts occasionally have provided relief. Dapsone, cyclosporin, and retinoids have been helpful in a small number of cases.

In the present patient, histopathologic study demonstrated the three typical characteristics of Hailey-Hailey disease. The secondary impetiginization was treated with systemic antibiotics, with moderate improvement. He was placed on low-dose oral retinoids and did well for 6 months. However, when the retinoid was discontinued, the disease recurred.

Clinical Pearls

1. Hailey-Hailey disease (benign familial pemphigus) is an autosomal dominant geno-dermatosis.

2. The primary defect in Hailey-Hailey disease appears to be disruption and dissolution of the desmosomal attachment plaques, with the adherens junctions remaining intact.

3. Systemic retinoids may produce remission.

REFERENCES

1. Berth-Jones J, Smith SG, Graham-Brown RA: Benign familial chronic pemphigus (Hailey-Hailey disease) responds to cyclosporin. Clin Exp Dermatol 20:70–72, 1995.
2. Hashimoto K, Fujiwara K, Tada J, et al: Desmosomal dissolution in Grover's disease, Hailey-Hailey's disease, and Darier's disease. J Cutan Pathol 22:488–501, 1995.
3. Hunt MJ, Salisbury EL, Painter DM, et al: Vesiculobullous Hailey-Hailey disease: Successful treatment with oral retinoids. Australas J Dermatol 37:196–198, 1996.
4. Metze D, Hamm H, Schorat A, et al: Involvement of the adherens junction-actin filament system in acantholytic dyskeratosis of Hailey-Hailey disease: A histological, ultrastructural, and histochemical study of lesional and nonlesional skin. J Cutan Pathol 23:211–222, 1996.
5. Tada J, Hashimoto K: Utrastructural localization of cell junctional components (desmoglein, plakoglobin, E-cadherin, and beta-catenin) in Hailey-Hailey disease, Darier's disease, and pemphigus vulgaris. J Cutan Pathol 25:106–115, 1998.

INDEX